EARLY PRAISE FOR

Blue Baby & Acute Coronary Revascularization

"Written by a loving family member and herself a surgeon about her uncle, an outstanding surgeon in his own right. It highlights the personality and professional drive that accounts for Dr. Ralph Berg's achievements in surgery and his total commitment to his wife and family. This is particularly applicable to Jason, his youngest son, born with cardiac anomalies that placed him in the category of blue babies.

"His constant search to find a 'fix' for Jason's problems was never far from his mind. His intense interest in cardiac physiology drove his desire to correct interrupted blood flow to the heart muscle, caused by said heart attacks. It became the basis for quick restoration of flow by emergent bypass surgery, which originated in Spokane and gradually became the norm throughout the world. A remarkable story about an extraordinary man, his family, his profession, and his passions."

—Julie Spores, CRNA

"A heritage of Spokane, Washington, of physicians both academic and nonacademics, of immigrants, of the American dream, and of family. A surgical master, Dr. Ralph Berg, facing rejection despite knowing he would be validated, continued to do what was right and saved lives. He continued to live his life. He struggled. He achieved both the correction of his blue baby, Jason, and validation of his acute coronary revascularization work.

"My favorite sentence in the whole book is 'With insight into what is frivolous and what is important and profound connection, I threw out the nomination, and we continued.' This is the moment my friend Tracy Berg, also the book's author, connected with her uncle, who was never going to tell this story, and this book began."

—Dr. Linda Harrison, family practitioner, PEO Chapter CL

"Especially because I am seventy-seven years young and those fifty-some years ago are now what I consider some of my most rewarding, Ralph Berg, a.k.a. 'Big Daddy,' had ideas and solutions about life that were somewhat questionable then but make a hell of a lot of sense now.

—Jim Kappen, RN and operating room manager, Valley Hospital

"You are missed, Jason Berg. Thank you for your big, beautiful heart. A toast to the legendary Jason Berg. To this day, one of the funniest, most crass and irreverent souls I have ever known. This weekend we would have celebrated your fiftieth birthday, and unbelievably today marks twenty-eight years since you so abruptly exited. Unforgettable and hilarious, I will forever miss your infectious laughter and that devilish smile. Thank you for adoring me all those years ago and reminding me to stay wild at heart. Love you, J. More than words."

—Erin Elizabeth Meenach

"Intimately involved with acute coronary revascularization, most of my education occurred in Philadelphia, Pennsylvania. Responding to an advertisement for an adult cardiologist, I interviewed with Dr. Ralph Berg, in Spokane, Washington. I accepted and worked with Drs. Berg and Kendall from November 1968 to February 1969. In March 1969, I set up my own practice in adult cardiology. I had great respect for the surgical abilities of both Drs. Berg and Kendall. However, I found Dr. Berg to be more approachable. In the summer of 1970, I discussed my theory regarding clot formation with Dr. Berg, and he agreed with my theory. The protocol emerged where he would perform emergency vein graft surgery on patients having a heart attack if I would do the coronary angiograms. If he felt, based on the results of the angiography, that he could effectively and safely perform the vein graft surgery, he would proceed. I obtained written permission to perform emergency coronary angiograms on several patients having a heart attack. What I learned was that coronary angiograms could be performed safely on patients having acute heart attacks. They did not have any significant complications from the angiography."

—Dr. Francis Everhart, cardiologist

"Dr. Tracy Berg's first book is a compelling story . . . about her famous uncle, Dr. Ralph Berg, the cardiac surgery pioneer from Spokane who was first to institute the open-heart program which cared for and repaired congenital heart blue babies."

—Nancy Rosenfeld, literary agent, principal of AAA Books Unlimited, co-author of *New Hope for People with Bipolar Disorder*

"Dr. Tracy Berg provides a surgeon's insight into how paradigm shifts in medical treatment take place as contingent, contentious, hard-won efforts accomplished by an interlocking network of researchers and practitioners. . . . This medical story happened in Spokane but is set in the national and international community of cardiologists and surgeons and has far-reaching implications."

—Betsy H. Bradley, PhD, historian

"As a blue-baby survivor with heart surgeon Dr. Ralph Berg, let me tell you how much I enjoyed this book. To read about the trials and advances that were made before the heart-lung machine was brought out of the dog lab . . . was interesting. This book is readable and easy to follow."

—Linda Childs, a blue-baby survivor

"As a blue-baby survivor, my favorite chapter was concerning Linda Childs and myself, Judy. We have been great friends for over sixty years now! The encounter we had at Whitworth University was divinely inspired, and Dr. Ralph Berg is the reason we met. . . .

"[Ralph Berg], shown as a respectful, caring, innovative and extremely generous man who never gave up, was loved by all of us patients. As a young adult he only charged me five dollars for an office visit.

"Diagnosed with congestive heart failure in 2017, I still work part-time and now have a new pacemaker. This long life is possible thanks to Dr. Berg, I am grateful."

—Judy Miller VanVoorhis, a blue-baby survivor

"This account of Dr. Ralph Berg's role in the development of open-heart surgical techniques for both children and adults, along with his dedicated team members, is riveting. . . .

"An important story, well researched and recounted by his niece, herself a general surgeon. Kudos to Dr. Tracy Berg for documenting this story, a significant contribution to medical history."

—Pauline Soehren, MSN, ARNP

"I had to quote a little Dead. May the warmth of *Blue Baby and ACR* wrap its arms around you, and like Jerry Garcia said, 'Every silver lining has got a touch of grey.' I love you, Jason."

—Estee Berg, emergency room RN

"Tracy Berg's *Blue Baby and Acute Coronary Revascularization* tells the story of a surgeon, pioneer, father, uncle, and role model on a journey to revolutionize cardiac surgery and patient care. This riveting story carries us through the personal and professional journey of this surgeon's life. Ralph Berg is what we all aspire to be, a hero. He was able to use his love and skills for family, medicine, and he contributed to the greater good. We all continue to benefit from his work. A must-read for any physician and every parent."

—Dr. Eric Strauch, professor of surgery, University of Maryland Department of Pediatric Surgery, Baltimore, Maryland

"*Blue Baby and ACR* is part memoir, part family history, and part chronicle of an enormously challenging aspect of modern medicine and surgery, with Dr. Ralph Berg at its core. The story of Dr. Berg is a vital thread within the fabric that is the history of surgical repair of complex heart defects. That his enormous skill and contributions to this field would ultimately be brought to bear in the struggle to save the life of his own beloved son, Jason, is [an aspect] rich in irony, drama, triumph, and tragedy. Woven together with the broader history of cardiac surgery, and told with unique perspective and insight that is both personal and professional, Dr. Tracy Berg has created an important and compelling work."

—Dr. Norman Lester, ENT surgeon, Atlanta VA Medical Center, assistant professor, Otolaryngology-Head and Neck Surgery, Emory University School of Medicine

"In the current environment, I could be struck down for saying this, but this story, *Blue Baby and ACR*, is more important to tell than the Bible!"

—Dr. John Shuster, orthopedic surgeon

"*Blue Baby and Acute Coronary Revascularization* by Tracy Berg is a genuinely gripping read. It is a fascinating story of Dr. Ralph Berg and his team in Spokane, WA, as they pioneered ways to mend hearts and save lives to the benefit of so many. Jason, the most raucous blue baby of all, showed no fear as he lived well."

—Cathy Berg Artesan, Jason's cousin

"When my dad, cardiologist Dr. Tom Mouser, returned to Spokane, Washington, in early 1973 to partner with Dr. Carroll Simpson, . . . he and Simpson worked closely with Dr. Berg and his talented surgical partners to perfect the care process even in difficult cases. . . .

"I enjoyed Dr. Tracy Berg's new book, *Blue Baby and ACR*, immensely as she described the Spokane Experience in detail. Perhaps even more significant is the story of the amazing Dr. Ralph Berg as he spends a lifetime training and improving the care of blue babies, culminating in the birth of his own son with severe blue baby syndrome."

—Bill Mouser, clinical pharmacist, MultiCare Valley Hospital (1990–present), Spokane, WA

"When I came to Spokane, Washington, in 1971 to join my uncle in private practice, my heart attack patients were going immediately to heart cath followed by the operating room for urgent coronary revascularization. . . . I did not realize this advanced treatment was unique to Spokane Washington. . . .

"It is my opinion that Drs. Ralph Berg and Frances Everhart's correct theory and two-tiered protocol that exploded its voluntary patient enrollment should receive the Nobel Prize for medicine. What they developed was a program that saved thousands of lives in Spokane and ultimately millions of lives around the world.

This book does an excellent job of describing the events regarding acute coronary revascularization for acute heart attacks. Tracy Berg deserves a great deal of credit bringing this information forward."

—Robert Hustrulid, MD, internal medicine, Spokane, Washington

"Family ties led me to move to Spokane, where I fit into the heart team in late 1985. . . . Although he could be difficult in the OR, I respected Dr. Ralph Berg for all he had done. . . .

"I think this book is an excellent narrative of a formative time in heart surgery, especially with understanding the mechanism behind myocardial infarctions, the groundbreaking treatment via acute coronary revascularization, [and] Dr Ralph Berg's . . . inner motivation to save his son."

—Dr. Christel Carlson, retired cardiac anesthesiologist, Providence Sacred Heart

"To get started, I was a bit skeptical, not having a medical background except assisting in the veterinary field. However, the story is told in a fascinating way that laypeople can understand and enjoy. Well done."

—Gail B Mackie

"This book is a well-deserved tribute to Dr. Ralph Berg and his Spokane, Washington, colleagues who safely pushed the boundaries of cardiac diagnosis and surgical treatment, advancing survival for so many patients then and now. It is both an insightful memoir of the Berg family and the personal pursuit of a cure for their 'blue baby' Jason as well as documentation of the advance in heart surgery procedures in mid-twentieth century Spokane. A great read for anyone interested in how an unlikely but supportive environment can create remarkable innovation. I was thoroughly enlightened and entertained by Tracy's first book."

—Julie Steury Reynolds, senior vice president of operations, Stem, Inc.

"Tracy Berg [is] amazing. I have always known that [she] rocked, but just add this accomplishment to [her] list. I loved reading [her] family's inspirational history and marveled at [her] uncle's courage and brilliance in development of the Spokane Experience. I was humbled to read about these very real people with their own lives, families, and struggles who went above and beyond to change medicine norms and save countless lives.

"The connection between [Ralph Berg's] work and the development of shock trauma at University of Maryland was crazy! . . . [Tracy's] detailed description of cardiac surgery made me want to go back to ECB Hall-Craggs's text for a refresher!"

—Mary E Pagan, MD, FCOG

Blue Baby and Acute Coronary Revascularization
by Tracy Berg, MD

© Copyright 2024 Tracy Berg, MD

ISBN 979-8-88824-565-1

All rights reserved. No part of this publication may be reproduced, stored in a retrieval system, or transmitted in any form or by any means—electronic, mechanical, photocopy, recording, or any other—except for brief quotations in printed reviews, without the prior written permission of the author.

Published by

◤ köehlerbooks™

3705 Shore Drive
Virginia Beach, VA 23455
800-435-4811
www.koehlerbooks.com

Blue Baby

& Acute Coronary Revascularization

TRACY BERG, MD

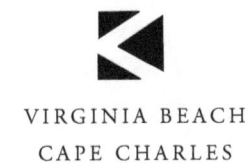

VIRGINIA BEACH
CAPE CHARLES

In memory of brothers Jason and Rory Berg and their parents, Ralph and Mary Berg. They taught us to live well by their will to live. For the Berg family, for Meridith Irena, and everyone touched by heart disease, may grief resolve and the path forward emerge.

TABLE OF CONTENTS

Introduction 1

Chapter 1: Revelation in the Operating Room, 1989 4

Chapter 2: Reasons to Leave 15

Chapter 3: Crown Prince, 1921 28

Chapter 4: A Six-Year Transformation, 1939–1945 41

Chapter 5: First-Year Surgery 59

Chapter 6: Thoracic Training 65

Chapter 7: The Road to Spokane, 1952 76

Chapter 8: Dog Lab and Hypothermia, 1952 80

Chapter 9: Sister Mary Bede and the Transition to
a Heart-Lung Machine 101

Chapter 10: Using the Heart-Lung Machine 134

Chapter 11: Acquired Heart Disease Intrudes 158

Chapter 12: Is It Fixable? 1969 183

Chapter 13: It Happened in Spokane for a Reason 189

Chapter 14: Acute Coronary Revascularization (ACR) 207

Chapter 15: Father and Son, the Anchoring Shot, 1973 ... 220

Chapter 16: Rejection ... 233

Chapter 17: Another Meeting of Minds, 1976 ... 246

Chapter 18: Marvalene's Paid Assassins, 1977–1980 ... 255

Chapter 19: The Jewel in the Crown of Hearts, 1980 ... 264

Chapter 20: Myocardial Preservation, Decades Ahead ... 273

Chapter 21: Jason ... 279

Chapter 22: The Governor, 1991 ... 309

Epilogue ... 318

Acknowledgments ... 320

Bibliography ... 321

INTRODUCTION

"In life, things start out one way and end up something else." As an adoring niece of Dr. Ralph Berg (1921–2017), I decided to let his words frame this book, a beautiful albeit brutal story that provides accurate medical history. A primer on blue-baby surgical repairs and the pioneering heart surgeons who did not succumb to fear as they developed each repair over several decades, the book also describes the precise nature of heart attacks, what they are, and how to treat them.

For my aunt and uncle, this story is personal—full of pain, grief, and loss. Dr. Ralph Berg's cutting-edge work and surgical success with blue-baby repairs by means of swift surgical technique and hypothermia attracted brilliant doctors from across the country, who arrived to work alongside him in Spokane, Washington. The first to arrive, in 1956, was Dr. Henry Lang (1923–1984), a Harvard-trained pediatric cardiologist. Also in 1956, the first heart-lung machine was purchased for use in my uncle and Lang's research lab, an indispensable step toward the human blue-baby defect repairs brought to Spokane in 1959. Dr. Ralph Berg credited Sister Mary Bede (1901–1988) for her support and insight with this purchase.

In the fall of 2006, during one of my usual visits with Ralph and his wife, Mary, my uncle opened up about Jason, a blue baby, and the close relationship between blue babies and heart attack patients. Retired yet full of vigor, my accomplished uncle explained the connection in surgical terms.

Prior to the pivotal decade of 1970 to 1980, blue babies had thankfully become rare, and the focus shifted to adult heart attacks. Ralph shared with me that in June 1970, he came across a wild and unconventional theory and treatment developed by cardiologist Dr. Francis Everhart: that of revascularizing the coronary artery during a heart attack. At the time, Ralph Berg's son was recovering from another heart surgery. Jason, a blue baby with no viable repair, having been born with a complex version of transposition of the great vessels, was doomed, and as part of the Greatest Generation, Ralph was stoic on the subject.

With the knowledge of what could and could not be done, Ralph Berg generated an environment of hope surrounding the possibility of a surgical cure for his son. Death was not an option. And so Dr. Ralph Berg agreed to do for heart attack patients what he desperately needed to do for his son, which was to preserve their myocardium.

The landmark scientific article published in October 1980 concerning this work in Spokane revealed the cause of heart attacks. "Prevalence of Total Coronary Occlusion during the Early Hours of Transmural Myocardial Infarction" was accepted worldwide. "Surgical Treatment of Acute Evolving Anterior Myocardial Infarction," which concerned the treatment, acute coronary revascularization of said occluded artery, was written and presented by Dr. Ralph Berg in May of that year and published in 1981 to further acclaim.

This body of work, nicknamed the "Spokane Experience," was carried out by dedicated private doctors—inspired by Dr. Ralph Berg—following a unique, voluntary, two-tiered protocol based on Dr. Francis Everhart's theory and an associated database. Exceptional teams of nurses, nurse anesthetists, and pump and OR technicians (from two public hospitals); a prehospital system developed by the Spokane Ambulance company; and education from Spokane's Heart Association chapter were being put to use in Spokane well before the pivotal decade. The work done in Spokane forever changed the treatment of heart attack patients.

When my uncle shared the story, he let me know he was content to take his grief-filled history to his grave. The story was hidden from the rest of the world and destined to remain so. Although the prospect was profoundly painful for Ralph, he ultimately agreed to let me share the story but requested it be told in "a kind and positive way."

In retelling this important story and the great work accomplished in Spokane, it is my hope to honor the acute coronary revascularization work of these cardiologists and heart surgeons and their deep commitment to family, and faithfully relay their gut-wrenching journeys. While his youngest son's heart defect remained without hope for repair, Dr. Ralph Berg worked throughout this pivotal decade to develop acute coronary revascularization. He struggled immeasurably but nonetheless maintained a calm and outwardly untroubled presence, continuing to perform his duties and treat patients.

Great surgeons have neither the time nor the wherewithal or personality to recount their own stories. What is obvious externally is remarkable, but what motivates someone to protect and reach back with ultimate care is beyond words.

CHAPTER 1

Revelation in the Operating Room, 1989

Having put off medical school's required surgery rotation for as long as possible, I was reaching the end of my third year in medical school. This was my last rotation before committing to a field of study. I felt vulnerable. Pediatric surgery rotation was about to begin. Would my aversion to surgeons and surgery hold?

A ten-year-old only child with attentive professional parents and a rare congenital metabolic disorder was admitted to the pediatric surgery service. I was the assigned medical student for this patient. Dr. Hill was the attending pediatric surgeon, as well as the chief of pediatric surgery. This child was being admitted for genital reassignment surgery. Her inborn error of metabolism (IEM) was familiar to me from my college courses. A 17-alpha-hydroxylase enzyme deficiency had resulted in severe testosterone reduction. The child was stuck between genders. Although the child had XY male chromosomes, the parents were raising their child female.

The child's fertility would be impaired with either gender choice, and the parents understood the overarching issue. As a male, this child would become severely underdeveloped because of the blocked testosterone. As a female, this child could appear normal. Genetically, the default position is female. Maleness develops in response to testosterone. The parents' compassionate, reasoned decision had been studied and reviewed by Dr. Hill's team. With this rare but fascinating case came a rare and fascinating surgery to correct the appearance of the child's private parts as puberty approached.

I was in awe of this family and this child—what they had been through and how they had determined to move forward. The surgical aspect of this child's care was to move the ambiguous external genitalia to a more feminine contour. Before the surgery, it was made clear that medical students were not allowed in the operating room. This was a pediatric surgery fellow and attending case, not a teaching case. There was nothing routine about it.

During the surgery, I kept checking on the progress, peeking through the window to the operating room. It annoyed me that I was not welcome to participate. Surgeons, so arrogant!

The day dragged on. First the pediatric surgery fellow left; he was needed urgently at Johns Hopkins Hospital across town. Next the senior resident left. He was needed elsewhere in the university hospital. Then the junior attending left, though she briefly stopped to chat, letting me, the medical student, know they had a long way to go to finish. No one was left in the room except the senior surgeon, Dr. Hill, operating alone. Worried that Dr. Hill had no help—after all, he could be tired, and the patient had been so long under anesthesia—I finally walked into the operating room.

The OR was quiet and tense. Dr. Hill was concentrating, seated with his head bent down. I stood quietly and close to watch, cautious of the sterile field. Finally, Dr. Hill looked up and said, "Can I help you?"

"I'm fine" was my instant reply. He stared hard at me.

"Go scrub," he said, and then added, "Do you know how to scrub?"

Well, I thought I did, and yet I did not really know how to scrub. Someone, one of the circulators, helped. As I sat at the operating table to assist Dr. Hill, it felt natural. He talked and showed me what he had done. The process followed what I had read, and yet it was wonderfully different and unique. He disclosed what needed to be completed and then continued with the surgical procedure on my patient. I assisted by holding instruments and tissue so he could see and work.

It was glorious: we worked and talked. Dr. Hill was calm and informative. I interrupted him with my opinion about how to create a specific tissue fold over the last portion of the case. He followed my advice. It did look better than what he was going to do. When the case finished, it was late, past 9 p.m. He sent me home.

The next morning, on rounds with the team at 6 a.m., the senior resident sternly sent me to Dr. Hill's office. I went without questions, certain I was in trouble for being bossy in the operating room, telling Dr. Hill what to do. A ball of tension, I was relieved when Dr. Hill was paternal and methodical with me. His office was pleasant. He said nothing about the case from the day before. He sat me down and graciously told me, "You are a surgeon."

I listened, unsure that I had heard him correctly.

He said, "You are natural with assisting and anticipating the case."

He was surprised I had not yet made a career decision. He said there still was time and laid out a plan. Reassuringly, he offered to help me. That day, I chose to become a surgeon.

After the residency match in March 1989, I landed a surgical internship at the University of Maryland. My first rotation was cardiac surgery. My uncle Ralph, forty years my senior, was a cardiothoracic surgeon in Spokane. He was a mystery to me, and I hoped this rotation—as notoriously difficult as it was—might shed some light.

Walking down the cool hallway of the university hospital's fourth floor, I was happy to see Norm Lester, a buddy from medical school, waiting. Funny, polite, and going into ear, nose, and throat (ENT), Norm was my partner on this rotation. Jumping right in, Norm commented on how demanding this rotation was going to be and ended with "Let's just get through it."

Dr. Alex Sequeira met us for orientation on the cardiac surgery service. It was a warm and beautiful June day in 1989. Norm and I were both nervous. The cardiothoracic surgeon attending (that is, not a fellow) was tall, dark, stunningly handsome, and spoke with an accent.

Originally from Nicaragua, he had a reputation for being exacting, and he detailed the surgical intern work and his expectations.

We walked around the post-open-heart surgery floor, two long, parallel hallways joined in the front and back. Patient rooms lined the exterior side of each hallway, with the waiting room at the back and the nurses' station at the front. In the middle were the storage rooms, supplies, workstations, and dirty utilities. Dr. Sequeira seemed calm but intense as he explained each facet.

The interns were to keep a notebook on the patients. One page per patient, including history, lab results, weight, procedure, days post-op, and other details. We were to work as a team, but we had separate sides of the hall and different patients. Dr. Sequeira explained how to cross-cover each other so that any attending cardiac surgeon could approach either intern to assist the cardiac surgeon in seeing their patients. We two interns were expected to be able to offer useful information on each patient, write daily progress notes, write orders as directed, identify and report problems with each patient, and learn heart surgery by assisting in the operating rooms.

The attending emphasized that coming to the OR was a privilege. Floor work needed to be done first. Beth and Jan, two quiet, professional women, were then introduced. They were physician assistants (PAs). Dr. Sequeira explained that Beth and Jan were there to make the surgical interns look bad. He went on to explain how much they knew about cardiac surgery postoperative care.

This did not make much sense to me. I was there to learn, and the PAs seemed like resources. Why would they try to make me look bad?

At the end of orientation, Dr. Sequeira told the interns how hard we were expected to work. He wanted us to be on call every other night but explained that the new chairman of the surgery department, Dr. Anthony Imbembo, thought every other night was too much. So, we would be "on call" every third night. Sounding like a slacker right off, I asked the question. Sequeira answered that the fellow would get the schedule and decide who was on call that night. He became irritated. Norm went quiet with his own line of questions to avoid further irritation.

At one point, Dr. Sequeira turned to me with a stern comment: "And I will make you cry."

Momentarily taken aback and concerned I had not heard him correctly, I sat mute but stared back. He repeated the statement. "You heard me. I will make you cry."

My temper flared at this jab, and I came back with "I can cry on demand."

Dr. Sequeira started to laugh. The orientation was over. Before walking away, he told me, "Present to the operating room when your work is done."

I saw it as a challenge. Norm said, "More like a threat and abuse."

Patient laboratory results were received on paper sheets once daily. Obtaining early results required a phone call and talking to lab personnel, who preferred not to be bothered. As did every rotating intern, Norm and I learned that getting early and additional results was important to patient care, allowing us to make accurate and quick interventions for patients whose clinical situations were changing more often than once a day.

It was a game. The surgical interns made rounds early each morning with the cardiac fellow. Occasionally, an attending cardiac surgeon would join in. The team would be brought up-to-date on each patient's condition and history and the plan for the day. Moving the patient's recovery from surgery forward, cardiac rehabilitation, and discharge from hospital was the daily goal. After rounds, the interns wrote up the progress notes, followed up on the orders, and checked the labs, addressing everything that had come up.

The PAs, Beth and Jan, worked well as a team, trading assisting in the operating room and caring for the patients. They were trusted by the heart surgeons. I watched them and learned from them. Norm and I, as interns, struggled against the lab and the slow results. Beth and Jan received results much sooner.

By the third day, I was ready for a visit to the operating room and walked in, per Dr. Sequeira's instructions. The OR team seemed surprised and asked about the floor patients. The floor work was done, and all was well. Plus, Norman was on the floor, covering my patients.

This case was a coronary artery bypass. I was instructed to scrub and work on the leg, from which a vein was being harvested. Beth moved quickly and efficiently and was soon ready to close the long wounds on the patient's leg, where the greater saphenous vein had been removed to be sent to the chest area and reused as a conduit for the coronary artery bypass. Beth seemed to be in her element, friendly and talking the whole time.

Timing of the vein harvest was important. Once the open-heart surgeon got the patient on pump, he did not want to wait another second for the bypass conduit. Each team member worked to move the case forward. It was amazingly well coordinated. Beth fitted me with instruments and instructed me on how to close the leg incision she had made. It reminded me of learning to sew when I was a kid. Beth and I chatted and worked together until the leg wounds were closed. Beth dressed them and wrapped a compression bandage around the limb. I was allowed to stay and watch the sternal wires go in; it was so cool to see. Then the chest was closed.

The next day, the same scenario. When the floor work was done, Norm happily remained on the cardiac surgery floor to cover my patients. He did not want any more abuse than necessary and made a point of staying away from the cardiac surgeons.

After reporting to the OR and getting grilled about my work, I was again invited to scrub into the case and learn the surgical techniques. Dr. Sequeira was sharp, precise, and demanding toward the team. I held the heart, which was stopped under slushy ice and cardioplegia so Dr. Sequeira could sew the distals. I loved it and wanted more.

I felt time-pressured to get into the OR. The steps of open-heart surgery were many, and Dr. Sequeira's room ran like a machine, coordinated, disciplined, and structured. Two teams worked at a near-frantic pace. Team A opened the chest cavity and installed the heart-lung machine before putting the patient on it. Team B obtained the bypass conduits from the patient's legs. Then Team A used Team B's vein conduits to bypass the blockages in the patient's heart arteries while Team B closed the long leg-harvest wounds. Both teams raced to finish first.

Around week three of the rotation, I strode confidently into the operating room, expecting another learning experience. It was hot outside in Baltimore, Maryland, but cool on the university hospital's seventh floor where the operating rooms were located. Upon my entry into OR 7, the atmosphere was tense. The cardiac surgical fellow was sitting in the corner of the operating room, facing the wall. *How strange, I thought.*

Looking around and noting that everyone was working intently and in silence, I greeted them casually. "Hello, the floor work is done, so may I scrub in?"

The usual inquiries about the floor patients and the work occurred, followed by heavy sarcasm and doubt from Dr. Sequeira. I responded only to the actual questions and ignored the dramatic onlay. The patients on the floor were being properly cared for.

Sequeira told me, "Go scrub," and I did.

Alone at the scrub sink, I thought about the emotional tone and not about why the cardiothoracic surgery fellow was being punished. I walked in with hands elevated and water dripping off my elbows. I was gowned, then gloved, and passed the team's critical once-overs checking for sterile breach.

"Can we give Dr. Fellow a second chance?" I offered, merely as a silence breaker. The room chilled, and the tension increased. Immediately, I became aware of how many professionals were in this operating room. Not one said a word as they glared at me, the cocky intern, the lowest person on the totem pole.

"Why?" Dr. Sequeira shot back.

"Whatever he did or whatever happened could be resolved" came flying out of my mouth. In the effort to save everyone, including myself, from further discomfort, I had now seriously erred in surgical etiquette. Dr. Sequeira exploded, throwing an instrument that bounced off the wall by the fellow. Then he shouted at the fellow, "Get out of my operating room!"

Now the angry surgeon turned on me.

"So, Miss Intern, you think you are the fellow?"

Having screwed up, I had no intention of excusing the fellow nor of doing his job. This fellow was eight years my senior in training, and I shrank back, trying hard to apologize and back down.

"I'm sorry. I didn't mean to—"

But Dr. Sequeira did not permit me to finish the sentence.

"If you perform, I'll work you like a fellow," he snapped.

At that moment, someone quietly nudged me into place across the table from this surgeon. I felt that I might have been better off working on the leg or with Norm.

The grilling began routinely but intensified as the case went along. Standing across the operating table from Sequeira, assisting him at the chest and not at the leg on Team B, I had an amazing view and watched intently as he prepared for the bypass. The heart and the aorta were big, beautiful, and powerful.

Pimping trainees is a classic surgical teaching method. At Maryland, it was sometimes called "leading you down the primrose path." Could you be intimidated yet stand on principle, or would you easily distract, cave in, or go with the flow? Sequeira fired through the questions about the Starling curve, basic coronary anatomy, and arterial disease, then electrolyte management. Sequeira relaxed a little as I answered his questions. The case was going well, now on bypass and waiting for Team B to produce vein.

Then he questioned me again. "Who invented acute coronary revascularization?"

Time slowed. That question sounded so official, so challenging. Dr. Sequeira was doing a coronary revascularization on a chronic angina patient. He was not treating an acute heart attack. It was the second case of the day, and he was being an arrogant jerk, so hard on the fellow and now turning on me, as if I could perform like a fellow. He thought he had me with this question, and he was clearly pleased.

I had expected to fail this exercise. Pimping always ends in failure, which is why it is such a successful teaching tool. Failure hurts but motivates. Although I was willing and I tried hard, I kind of wanted to fail quickly and get the torture over with. However, I could hardly believe this last challenge. As the room anticipated my downfall, I experienced a moment of calm.

"I know this. It is Dr. Ralph Berg, my uncle, from Spokane, Washington."

Poised and confident, I sat there thinking, *And he is like you, Dr. Sequeira. Arrogant demeanor, with high expectations wrapped in anger at the hint of failure.*

Sequeira stopped in his tracks. He laid his instruments down. The room went quiet but was not so tense. He stared at me before posing a few confirmatory questions about my genetics. He was obviously affected, and he could not understand why I had changed my last name. Then he asked, "Can I touch you?"

It was a moment of awe over an eminent heart surgeon. It was not negative. At that time, I had no idea of the impact that Uncle Ralph had had upon the world of cardiothoracic surgery—sufficient for an attending surgeon to stop an open-heart operation midstream and ask if he could "touch" the man's niece. We began to work again, in lovely silence.

Finally, I asked, "So, can I do the proximals?"

I felt like I had passed the test. Fellows do the proximals. Dr. Sequeira relented. I did one proximal anastomosis that day, with his immediate supervision and guidance—the circular punch cutting into the aorta, the tiny blue interrupted sutures, which he had to tie down once I laid each in. Sewing from the saphenous vein conduit into the aorta in a neat little circle was heavenly. Exhilarating.

At that moment, Dr. Alex Sequeira became my mentor.

Sitting in Dr. Sequeira's office that evening, reading Dr. Dwight Magoon's (1925–1999) book chapter on Dr. Ralph Berg and acute coronary revascularization, a major scientific advance that forever changed how heart attacks are treated, I experienced a mix of emotions. I had questions. What about my cousin Jason? How did his struggles relate to his father's work?

Inevitably, life goes on. Surgical residency was an amazing time. Inside of a single moment, everything could and would change. And yet residency was structured, and each year I grew closer to becoming a general surgeon. Understanding Dr. Ralph Berg, his accomplished scientific contributions while parenting Jason, took much longer. This story was to remain hidden, its grief overwhelming for my uncle, who had been so entwined in the surgical blue-baby repairs and then with Jason.

For millennia, blue babies had been doomed. There was no hope, no knowledge of what was happening, and no expectation that a cure was coming. Niels Stenson—a scientist, a highly intelligent seeker of the truth, and then a saint—described a common blue-baby defect in 1672, cared for these children, and grieved for their short lives.

As an embryo, the heart starts as a tube and develops four in-line separations to form four valves and four chambers. The tube folds, maintaining its in-line flow and retaining low-pressure inflow at both atria (the upper chambers) and higher-pressure outflow at both ventricles (the lower chambers). A normal heart has two upper and two lower chambers. The atria receive incoming lower-pressure blood. The right atrium receives venous blood from the body via the vena cava. The left atrium receives clean, oxygenated blood from the pulmonary veins. The valves, tricuspid (right) and mitral (left), are gates between the upper and lower chambers. The muscular ventricles pressurize and pump blood out. The valves with the lower chambers, pulmonary and aortic, are exits to the lungs for the pulmonary valve and right heart and to the systemic circulation for the aortic valve and left heart. These two valves are very close to each other. The right-sided circuit to the lungs is much smaller than the left-sided circuit to the rest of the body, and thus the right ventricle has less work compared to the left ventricle.

In blue babies, the holes between the heart chambers occur between upper atrial or lower ventricular chambers. The valves can be stenotic or underdeveloped or fail to act as a gate. The great vessel defects include a patent ductus, transposition of these vessels, and underdeveloped or absent valves and chambers.

The struggles to develop a repair, to improve techniques and share the latest advances so other heart teams could provide safe surgery for the blue babies, came in fits and starts in the mid-1920s. Repairs of blue babies with a single defect, such as a patent ductus, a single opening between either but not both the upper or lower chambers, or one heart valve closed with calcified adhesions, were being performed successfully without opening the heart. With the heart-lung machine, by the mid-1960s only the rarest and most difficult defects remained without a durable surgical repair. Jason, born in 1969, had such a defect. With prenatal care, better medical imaging, and vaccines, the incidence of blue babies thankfully decreased.

CHAPTER 2

Reasons to Leave

For the Berg family, the old country is Norway. Ralph Berg's father, Thoralf, came to America with his father, Anders Magnus Berg, in 1908. In the old country, when times were good, the first son would take over the family business. When times were hard, first sons could be sent away, even sold to afford families the small benefit of struggling on. Times were hard in the old country.

Anders, from a small, landlocked Swedish farm, was the second child and first son, born in 1862. The family continued to grow. After his schooling, the family, now with seven children, did not need Anders to take over the farm as was tradition for first sons. Nor could the family keep him on, with such limited land and younger children to care for. Thus, Anders was sent away at age thirteen, apprenticed to a craft. Guilds and the master craftsman were entitled to contract for young apprentices. This was the backbone of the Scandinavian economy. Sanctioned by monarchy and town government, contracted apprentices exchanged inexpensive labor for lodging, food, and formal training in the craft.

For seven years, Anders lived and worked with master baker Ostberg at his bakery and developed a love of baking. With approval from the bakers guild, Ostberg sent Anders to work in the city of Kristiania, the then capital of Norway. Joining Anders was his new wife, Ostberg's youngest daughter. When Anders checked in with the city registrar, the registrar complained, "Anders Magnus Olson—so many with this name"; so Anders gave his last name as Berg: Anders Magnus Berg.

The population of Scandinavia expanded rapidly. By 1882, the economy, government, and population were unbalanced, and times grew difficult.

Anders and his wife took up residence in the living quarters of the guild bakery, attached behind its storefront. Anders hoped to become a master baker and imagined a day when Norway would become independent from both Sweden and the Dutch. His wife, Christina, managed the store and sold bakery items to the public. A diligent storekeeper, neat and tidy, she ran off customers who stopped in for a sample before buying. Always hopeful, Anders wanted this group to become regular customers. He baked and developed repeat clients.

Their first and only child, Anna Louise, came along in 1887. A healthy and vibrant child, she grew up strong like her father and was a natural with customers and orders.

No more children came. Christina faded and then died.

Anna had just started school, and the practical needs of everyday life clashed with the little family's grief. A bread baker but not a bakery owner, Anders was making a living. Soon it was settled that he should marry again.

The dark and beautiful Torina Nee had recently arrived in Norway from the Far East. Family lore is that Torina's father, a Finnish Viking with fiery red hair and blue eyes, had become a Norwegian sea captain. After an excursion to the Far East, he brought back a family—an Asian wife and their two daughters, Torina and Camilla. Both Anders and Anna became devoted to Torina. She was beautiful, social, and fun. She soon married Anders. The match was strong. Anders, a decade older than Torina, was a stable, established husband and provider.

Torina gave birth to a girl, Olga, in the winter season. Olga died. With the land frozen, burials had to wait. Olga was buried properly in the spring. Young Anna had worried all winter about rats coming near her dead baby sister, on hold in the basement.

Anna was joyful when Torina brought home her second child. Kitty Marie was born mid-September 1895 in Moss, Ostfeld, Norway, surrounded by Torina's family for support. Anna was nine years old.

Anders's third child and first son, Thoralf, arrived June 1897, born at the bakery. Robust and precious to his mother and father, Thoralf would bear a heavy burden. If times were good, he would stay and run the family business. However, Anders was not the business owner, and times were getting harder.

A second son, Olaf, was born September 1900. Torina was an engaging and kind mother with her beautiful children: Kitty, with her auburn hair; Thoralf, with his thick black hair; and Olaf, with bright-red hair. All had skin darker than their father's and blue eyes. Torina and her three children were called "dark Swedes." Anna helped with the bakery and with the new baby and was still in school. In the tough economy, Thoralf began to learn the workings of the bakery from his father.

When Olaf was two and Torina was again with child, he came down sick with fever and was ill for many days. The family held vigil over him. The doctor was called. Olaf, a tough fighter, held on. He was affected but did not die. Though he was almost deaf and a little slower after the illness, the family was forever grateful he did not pass, and they protected him fiercely. Anders and Torina knew he would always need family to care for him, which strengthened their resolve.

A third son, born January 1903, was named after Anders and affectionately called Andy. Torina developed bed fever shortly after delivery. She was so sick that Thoralf and Olaf were sent away, back to the family farm. With her new baby and her daughters tending her, still Torina could not recover. She died. It was devastating for Anders, for the children.

At forty-one years of age, Anders was a widower again. He had steady work, yet he was unable to move into the master craftsmen guild and gain ownership of the bakery. Now a single father with five children, the youngest a baby, he was in a precarious position. Beyond Anna, who had finished her schooling and a year of catechism with the church, there was little support for his family. To survive, the grief was turned to work, the resolve to carry on. Anders's beloved city of Kristiana, still a territory under the Swedish government, gave Thoralf a tattoo—a mark along the inner left forearm to dissuade Anders from selling him. Selling children was outlawed in Scandinavia in 1900.

Kitty and Thoralf went to school. Thoralf played violin and was a diligent student and a loyal friend. Thoralf's tattoo and bakery work gave him a certain status among the street kids, many of whom were his friends. Some attended his school. Coming into the bakery store, which was always warm, and a bread scrap here and there went a long way. Olaf followed his brother into the bakery business. Both young brothers were strong workers.

Anders honored Torina with steadiness and hard work. He never remarried.

The taxes were steep in Norway, but the tithe, 10 percent of Anders's earnings to the state church, became a bitter link to the Swedish government. Anders decided to leave the old country; soon the Berg family would become part of the mass Scandinavian emigration (Hendron 2011). However, for health and safety, children had to be at least three years old for ship travel over ocean. Baby Andy would turn three in 1907. Plans were made. The family continued on with little outward sign of their intentions while saving money for travel. They were all vulnerable.

Kitty and Anna cared for the store. Anna stayed with her father and the young family and did not marry, instead getting extra work as a servant to save up for the upcoming journey. The family worked as a team, honoring Torina, as they focused on the free land in the new country. Consequently, sweet baby Andy grew up with the idea of farming homestead land. With each birthday, he marked the countdown to leaving Norway. His anticipation for the adventure helped them all.

Anna left for the new country late in the summer of 1907. Age twenty, she traveled to Liverpool, England, where her ship, the *Virginian*, was boarding. The cabin next to her housed a recently widowed Russian Hebrew man. On the transatlantic crossing, Anna enjoyed talking and sharing his company. He knew her language and taught her some English. When the ship landed in Quebec, Canada, on September 20, they parted, and Anna entered the new country through the northern state of Vermont. She took a train out to Creston City, Washington. Guided by an immigrant cousin, Anna applied for a homestead, the most amazing benefit offered by the new country.

In February 1908, Anders packed up and left Norway on the ship *United States*. His younger children—Kitty, eleven; Thoralf, ten; Olaf, seven; and Anders, now four—had no problems on the weeklong ship ride. There was lots of eager talk about the new country and the land. Young Andy's excitement brought smiles to all. They arrived at Ellis Island on February 27, 1908, then traveled the rest of the way to Creston City by railroad car.

The new country had low taxes. State and church were separate. There was no monarchy, and land was available; it seemed too good to be true. Anders enjoyed the travel, the train ride, and the beautiful land rolling by his window, his inability to speak English relegated to a minor concern.

When the family reunited at their cousin's home, Anna was already speaking the local language and welcomed them with an announcement: She had gotten two homesteads. The first eighty acres, near the town of Locke and the Tacoma River, as planned, was for her father. The second homestead, with her new husband, Martin Matson, a young Norwegian immigrant, was close by in Boulder Basin. The rail line had already been surveyed and was being completed in stages. Soon both homesteads would be connected by rail to the city of Spokane. It was a great surprise for Anders. He was so pleased that they were together in this land of opportunity.

During the mild winter in 1908, the reunited family spent little time cramped in their cousin's small house. Anna's new husband had gotten right to work and was building two cabins, one at each homestead. Anders worked alongside him. Before too long, they all moved to Anders's newly completed homestead cabin.

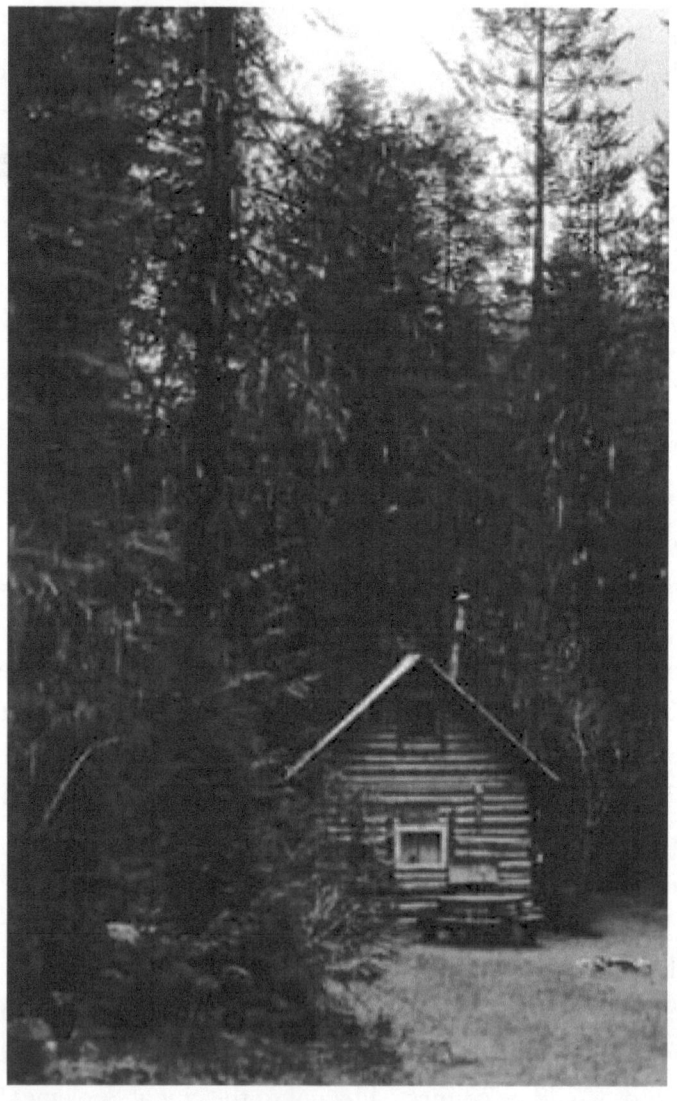

The family all moved to Anders's newly completed homestead cabin, 1908.

The young couple, set on farming and living on their land, enjoyed this time with Anders and the children. They could take longer to finish their cabin.

A spring crop was not possible that first year. The heavily timbered, rocky land on several slopes needed tree and rock removal before it could be plowed and seeded. With an immediate need to feed the children, Anders decided to visit Spokane. Anders walked to the railroad track from his cabin and hopped a train into town. He found a growing, vibrant city and quickly picked up a job baking bread.

The children stayed at the homestead and were always anxious for his return. He came back between jobs. On one return trip, he discovered Kitty and Thoralf had been fighting—with knives. They were also cold and ended up burning the front steps of the cabin for firewood. Anna was at her own cabin, finishing the build with Martin and neighbors. The children felt they had been left to fend for themselves.

Anders, pressured to decide, knew homesteading meant farming, which was not easy or simple. His land needed so much work; meanwhile, there was immediate opportunity in Spokane. His baking skills had already proven useful for jobs that paid, and the bakery where he was currently working had just been put up for sale. Located in the Lidgerwood neighborhood, it was close to a lumber mill.

Spokane was an advanced city. It had hydroelectric power and electric cable cars that connected all the neighborhoods. The Lidgerwood bakery had long, thin brick ovens that were sound. The storefront had large windows facing a main cable-car-equipped street. The rooms above the bakery were much larger than he was used to. There was no master craftsmen guild with rules on supplies and marketing his bread that would keep Anders out. In fact, there was a strong Scandinavian business community who welcomed and encouraged Anders (Hendron 2011). What an opportunity to do what he was unable to do in the old country!

Anders went to the land office to put his homestead up for sale. He was lucky; his eighty acres were deemed submarginal for farming.

Because of this, he could sell it back to the US government. The homestead with its improvement—the house—was valued at $219. Anders did not hesitate. He sold it. The money had a purpose. Anders was to be master baker of his own bakery. It was June 1908.

When Anders returned to the homestead cabin with his receipt and his proceeds, Anna was very happy for her father. She and Martin agreed to help. They would stay in Anders's homestead cabin with the younger children, at least until fall. Anders needed Thoralf in the city to work.

Anders bought the Lidgerwood bakery—north side of Spokane, southeast corner of Nevada and Bridgeport Streets—from the old couple who owned it, Mr. and Mrs. Shuster, for $100. Anders's dream was now real.

The former owners and bakery clients liked Anders and remained loyal to him as the new owner. Every day, Anders walked from his bakery and down the north hill into the business district of Spokane. There were several flour mills along the river where he could purchase flour. He would pick up a 100-pound bag from the north side of the river and carry it over his shoulder to the trolley cars. He would then pay to ride the trolley up the north hill. From the trolley stop, it was a short walk to the bakery.

Keeping the brick oven in the center of the bakery going was essential. There was wood on the lot that came with the sale and a wood mill down the hill—another pleasant contrast to the old country, where wood was only available through the guild, hauled in by carriage. A cord of wood was needed each day. Thoralf split and hauled it into the bakery. Both men stoked the oven. Anders baked one bag of flour at a time (Hendron 2011).

Mixing bread dough is a simple task, but turning a batch of dough into loaves requires kneading. A failure here would end an apprentice's career quickly. Done by hand, kneading makes for large, muscular arms and shoulders. This work can be exhausting and requires timing, speed, strength, and knowledge of the dough's chemistry. Anders had taught Thoralf the bakery tasks in the old country. Thoralf picked it up easily.

Loaves, rolls, and pastry were all for sale to customers in the storefront, and large orders were delivered by trolley or horse-drawn cart. Without further help, though, they struggled with the storefront; on the next trip to the homestead, Anders brought Kitty to Spokane. The younger sons were to stay with Anna and Martin. However, the boys preferred their own homestead. Young Andy loved the land and was set on being a farmer. Olaf was content when everyone else in the family was content. They promised that if a new homesteader arrived, they would leave then.

Kitty and Thoralf entered public school in Spokane that September. Because they did not speak English, the school placed them in the first-grade classroom. Thoralf, eleven years old that summer, was academically competitive. Kitty, at thirteen, was close to the end of her education. Annoyed by the young children in the classroom, she zeroed in on a girl named Leila, who was attentive and not bawling. Kitty and Thoralf both befriended Leila. Leila was particularly struck by Thoralf, so handsome with his blue eyes.

The language barrier was more difficult for Kitty, but soon both children were placed into a higher-grade classroom. English became their language. Thoralf excelled at school, though he continued to speak Norwegian as well, not wanting to lose his first language. Kitty would finish her schooling that year.

As a hired baker, Anders had introduced some of his breads at the Lidgerwood bakery, and they were well liked. The bakery soon had new customers who came for the Scandinavian hard rolls and bread loaves. They also sold pop and ice cream. The previous owner's wife, Mrs. Shuster, would come in and order from Kitty at the counter, and together they enjoyed many a pastry and "pop on ice."

By October 1908, the Matson cabin was up and shingled, but it needed flooring, chinking, and mudding. Though the weather was bright and beautiful, Anna wanted to get on with the work before the season changed. A hard worker herself and tough on everybody else, Anna kept after an older homesteader to start the mudding. He wasn't ready. He went home on Saturday night to take care of his cats. When he came back the next day, the weather had changed to one of those cold, clammy fall days with low-lying clouds, and the chinking was about done, with Anna doing a big share. She could split cedar and drive nails like a man. The homesteader, one of the originals to the area, was mad from all her ribbing. When he started mudding, mud flew clear through the cabin from wall to wall. Anna yelled, "Not quite so much power there." His answer: "This is a helluva job for an old man with rheumatism."

Olaf and Andy were as happy for their father as possible, but there had been so much hopeful talk about homesteading, farming the free land. To young Andy especially, baking bread had been difficult and bitter back in Norway. To break up the family—at least temporarily—was understandable; however, to the boys, the homestead cabin was their place. Andy and Olaf were to move to the Matson homestead that fall with their older half sister, whom they called Mrs. Matson. As far as they were concerned, though, the land and the cabin were always waiting for them.

By the time the census man came around in the early spring of 1910, the Berg family was settled, able to look forward. The last leg of the railroad came through that summer. With a train ticket and the rail stop at Locke, the separation distance was manageable.

Anders hired a worker for the bakery leading up to July 4, 1910. He wanted to be with all his children, together, for Independence Day in the new country. They celebrated at a neighbor's homestead. It was a beautiful day. The menfolk fished with cane poles, and the ladies fried up the fish. These neighbors were the first to have a cow, and the ice cream, milk, and strawberries were big treats. After the picnic, it was decided that Kitty would stay with these neighbors as they had a new baby that summer and a three-year-old son. This arrangement would allow the lady of the house to go out and harvest. That was the customary way to make a homestead stake in those days.

Andy and Olaf still spent most of their time at "their" homestead cabin. They fished out in the backwoods, played baseball, and shot pine squirrels. Then, late that summer, everyone was evacuated due to fire. The Great Fire of 1910 burned a swath of land straight up the mountain from one of the settlers' barns on Tacoma Creek. There was also a fire in Spokane that burned the downtown area. The bakery up on North Hill was fine, and so were both homesteads. The fire had been set off across the Northwest by lightning strikes, fueled by heavy winds and a dry spring.

After that fire, both Olaf and Andy started school in Spokane. Olaf did remarkably well. He kept up with his younger brother and even went into the grade ahead.

Soon new settlers came into the area by way of the fire trail. The trail led them to soft sand hills above the south fork of Tacoma Creek. Easy clearing of the trees in the burn path helped with rapid settling of that area. Spokane also grew rapidly after the fire (A. Berg 2002).

Thoralf, now taking night classes and working the bakery, kept the accounts and filled orders. For a break, he would take a fresh loaf from the morning batch and go outside. If it was cold, he would climb out his bedroom window, sit next to the warm brick chimney, and enjoy the view over the river and downtown, munching on his bread and hard cheese (Hendron 2011).

The Davenport Hotel opened in Spokane in September 1914. It was the first hotel with air-conditioning, a central vacuum system, and housekeeping carts. The *Spokane Newspaper* introduced the hotel to the public with a special Sunday ad trumpeting "the new two-million-dollar hostelry of Spokane." At its opening, the Davenport Hotel was also the largest private telephone branch exchange in the entire Pacific Northwest with 450 handsets. It had the largest and most complicated plumbing—thirty miles of pipes delivering hot and cold drinking water to every one of its 405 guest rooms. Gilded in gold, sparkling with crystal and a huge glass ceiling over the atrium, and illuminated throughout with "electroliers," the hotel was as grand as the finest ocean liners of the day. Anders began to sell his bread there; Thoralf made the deliveries in a new truck. Anders also belonged to a group of Scandinavian merchants who met quarterly at this hotel.

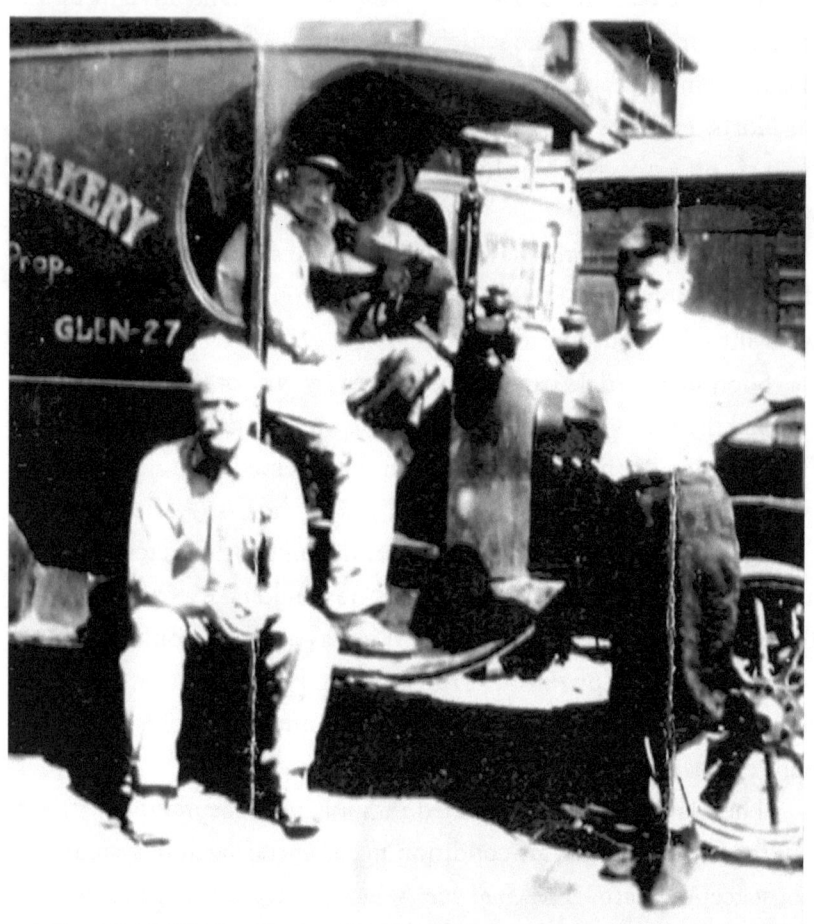

Thoralf made the deliveries in a new truck

Around 1916, with both of his girls married and doing well, Anders insisted his three boys work with him. But the boys did not want to bake bread for a living. Young Andy talked of being a weatherman and Olaf a prospector. Both Olaf and Andy loved rocks and filled the basement with them. Thoralf wanted to be a machinist; intelligent, he had taken a second job with the railroad roundhouse, and he wanted to get an education—high school, trade school, even college.

Then, one day in September 1918, Thoralf received draft papers. His friend Stewart, also twenty-one years old, got the same set of papers. Together the two friends talked about being drafted and serving the country in the Great War. In preparation for service, they took off together and spent a couple of weeks camping up at Priest Lake, enjoying their last days of freedom. By the time they returned to Spokane, ready to report, the war had ended. All were thankful.

CHAPTER 3

Crown Prince, 1921

When the war ended before his draft presentation date, Thoralf decided this was his opportunity to see what life could be. Returning from Priest River to this news, he found his father and brothers prepared for his military absence, running the bakery without him. So Thoralf took off on his Indian motorcycle and headed to the west side of the state. He loved riding the open road. He had a bedroll and slept along the roadside in grass fields. He visited his sister Kitty and her husband, Roy, in Tukwila, Washington.

Roy got Thoralf a factory job where he was working. Together they rode the Indian up and down the inner urban highway to the factory and then home. Roy and Thoralf spent hours in Roy's garage after work. Roy was interested in brakes. With automobiles getting heavier and moving faster, the caliper brakes used with horse carriages were inadequate. The two men repaired many of these brakes in Roy's garage. They designed a disc brake, tested it, and modified it, and it worked. They talked about getting a patent. Kitty enjoyed this time with her younger brother.

Thoralf was surprised but happy when a letter arrived from Leila. She had missed him terribly during the half year he had been gone. In no uncertain terms, she asked him to return to her and Spokane. At eighteen, she was ready to marry. Thoralf finally knew what he meant to Leila.

She had been enthralled by him since they first met in the fall of 1908. Thoralf, out of place with his broken English, had been shy and quiet back then. His contained demeanor initially had Leila concerned he might be dumb. Thoralf played violin and Leila the piano; they played together, and it drew them closer. As their friendship grew, Leila learned about the death of his mother, his tattoo, the family's decision to leave the old country, being an immigrant, and having to work and put school second. Leila found him kind.

Thoralf would regularly visit Leila at the house her father had built, a nice break for Thoralf. Living above the bakery with his family and working every day was a crush. Leila made lunch and carried it to her father daily in the summers—a short walk down North Hill to the Exchange Lumberyard at Buckeye and Hamilton Streets where he worked. Then, in the summer of 1914, Leila discovered men gathered around her father as he lay on the ground, hurt by a large timber on a pulley.

Through the commotion, Leila comforted her father. He was able to limp home with her help, bent over in pain. Sick for many months with weakness and infection, he could not work. Eventually, a stooling wound in his right lower abdomen developed. Her mother had to get work, as there were young children. Leila dressed the stooling wound, which caused her father pain. Washing and bleaching the dressings nearly overwhelmed her, and she became sensitive, almost defensive about his illness.

Her father slowly got better. Leila took a job after school. The money helped. Leila's friendship with Thoralf was stabilizing for her. He was supportive of her efforts to work and go to school. He checked on her often.

It became too much for Leila when she entered high school. She reluctantly quit school to work full-time at the phone company. When her mother announced another child was due, well, this seemed irresponsible to Leila. Her dreams of college were shattered. She formed an agreement with her parents that she would help with money from her work at the phone company, but Leila would not take care of this baby. She did not want to be a mother's helper.

After receiving Leila's letter, Thoralf returned to Spokane. When Anders heard his son's news, he was hopeful. The bakery had suffered while Thoralf was away. Thoralf's skill kneading the bread and dealing with the accounts and the customers was needed. But Anders understood Thoralf had a choice. The first son talked with his father and, at the age of twenty-two, agreed to take over the bakery. Then Thoralf asked Leila to marry him. She said yes to her handsome and intelligent man. Bypassing his dream of being a mechanic was a sacrifice Thoralf made willingly.

In late May 1919, Anders set the will. His first son, Thoralf, would take his place upon his death.

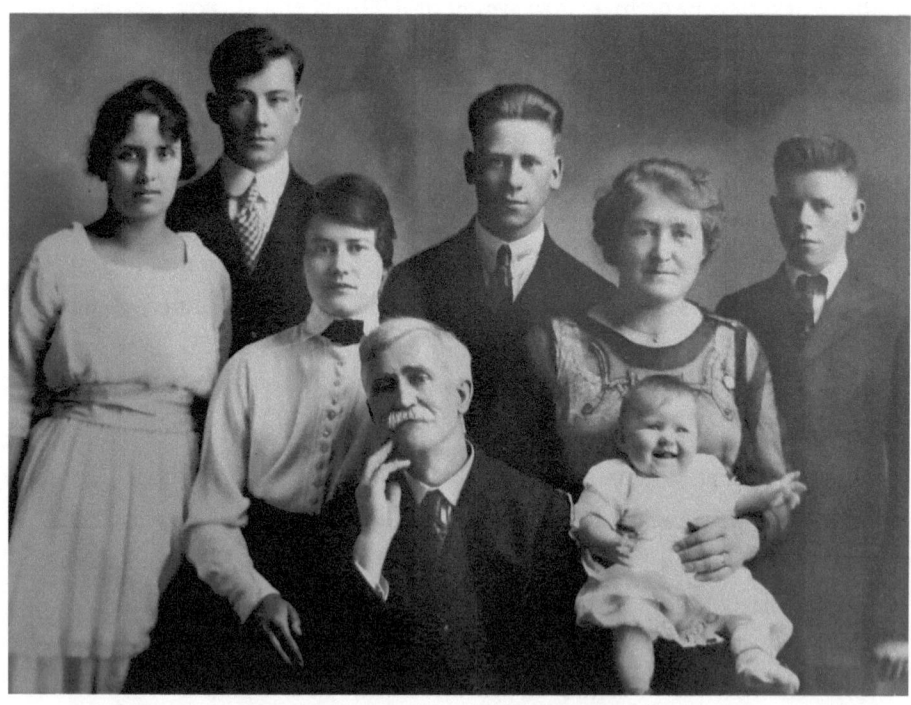

Wedding of Thoralf and Leila with family, 1918. After the wedding, Thoralf and Leila moved into a small house close to the bakery.

After the wedding, Thoralf and Leila moved into a small house close to the bakery. Thoralf continued with night classes.

The Berg family's decisions and hard work led to productive lives. Kitty and Roy moved forward with a patent for the disc brakes. Anna divorced Mr. Matson after their homestead burned to the ground from moonshining. She adopted a young girl, her only child. Anna then found and happily married the kindest man. Anders remained single, attended church services, and honored his beloved Torina. He lived at the bakery, dedicated to his work and family, especially Olaf.

Leila became pregnant and gave birth to a boy, Ralph (the American version of "Thoralf") Berg, on May 22, 1921. Thoralf could not believe how beautiful his new son was. He dreamed of great things for the infant. First child, first son, and first grandchild.

It had been an easy decision to take Leila to the Park Hill Hospital for the delivery. She was attended by Dr. McCoy; for many years, Kitty had worked for this doctor's wife as a mother's helper. Sitting across the river on the south side, the hospital was owned by the doctors. Thoralf was thankful for a healthy son and that his wife had not died in childbirth.

Historical Note 1, 1921

Insulin was discovered by Canadian Dr. Fred Banting (1891–1941), a WWI surgeon who returned from war and struggled to establish a surgical practice.

The worldwide flu epidemic left tens of millions dead. Many flu survivors were children who then developed diabetes, with a slower death. Prior to the discovery of insulin, most doctors' approaches to these diabetic children was to advise letting the child eat whatever they wanted and die in a timely manner. The only therapy, offered by one rare doctor, was a disciplined and draconian diet under medical supervision. This diet method offered these children more time, up to eighteen months, with the hope that a therapy would be forthcoming from the medical researchers.

The idea to ligate—or tie off—the pancreatic duct to shrink and remove the exocrine pancreas cells, leaving the elusive endocrine cells, was not originally Dr. Fred Banting's idea. However, he learned the postligation extract was collectable and contained the elusive islet cells that produced hormones to regulate blood sugar. His team established postligation models of diabetic animals, rabbits, and sheep. The extract could be delivered back to the diabetic animal models in the research laboratory, and it would bring the animals' blood sugars down.

Next, they extracted volumes of insulin from freshly slaughtered commercial animals. They injected the islet extract/insulin into the diabetic animals and effected a benefit. When Dr. Banting brought insulin to these starving diabetic children, he personally injected the insulin. Because he was unable to test blood sugar levels, several of the children died of overdoses. These overdose deaths nearly overwhelmed Dr. Banting with grief. But ultimately, insulin for diabetes was a huge success. Over the years, technology continues to improve the outcome of this illness (Ainsberg 2010).

Historical Note 2, 1923

Using a tenotomy knife where the sharp blade could be fired from its sheath when needed, surgeon Dr. Elliot Cutler (1888–1947), at the Peter Bent Brigham Hospital in Boston, was able to successfully open a stenosed valve leaflet on a patient with rheumatic mitral heart disease. His cardiologist, Dr. Samuel Levine (1891–1966), was well known for his plan of care for heart attack patients: rest for six weeks and then slow advances to a sedentary lifestyle in an armchair (L. Cohn 1993).

At the North Hill bakery, the Berg family was happily settled, with Thoralf, Olaf, and Andy working with their master baker father. The brick building was solid, the storefront had big, inviting windows, and it was on a busy corner. Its reputation for fresh breads and sweets steadily grew its clientele.

After twenty years of struggle, it seemed a fitting time for Anders to return to the old country for a visit. Family there was dwindling, as so many had left. He traveled to Norway by himself over the summer of 1927, journeying by railcar across the country and by ocean liner across the Atlantic. When Anders returned to the Northwest, he shared how pleased he was that Norway was no longer a territory; Kristiana was now called Oslo. Anders brought home baskets filled with gifts for his grandchildren. He had also arranged for his younger brother's daughter Karina, studying to be a nurse, to come the next summer for a visit.

Not far from the brick bakery, another bakery came up for sale. Thoralf liked the modern electric mixers. The building had a brick oven and a house attached in the front, with a lawn. A porch ran from the back kitchen door to the bakery. A third lot was used for firewood. Anders and Olaf could move into the house. Thoralf, with his father and brothers' approval, sold the old bakery and bought this one in the fall of 1927. The electric mixers allowed them to make more dough, and soon they were selling bread, hard rolls, cake donuts, raised donuts, cinnamon rolls, snails, and maple bars—all downtown, as there was no longer a storefront. Thoralf ran the business and made the daily deliveries in the truck (Hendron 2011).

Thoralf and Leila's children grew sick in the late spring of 1928. Their daughter recovered from the chicken pox in a few days, but Ralph developed shaking chills and was talking out of his head. The extended family gathered, and all thought Ralph was going to die. Thoralf sat by his son's bed, himself sick with worry.

Anders's niece Karina arrived from Norway as planned. When she found young Ralph so ill, she took it upon herself to tend him. She never left his side. She slept with him, fed him, and washed his brow when the fevers came. Thoralf finally called the doctor, who noted an ear infection had progressed to the mastoid bone, which is filled with air cells. Ralph was taken to the hospital, and the mastoid abscess was surgically drained.

During recovery, Thoralf played his violin for Ralph. He sang to him. He talked to him and read to him. Sir Alfred Tennyson's book of poetry was a favorite. Ralph would muster a smile whenever his dad got to the line, "Men may come and men may go, but I go on forever" from the poem "The Brook." Ralph slowly got better, but worried, "I messed up Karina's vacation."

His energy and willfulness steadily returned. Leila's youngest brother, who was six years older than Ralph, came over and took Ralph out for a bike ride. He put Ralph on his front handlebar and rode him up and down the street. When they came flying back, laughing at the youngsters chasing them, the elders knew Ralph was to be okay.

Young Ralph started work with his grandfather once he was well enough. He would walk the mile from his parents' house to the bakery. Anders had his grandson grease the pans to be ready for the next day. Then he added the task of sweeping out the hardwood floors. Soon young Ralph was helping with the wood. The brick oven demanded a cord of split wood daily. Ralph performed these duties until he left for college.

On weekends, Thoralf drove his family out into the country. The young family was mesmerized by the beauty of Lake Coeur d'Alene. First stop was Spokane Point, a five-mile drive on a dirt logging road from Worley, Idaho. Ralph would eagerly call the ferry from Spokane Point by raising a flag on the float house. Across Lake Coeur d'Alene, the ferry boat captain would see the flag and head over, mooring on Spokane Point. Being out on the water, their car on the ferry, was exhilarating to the entire family. Once their time across the lake was complete, usually involving a picnic and ice cream, the drive back to Spokane would take them around the north part of the lake, through the town of Coeur d'Alene. It was a stunning and beautiful road trip.

Ralph started school in the fall of 1929, going into third grade at the local public school. He was an excellent student, which pleased his father, but there was little else to be happy about. The Great Depression took its toll everywhere. Fathers looking for any work in exchange for day-old bread loaves resonated with Leila. She knew the challenge of a father out of work. She handed out as many bread loaves as she could. Thoralf always had the day-old bread up for discount; he too remembered the hard times in Norway. Soon some of the neighborhoods became rough, but overall, the bakery held steady during the Depression and its aftermath. Thoralf and Leila were thankful for the work.

In the late fall of 1930, Leila got a phone call from the hospital. Her father was ill, and she should come right away. Thoralf was out in the delivery truck, so she ran the mile to the bakery. Olaf and Anders were there. Anders did not drive, and Leila did not like to drive and was too distraught to do so, so Olaf drove her to the hospital. At five miles per hour, deaf as a post but not dumb, he got Leila there safely. Unfortunately, when they rushed into the hospital room, Leila learned her father had died. On autopsy it was discovered that her father had colon cancer in his stooling abdominal wound from fifteen years earlier. He was barely fifty years old.

Olaf felt terrible that he had not gotten Leila to the hospital sooner, "so she could see her father and say goodbyes."

Historical Note 3, 1930

Dr. John Gibbon (1903–1973) was a research fellow at the Harvard Medical School, working with the surgical team after completing his surgical training at Pennsylvania Hospital. A patient with a massive pulmonary embolism—a blood clot in the lung—after a surgical procedure was deteriorating hemodynamically, approaching death. At this time in history, the dramatic pulmonary embolectomy surgical procedure was high risk, performed only as a last effort to save a life. Young Dr. Gibbon was on watch and called for Dr. Edward D. Churchill (1895–1972) at the moment this patient's life was on the line. Dr. Churchill performed the embolectomy. The patient died, and Dr. Gibbon was deeply affected. He conceptualized a machine that would help in such a surgery where the heart and lungs were not able to perform. He began his research into a machine that could stop the heart while performing its functions so surgeons could efficiently perform lifesaving operations (L. H. Cohn 2003).

Ralph, done with eighth grade, went on a trip with Anders to Yellowstone Park in the summer of 1932. They drove and stayed several weeks, with a five-day camping trip in the middle. It was beautiful and special. When they returned to Spokane, they were surprised to find Kitty and her children living at the bakery.

Roy, Kitty's husband, had last been seen at the boat docks north of Seattle while on a trip to visit family in Canada. He never made it to Canada. Kitty had no money and a new baby. Responding to a series of escalating wires, Anna sent her husband to fetch her sister. After paying bills and arranging a moving van, he drove Kitty and her four young children home to Spokane. They moved in with Olaf, who was pleased. A distraught Kitty planned to go on "relief," a state program for single mothers with children, but Anders would not let her. He wanted to care for his daughter and thought he and the Berg family could do so. Retirement or even slowing down was not in Anders's constitution.

Kitty was soon working at the bakery. There was no storefront, but there was work. Olaf loved caring for them. Thoralf was less enthusiastic.

All held out hope that Roy would come back. Kitty never divorced, never saw her husband again, and never remarried. Anders learned the patent for the disc brake had not been secured, paid the fee, and secured it for ten years. The family carried on and took care of each other.

Every Sunday evening, Thoralf and Leila came to the bakery. They visited and did the orders for the next week, coordinating supplies, production, and deliveries. They took orders from and sold to the Post Street market, Desert Street Hotel, open-market vendors, and the Davenport Hotel. The open markets were Ralph's favorites. He and his dad would make deliveries early in the morning to the booth vendors, who would sell the breads and reorder for the next week. The Scandinavian loaves, etched on top with three marks made by Olaf and his razor blade, were in demand.

At the end of summer, Thoralf's niece and his daughter, ages five and seven, were running through the bakery. His niece slid on the wood floor, fell, and hit her mouth on the flour stand, knocking her two front teeth into the roof of her mouth. At the dentist the next day, her baby teeth were pulled out. This event so upset Leila, tidy and rigid in her standards, that she stopped coming over on Sunday evenings, and whenever Thoralf met up with his family, she refused to join him (Hendron 2011).

Ralph, nicknamed "Crown Prince," was big, smart, strong, and handsome, with dark, curly hair and bright-blue eyes. Thoralf explained the nickname to his nieces and nephews: "I never have to spank him." When asked seriously by his young niece about what made Ralph so special, Thoralf said, "Ralph has a sound mind and a calm demeanor. He is a hard worker, and talented. Curious and engaged in everything, he has an innovating, figure-it-out-and-fix-it personality."

Thoralf continued his education with night classes and enjoyed his son's academic success. He bought a piece of land on Lake Coeur d'Alene by the ferry dock. His brother Andy bought their father's original eighty-acre homestead up north that same year, 1933, fulfilling a lifelong dream (A. Berg 2002).

Ralph, at age twelve, hardly knew of the homestead. He loved to be at the lake. With every arrival at Spokane Point, Ralph performed his task of setting up the flag. Mr. Ketchum, the ferry operator, would start up the boiler engine and come the mile across the water to get the family, making several trips a day on the weekends. The nearby pheasants, scared out of hiding by the ferry, would attempt to fly across the lake to escape. Some would drop into the water, exhausted. Ralph paddled out to save as many pheasants as he could. Some did not make it (R. Berg 2006).

The lake was quiet on the weekends during the winter holiday, so the men got wooden skis, drove to Mt. Spokane, hiked up the slope with their skis on their backs, and skied down. They would do this until they were exhausted. Leila stayed home with her daughter, cooking and cleaning. Then she would go out shopping with Kitty.

A gun-shooting range opened in Spokane. Ralph had long hunted with his dad and uncles. This was how the family survived on the homestead. Thoralf and his brothers shot deer, squirrels, and marmots for meat, but Thoralf was leery of skeet shooting at this range. The precision shooting was expensive and not directly tied to a practical need; it was just a sport. But Ralph was an excellent shot and would not let the topic go. Another man asked Thoralf if he could enter Ralph into the skeet-shooting competition. Thoralf agreed to this, curious how the youngster would do. Ralph shot his father's side-by-side Fox rifle and took first place. Hunting and precision shooting as a sport became a passion of Ralph's.

When the summer of 1934 rolled in, Thoralf and his son built a cabin on the lake property using some logs that had come loose from tugboats moving huge log booms down the waterway. They added an outhouse, a welcome luxury to Leila. A local hardware store in Worley, Idaho, had opened the summer before, and Ralph and his dad were frequent customers with the new cabin and long weekends at the lake. Father and son also built a boat with an outboard motor and boated all over the water. Before too long, Ralph was boating alone. He particularly liked to go up the St. Joe River and into all the little lakes that channeled into the river.

As a willful child who had survived a childhood illness, Ralph pushed the limits. His parents were not inclined to reprimand him. A young teenager during the summer of 1935, he made a bow and arrows and shot the neighbor's cat. The police came. There was much upheaval over this. Another time, he was fooling around with a .22 pistol and accidentally shot himself in the hand, developing an infection at the site. Luckily, a doctor came on a house call for his sister. The doctor determined she had strep throat and gave her a new sulfa antibiotic. Ralph, lying on his parents' bed and moaning with his throbbing hand hanging over the edge, soaking in a pot, caught the doctor's attention. The doctor took Ralph to the hospital and lanced the abscess in his hand, in addition to administering sulfa drugs (Gayda 2011).

Ralph started at the new John R. Rogers High School that fall. Thoralf was impressed by his son's natural talent. Ralph got a job offer from a neighbor and was excited and eager to accept it, wanting to help the family. But his dad told him, "No, you are going to college." Thoralf wanted Ralph to reap every advantage of this new country. He knew Ralph would become something important.

Ralph played football, as did his younger cousin Andy Berg Jr., who would go on to play football at college. Leila got upset watching Ralph limp home with his football friends, laughing and talking about the team. Despite Leila's worry and obstruction, she could not influence her son. So she threatened the football coach, but it came to nothing. Fortunately, Ralph never got seriously hurt or had his teeth knocked out. He was elected student body president in his senior year.

Historical Note 4, 1938

Dr. Robert Gross (1908–1988) successfully ligated a patent ductus, the intrauterine connection between the aorta and the pulmonary artery—the two great vessels that keep blood flow out of the lungs—that closes at birth to vitalize the lungs, in a symptomatic seven-year-old girl at

Boston Children's Hospital associated with Harvard Medical School. He performed a second successful operation within a short time.

Dr. Gross, thirty-three at the time, was fired for this success by the skeptical senior surgeon Dr. Ladd upon his return from vacation. Dr. Gross had intentionally waited until Dr. Ladd was on a ship to Europe before operating outside the dog research lab on the young patient with a blue-baby defect. These two surgeons had a tense relationship, as the older Dr. Ladd had difficulty controlling and little appreciation for the younger, brilliant Dr. Gross.

The patent ductus was the first blue-baby defect for which a repair was scientifically developed in an animal research lab. When the ductus fails to close, it steals blood flow from the lungs. Located outside the pericardial sac, the ductus causes a shunt where blood from the aorta, a high-pressure artery, goes directly into the pulmonary artery, a lower-pressure artery, and back to the left atrium and ventricle, bypassing the lungs and causing extra work for the heart. When successfully ligated, the heart is helped by decreasing its workload (Chaphin 2014; L. Murray 2013).

When Ralph graduated high school in 1939 with honors, Thoralf was pleased. When Ralph started college with a scholarship, he was proud; but the expense was difficult. It was more money than Thoralf had spent taking night classes and more than he could muster. Still, he gave $500 to Ralph and enjoyed discussing the topics Ralph was learning whenever he came home from Pullman and Washington State College.

CHAPTER 4

A Six-Year Transformation, 1939–1945

That day was special. Mary Lenz was standing by a tree in the schoolyard, waiting for her family after school let out for the day. She was also hoping to see him. She really liked him. He was so handsome.

Ralph approached her. She anticipated only a conversation, as he was dating her friend, and Mary could understand why. Her friend was cute, an outgoing cheerleader whose mother was adored by both Ralph and Mary. Mary was reserved, serious. Ralph did not say anything when he got close to Mary. Then he kissed her.

With that kiss, Ralph chose Mary Lenz, and she was thrilled. She was sixteen years old, and it was the late spring of their junior year in high school. Ralph never looked back. Mary, tall, elegant, and beautiful, had known from the start of eighth grade that Ralph was for her. He was so very smart. Initially, while in middle school, Mary had a concern about his character. But she came to know him. He was solid. She waited for Ralph.

As they dated over the summer, took trips with Ralph and his family to the lake, then started their senior year at the high school, it was obvious to friends and family that Mary was for Ralph, though Thoralf and Leila worried that she might distract Ralph from his studies.

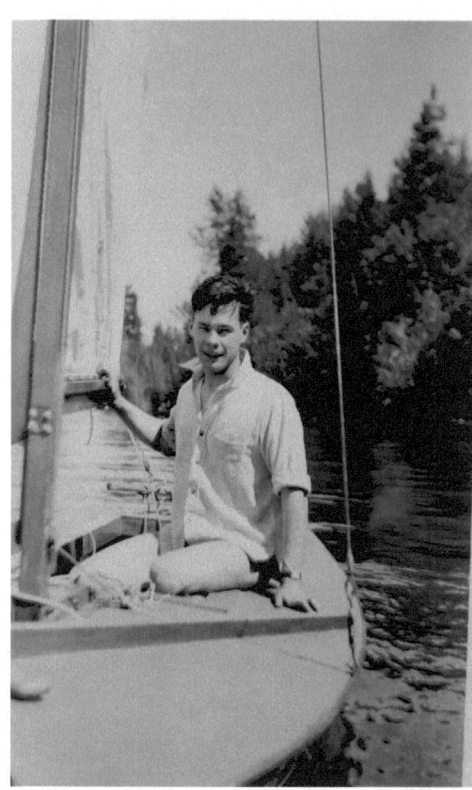 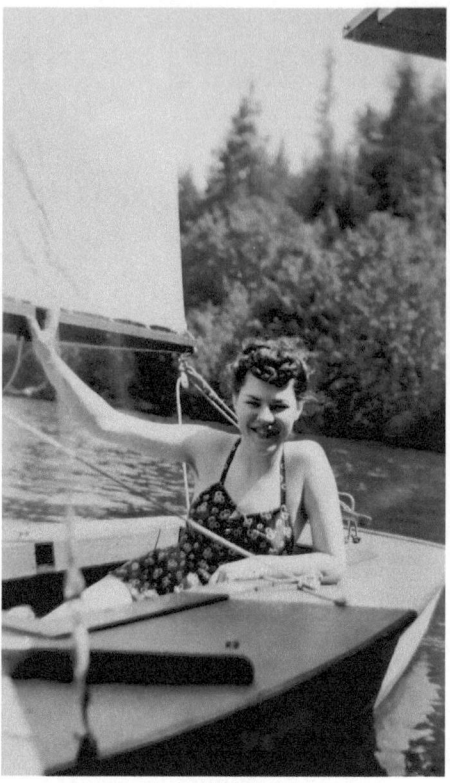

Mary and Ralph in the sailboat at lake CDA summer after high school graduation 1938. The trips to the lake were favorites.

The following spring, 1939, Ralph and Mary graduated from Rogers High School, Ralph with honors and an academic scholarship to attend college the next fall. Mary had enjoyed high school. She started work right after completing her diploma and saved her money, with plans to attend college in the future. She and Ralph were both hard workers.

Mary's mother, Jesse, had adopted young Mary from her widowed and pregnant sister when Mary was just two years old. Edward and Jesse Lenz were stable and caring parents. In time, Jesse developed a goiter, which slowed her down. Mary picked up her mother's work—dishes, laundry, sewing, cooking. Mary was the caregiver at her home. She got her family through the difficult times.

For Ralph, college started as one thing and ended as something else. When he left home for Pullman, Washington, in the fall of 1939, he was the first in the family to attend college. The first to truly enjoy the fruits of the family's efforts to provide stability. It was exciting and special. Ralph was challenged, and he excelled, looking forward to his science and physiology courses and leaning toward advanced studies in medicine.

Visiting home meant an eighty-mile drive on a dreadful road. For Mary, so happy to see Ralph on an occasional weekend, the separation when he left was difficult. She missed him and wanted to be in college with him.

Europe was at war once again in the fall of 1939. The impending American entry into this war kept Thoralf and Anders engaged with world politics. Then Anders came down sick in early spring 1940. He had gotten thin, and a bad cough set in after getting caught in a rainstorm following a downtown Norwegian music concert that he attended with Kitty. Anders continued to work until he was too weak to get out of bed. He died in early April. The autopsy showed Anders had stomach cancer.

Germany invaded Norway the next week, and everyone in the family agreed it was a blessing that Anders had not had to suffer with that knowledge.

Things changed even further. Ralph heard bits and pieces when he could arrange to come home. In the end, the family's financial stability was diminished. Anders's last will and testament left the bakery to Thoralf. Ownership did not change Olaf's view of the bakery and his role there. He continued to work and care for Kitty and her family. For Thoralf, there was no surprise in this document outlining his life. He too continued his work. Without Anders's efforts, though, money to support Ralph at college remained tight. Their younger brother, Andy, left the bakery (A. Berg 2002).

Over that summer, during work at the bakery and visits to the lake, Ralph recognized the rising turmoil in his family.

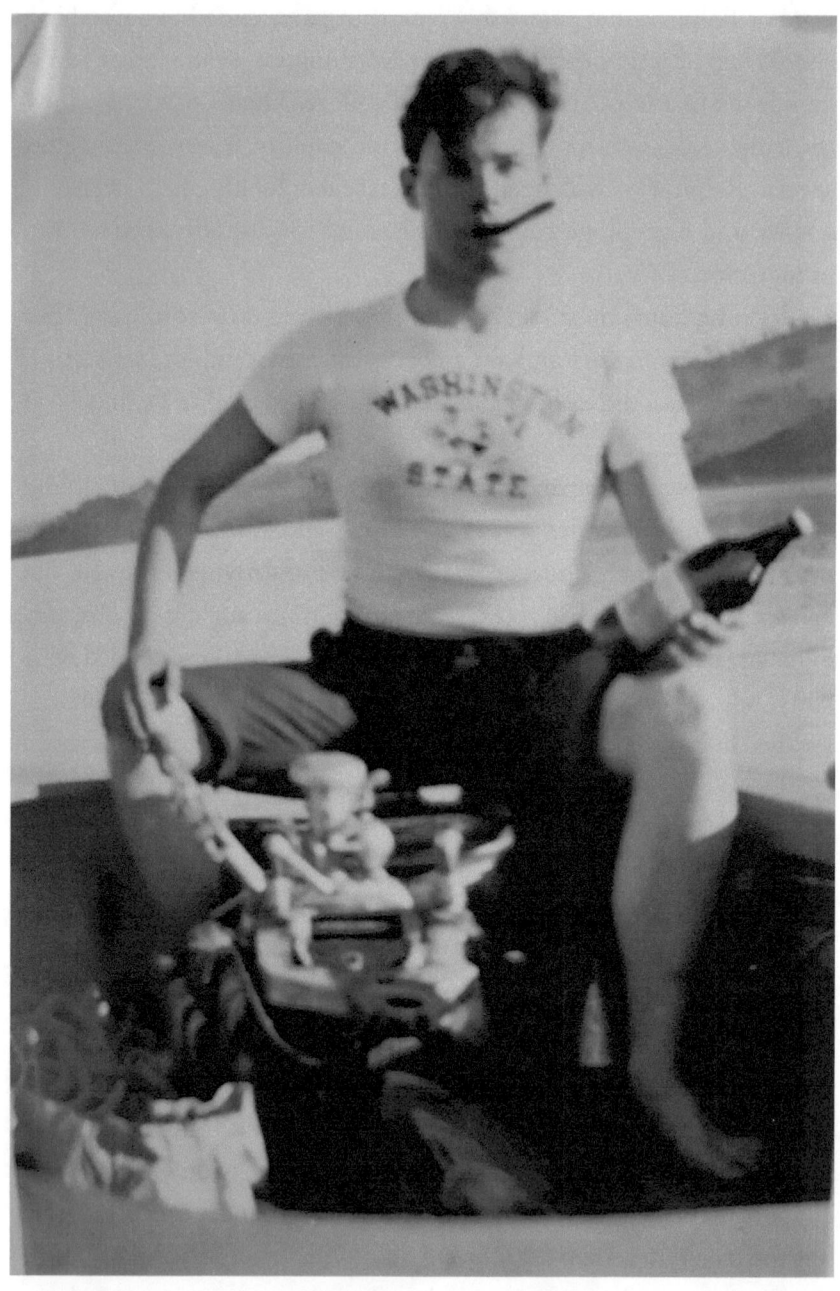

Ralph in motor boat with beer, cigar, and WSC T-shirt, summer after his first year of college, 1939.

His two aunts, Kitty and Anna, were at odds, with Anna blaming Kitty for exposing Anders to the cold elements. Meanwhile, Ralph's mother, Leila, was looking larger and acting secretive. All assumed she had cancer, so it was quite a surprise when Ralph's parents, now forty-three and thirty-nine, revealed a pregnancy.

Dr. Herb Eastlick, a new professor in the Department of Physiology, arrived at Washington State College when Ralph returned to campus in the fall of 1940. With a PhD in cell biology from Washington University in St. Louis, Missouri, Dr. Eastlick was a taskmaster and an autocrat in the classroom, holding his students to a high standard. Ralph was impressed. In turn, the professor was impressed with Ralph, a diligent student whose mind was logical and sound. The two young men became close.

Dr. Eastlick facilitated Ralph's getting a much-needed job. On weekends, for thirty-five cents per hour, Ralph made galvanized metal replicas of ear cartilage in the taxidermy museum. The taxidermist would finish the mount by stretching the hide over the metal ear form. Being a hunter of fish, deer, and birds, Ralph really enjoyed this artistic work.

Toward the end of his sophomore year, Ralph came to Spokane more frequently. When the spring semester was done, he moved back. The first thing he did that summer in 1941 was ask Mary for her hand in marriage. Ralph was ready and longed for a solid relationship. Mary, smart, calm, honest, and loyal, said yes without hesitation. Because his parents were focused on their new baby son, he did not mention his engagement. Mary made herself a beautiful wedding outfit. On September 19, 1941, at the small wedding chapel in Coeur d'Alene, Ralph and Mary were married. Mary's parents were present. When the newly married couple returned to Spokane, they celebrated with Ralph's new in-laws.

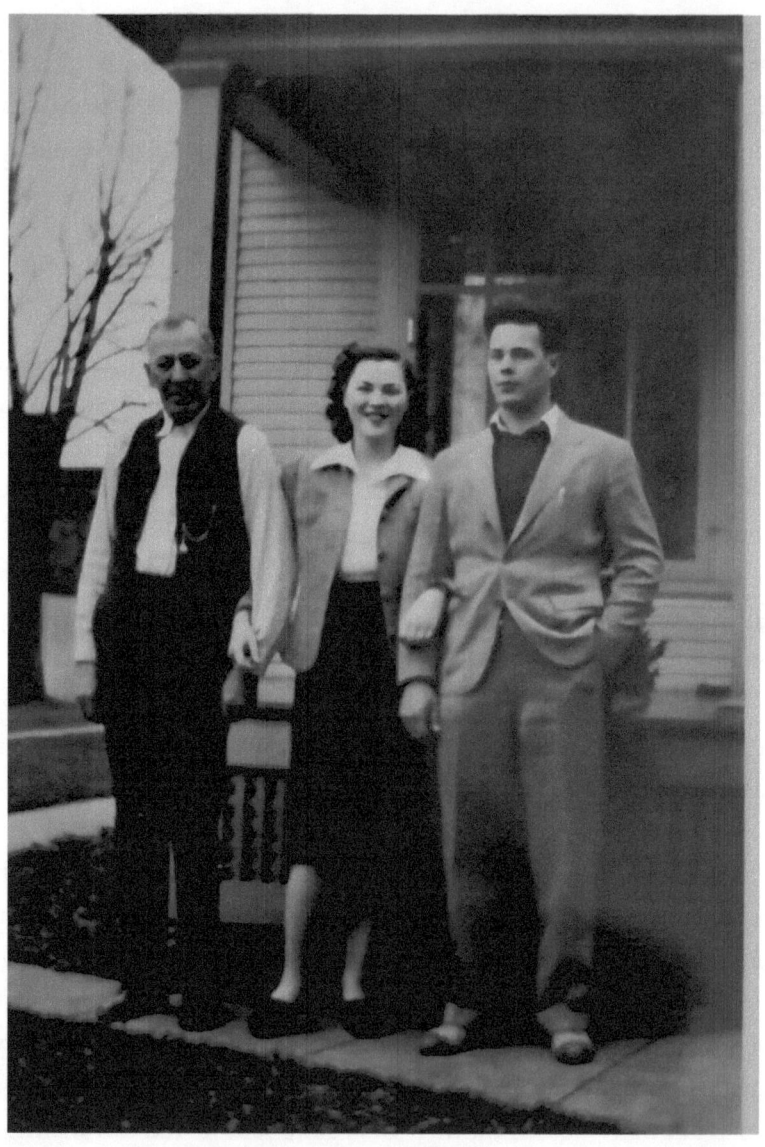

Ralph and Mary standing with her father at his house in the fall of Ralph's second year of college, 1940.

Then they told Ralph's parents their news. Thoralf and Leila were not prepared. Still worried that Mary could distract Ralph from his studies, and with Leila particularly unsettled with her latest child, their advice to the young couple was "Don't expect help from us with any children."

Ralph and Mary laughed it off. Ralph could see that his new brother, Mike, made his father happy.

Ralph registered and entered his third year of college. Mary, just starting college, signed up for general courses. They rented an apartment. Mary got a job making four dollars a day, typing and editing letters with the Agriculture Extension Service. They soon realized their situation was untenable, so they poured their efforts into helping Ralph finish his education. Mary stepped out of her courses.

At the Agriculture Extension Service, Mary was the most junior employee in a poorly run office where the bosses sometimes played cards. She tried to improve the office's efficiency. Ralph and Mary, both children of the Great Depression, saved every penny and were frugal and somewhat disturbed by this brewing war concern. The amount of money being spent for an inefficient office seemed wasteful to both.

Ralph made plans for medical school. Dr. Eastlick advised him on professional school entrance and application, highly recommending his alma mater, Washington University. The young couple visited the home of Dr. Eastlick and his wife, where the two couples discussed professional school and the Eastlicks' life in St. Louis. Ralph and Mary both liked and trusted Dr. Eastlick immensely. Dr. Eastlick wrote a letter of introduction and recommendation to support Ralph Berg's applications, and Ralph soon sent them out.

He was accepted to Harvard Medical School; however, he was advised that unless he had enough money, he would be better off choosing another school. At the time, medical schools were filled with "sons of wealthy men."

The surprise bombing of Pearl Harbor on December 7, 1941, brought the United States into World War II. Most of the lumberjacks were drafted, and wood became scarce. Thoralf switched both his house and the bakery house to coal furnaces. The bakery oven could not be converted.

The letter from Washington University's School of Medicine in St. Louis arrived. Ralph had been accepted to Dr. Eastlick's alma mater. Mary was pleased. Dr. Eastlick was pleased. Ralph accepted this offer. Shortly after accepting, Ralph and Mary learned he could start medical school that fall instead of the following year. All over the country, the war demand for young men was creating a domino effect of change. Colleges, universities, and professional schools were compressing their curriculums to fulfill education requirements and graduate men on an accelerated timeline. In many cases, positions were left void as men in training and with academic appointments left for war (R. Berg 2006).

Washington University was starting the next medical school class early, by a year. And Washington State College agreed to compress its four-year degree into three years by accepting the medical school's anatomy course as a fulfillment of senior-year requirements for the undergraduate students. Ralph would send the anatomy course credits back to Washington State College and receive college credit. His Washington State college diploma would be received at the end of his first year at Washington University.

Ralph's career in medicine was met with encouragement and reassurances. It was a natural continuation of his successful academic career. His degree, a bachelor of science, cum laude, would be awarded the following year. It was more than Thoralf ever expected.

Mary's support of her husband was constant. The young couple left Pullman and Washington State College with high hopes. Work and some welcome vacation time in Spokane and Lake Coeur d'Alene filled that summer. In Spokane, the older Berg aunts were finally reconciled, as Kitty was now sick with cancer. Ralph's younger sister, Margaret, had graduated high school and struggled to find a job. It was a hard reality. There were no scholarships that year due to the war. Margaret was expected to put herself through college. She failed the typing test, a skill she had neglected to learn, believing she would not be a secretary if she attended college. Finally, she got a job key-punching cards for IBM at the air depot. Living at home, working, and helping with her new brother, she saved for college, as Mary had done (Gayda 2011).

Late August 1942, Ralph and Mary left for St. Louis on the train. "It is an honorable profession" were Thoralf's affirming words as his oldest traveled to start medical school. Ralph and Mary moved into an apartment close to Barnes Hospital and the medical school. As Ralph started his medical training, Mary got a job with the Time and Leave Department, a war effort department (M. Berg 2011).

Ralph's aunt Kitty died that September. Her children stayed with Olaf at the bakery. Andy and Olaf took the disc brake and the ten-year patent to Seattle and showed it to Studebaker and Ford Motor Companies. The patent was due to run out. Studebaker was interested, but no sale was made. The patent ran out a few weeks after Kitty passed (Hendron 2011).

Before long, the heat of St. Louis, Missouri, grew uncomfortable. Mary went looking for a cooler living situation. Out on Olive Street, a road lined with big shade trees and close to the university, she found a nice brick house with beautiful wood floors, two bedrooms, a bath, plus a back porch and full basement. With a small loan from her mother, Mary bought the house for $5,750 with a mortgage. Through her work connections and neighbors, she put together enough furniture to fill the house. She made the draperies. An excellent seamstress, Mary set another goal. Her husband would be the best-dressed doctor ever and always. Every day, they made dinner a special event for themselves. Then she would fix up the house while he studied.

The Washington University School of Medicine was progressive. Dr. Mildred Trotter had become course master the year before. An excellent professor, passionate about anatomy and teaching, she was the first woman to achieve full professorship at Washington University. Ralph enjoyed her course. His performance in anatomy was excellent, and he qualified for Phi Beta Kappa in an academic year where he was both senior college student and first-year medical student. Ralph sent his anatomy coursework back to Washington State College to complete his college degree.

Mary's job in the Time and Leave Department was to track hours for the military's commissioned personnel. Mary noted that the war caused everyone to appear busy, but this appearance was occasionally disingenuous. At the office, Mary avoided the typical office drama and worked from 8 a.m. to 6 p.m. daily. She looked out for details and occasionally discovered ways to make the department more efficient.

At Washington University, the adoption of aseptic technique was absolute. The science of bacteriology was well accepted, and the university was on the forefront of every medical topic with their husband-and-wife academic teams. The school was filled with clinical professors from a broad scope of practice. Ralph was not limited and enjoyed his studies.

At first, there was talk. The war continued to intensify, and by January 1943, the need for men was a universal strain. Voided positions were often left vacant. In the fall, with the start of a new academic year, the medical school curriculum at Washington University was further compressed. Aiding the war effort was important. Ralph's entire medical school class was commissioned into the military as Army officers. They would graduate in three years instead of four. Clinical rotations were to start in place of summer break. The doctors covering the rotations were often senior medical students.

There was a benefit to being commissioned into the Army as Ralph's second year of medical school started. New doctors were being drafted into service and sent to Europe or Africa. Being commissioned by the Army in some small way offset Mary's fear of her husband being drafted. The military stepped up and paid for medical school tuition. Each officer would pay it back with medical service after graduation. Additionally, Ralph's military medical service could count toward advanced postgraduate training. These changes and the war were dramatic. However, for Ralph and Mary, medical school was quiet.

They both worked, both enjoyed their work, and together they kept a steady routine. Ralph particularly liked embryology and continued to excel in each class.

With the New Year, 1944, Ralph became a member of the medical honor society Alpha Omega Alpha. In the spring, Washington University's graduating medical school class included Dr. Edwin Gerhard Krebs, a biochemist who would go on to discover how reversible phosphorylation acts as a switch to turn on or activate proteins as they regulate various cell processes. He won the Nobel for Medicine in 1992.

Ralph started with surgery service in the summer of 1944 under Dr. Evarts Graham (1883–1957), who ran the service at Barnes Hospital in St. Louis and the academic surgical training program for Washington University.

Dr. Graham was heavily involved in the war effort, pushing to make more doctors and surgeons available. He was also suffering acutely from the void left by his own trained surgeons. Several had been drafted and were overseas. Chest surgeon Dr. Thomas Burford (1907–1977), who had recently completed the chest fellowship, was drafted and left for Africa. Dr. Graham could not slow down. He was toward the end of his career but still took calls at night, ran the department, operated, and trained the medical students and surgical trainees. A rotating medical student with the compressed curriculum caught his attention. Ralph Berg was smart, good with his hands, and calm.

Ralph learned that back in 1923, Dr. Graham had developed gallbladder cholecystography, a diagnostic imaging test that enabled surgeons to diagnose diseased gallbladders before life-threatening complications set in. Surgical removal of the gallbladder was the treatment. However, Dr. Graham's special interest was chest surgery. The crush of tuberculosis patients over his career had led this staunch advocate of general surgery to launch a chest service as part of general surgery training at Washington University. Surgical treatment for tuberculosis was thoracoplasty, a common surgical procedure performed under anesthesia where the affected chest wall is opened with an anterior lateral thoracotomy incision, the affected lung is collapsed, and the chest wall, i.e., the ribs, are contoured so the lung cannot reexpand. The general surgical team met weekly for chest conferences and case review.

Dr. Graham had performed the first successful pneumonectomy in 1931, on one of his surgical colleagues. Like a thoracoplasty, the chest on the side with the large mass was opened. The lung was removed by dividing both the airway and the arterial and venous return with sutures. The chest was closed without contouring the ribs. Dr. Graham's patient and colleague did well with this surgical first. The pathology confirmed lung cancer. Both surgeons were cigarette smokers. In addition to the significant advance in surgical treatment of lung cancer, the scientific search for a link between smoking and lung cancer started with this case. When Graham, instrumental in founding the American Board of Surgery in 1937, was awarded the Lister Medal for his contributions to surgical science in 1942, his acceptance oration, "Some Aspects of Bronchogenic Carcinoma," discussed the link between smoking and disease.

The chest service was desired by the serious surgical students at Washington University for its intensity and scientific orientation. Medical student Ralph Berg was deeply influenced by Dr. Graham during this rotation.

That fall of 1944, Mary learned she was pregnant with their first child. Due in the springtime, she continued to work. She felt fine. The young couple was pleased and made plans. Mary liked the idea of staying home after the baby came.

In the meantime, surgical advances were constantly being made. Dr. Dwight Harken (1910–1993) started his series of heart surgeries in June 1944. His WWII experience at a British hospital where wounded soldiers with chest shrapnel were treated was documented in 134 cases. These men had not died in the field nor on the way to hospital (Johnson 1970). Therefore, by default, these wounded soldiers were more stable than the soldiers who could not be transported due to being unstable. Dr. Harken, with his team monitoring intraoperative EKG, successfully removed shrapnel from all positions in the chest and mediastinum, including intracardiac. He learned the heart was tough and could easily withstand surgical techniques. He used simple chest X-rays, manual palpation, magnets, stay sutures, and long, grasping instruments to remove the shrapnel. This was a major new finding. Previously, the heart had never been approached surgically, and death from all forms of heart disease, mostly among blue babies, was inevitable (Dwight E. Harkin 1946).

Elsewhere, Dr. Clarence Crafoord (1899–1984), wanting to learn about clamping the aorta, visited Dr. Robert Gross in Boston, who had learned the aorta could be clamped for short periods of time with his work on patent ductus repairs. Dr. Crafoord then successfully operated on an eleven-year-old boy at Staatsburg Hospital in Stockholm, Sweden. Intraoperatively he confirmed the stethoscope diagnosis of coarctation of the aorta at the location of the ductus remnant—a severe narrowing of the aorta close to the heart. He clamped above and below the short segment coarctation and resected the narrowed, diseased portion of the aorta. Dr. Clarence Crafoord performed an end-to-end anastomosis to bring the healthy ends of the aorta back together. The clamps were removed. The child did well and left the hospital two weeks later, without disparity of blood pressure between his upper and lower extremities. The report came out October 19, 1944 (Johnson 1970; Goran Wettrell 2023).

On November 29, 1944, Dr. Alfred Blalock (1899–1964), chief of surgery at Johns Hopkins in Baltimore, Maryland, successfully performed the first subclavian-artery-to-pulmonary-artery shunt on a child with the congenital heart defect tetralogy of Fallot, first described by Niels Stenson in 1647. Tetralogy of Fallot, a combination of four defects—stenosis (narrowing) of the pulmonary valve, a ventricular septal defect (VSD), aorta shifted off its valve toward the VSD, and a thick right ventricle—was common and well studied. The subclavian and pulmonary arteries are located outside the pericardial sac containing the heart.

Dr. Alfred Blalock was assisted by surgical residents Drs. William Longmire (1913–2003) and Denton Cooley (1920–2016). The procedure's development team included lab supervisor Vivien Thomas (1910–1985) and pediatric cardiologist Dr. Helen Taussig (1899–1964). Vivien was masterful with his surgical skill in the well-established dog research lab and was called in to assist Dr. Blalock with this first case.

To develop this procedure, Dr. Taussig presented the problem and her proposed repair to the surgical team. She had collected and studied hundreds of blue-baby hearts at necropsy. This surgical repair and its success launched a flood of positive media. Over the following weeks, months, and years, desperate but hopeful parents brought their doomed blue-baby children to the Johns Hopkins Hospital for this procedure (V. T. Thomas 1985).

The success of the Blalock–Taussig–Thomas shunt and significant worldwide media attention on the plight of blue babies gave hope and an option to parents with a blue baby. There was a different impact on the surgical service at Barnes Hospital. While this shunt was exciting, surgical shunts to correct congenital blue-baby hearts were technically challenging surgical repairs with high mortality. The Blalock–Taussig–Thomas shunt, simple in concept, was critiqued for being small. Starting with the small subclavian artery being sewn to the pulmonary artery and carrying its flow into the lungs, the shunt would shrink, then clot off over time. Dr. Graham preferred the larger Potts–Smith shunt, developed at Harvard Medical, which connected the thoracic aorta and the pulmonary artery, which were close together. He thought it would be a less challenging surgical shunt to perform.

Holidays and vacations continued to be stressed by the war-induced doctor shortage. In the winter of 1944, medical student Ralph Berg was pleased to fill in for general surgery resident Dr. Karl Poppe, due for a much-needed two-week break. While covering the surgical duties, Berg lived in the hospital. Mary hardly saw her husband. One early morning, while outside getting the newspaper, she slipped and fell on the ice, hitting her back hard on the concrete front step. It hurt her so badly that she could not move.

With great effort, she finally crawled back into her house and got into bed. She called Ralph, hurt, cold, and pregnant. He came home and determined she had torn the underlying fascia but not the skin on her back. For the rest of his time covering for Dr. Poppe and interning at the hospital, Ralph came home early every morning, started the fire for Mary, and brought in the newspaper. Her injury left a huge bruise, but she recovered, and the scare was soon a memory about sacrifice. They both carried on.

A Texas oilman was admitted to Barnes Hospital with skin lesions. This wealthy gentleman was looking for another opinion and some hope that he might recover. Since he was a private patient, he was housed in the private pavilion of the hospital. The medical team gathered data about his lesions before consultation with a dermatologist. They ordered a gram stain with culture to evaluate for infection. Young medical student Ralph Berg, the covering surgeon, was called to do the gram stain.

First, he read this patient's chart. When he walked in and introduced himself, the skin lesions were open, weeping sores all over the patient's body. This patient was a mess. He told Berg he had already been to several medical centers, looking for a diagnosis and cure. No diagnosis had been made. He was getting worse, and to date, all had told him his condition was serious. He had already been to his hometown funeral home to make arrangements.

Berg took a sample from one of the pustules on the patient's skin and took it to the lab. He prepared a gram stain and a slide. The microscope revealed an organism, a rod that was not staining. Ralph knew tuberculosis is a gram-negative rod, so he set up and precisely swabbed the culture plate to attempt diagnosis of tuberculosis with an acid-fast stain. Berg also did a second gram stain. After all, maybe the first was an error.

The acid-fast stain takes a little more time, so he left to attend his patients on his ward. When he was called down to the laboratory about two hours later, he learned the ailment was not tuberculosis, as the acid-fast stain was also negative. These rods were again not staining, not on acid-fast and not on gram stain. Therefore, it had to be leprosy, a bacterium rod that is not tuberculosis and does not gram stain. Without the verification of a repeated gram stain, he too would have been unable to make the rare diagnosis.

Berg wrote the diagnosis—leprosy—in the patient's chart. The patient was then moved to isolation. The dermatologist visit, although moot, still occurred. When covering surgeon Berg visited him the next day, the patient complained, "They are treating me like I am a leper!" It was still sinking in that he in fact had leprosy. Fortunately, leprosy was treatable with a newly developed intravenous antibiotic drug. Berg reassured the patient that his grave reservation could be released, the leprosy sanatorium avoided, and he would have treatment and recover. This appreciative patient seeking a second opinion was thankful and impressed (R. Berg 2006).

By late February 1945, most involved knew the Americans were winning the war. Dr. Evart Graham invited senior medical student

Ralph Berg to be his surgical intern for the next year. Ralph would start directly after graduation.

Mary delivered a healthy baby boy on May 5, 1945. She was doing fine and so was the baby. Ralph and Mary planned for mother and child to rest and recover in Spokane with Mary's parents that summer. It was officially decided that she would stop working outside their home. On May 8, Victory Day in Europe was announced.

The Blalock–Taussig–Thomas shunt being performed at John Hopkins hospital continued to help blue babies. Families brought their babies to Hopkins from all over the world, and other academic institutions were sparked to address blue babies and congenital heart defects. The chest conferences at Washington University remained focused on these emerging surgical procedures—the shunts performed inside the chest and mediastinum. The concept of open-heart and a machine that could take over the heart's pump and oxygenation functions was batted about. To allow operative procedures inside an empty, still heart would be a big assist in developing and repairing congenital heart defects.

Leading up to Ralph's graduation, Mary put their brick house on the market, hoping it would sell quickly, and moved all their belongings to storage. Ralph's parents and his little brother were coming from Spokane by train for the ceremony. The graduation of his first son from medical school was a defining moment for Thoralf.

The graduation ceremony occurred on a beautiful, sun-filled day in June 1945. The entire medical school class—military officers with their graduation robes covering their military uniforms—were thankful the war was ended. Now an Army officer and a doctor of medicine, cum laude, with Alpha Omega Alpha honors, Dr. Ralph Berg had a bright future. At twenty-four, he would be starting surgical training with Dr. Evarts Graham, the father of chest surgery (R. Berg 2006).

After the celebrations, Mary and the baby headed back to Spokane in Ralph's Buick with Thoralf driving. Ralph's young brother, Mike, now four, was also in the back seat with the mother and child.

Fascinated with Mary and his new baby cousin, he marched on the seat and commanded the car. Leila later remarked, "Mike walked home from St. Louis after Ralph's medical school graduation."

Dr. Ralph Berg had finished college and medical school in just six years.

CHAPTER 5

First-Year Surgery

In June 1945, Barnes Hospital and the entire surgery department for Washington University had a depleted surgical staff. The chest service did not have a thoracic fellow nor an attending surgeon that summer. Dr. Graham, working full-time himself, was using his younger surgeons to fill in and move up. He anticipated that some of his former trainees would return to his department postwar. Notable in this situation was handsome and pleasant surgical intern Dr. Ralph Berg. He had performed well when covering for surgery residents as a medical student, his hands steady in the surgery room, always conveying a calm, thoughtful demeanor. Keeping Dr. Berg on as a surgical intern was natural.

Ralph liked his work with Dr. Evarts Graham. As an intern, he lived in the hospital and became Dr. Evarts Graham's right-hand man that summer. Together they ran the surgery service and the chest service at Barnes Hospital. Dr. Berg led the weekly chest conference.

Research, important to Dr. Graham, was also impacted by war shortages. Time strapped, Graham explained the surgical research project and how he would supervise Berg. A congenital anomaly called esophageal atresia, involving the absence of a segment of the esophagus, was the research topic. The esophagus normally runs behind the mediastinum, connecting the mouth to the stomach, explained Dr.

Graham. Children with esophageal atresia could not swallow food into their stomach. To buy time for these children, a feeding tube would be placed through the abdominal wall directly into the stomach. A surgical repair was in development in the dog research lab.

There was a young man, the lab diener, who washed the surgical instruments and kept the lab tidy. Ralph immediately liked him. The diener also took care of the dogs and the autopsy room. The dogs were treated well in the research lab.

Following one operation in the lab with Dr. Graham, Ralph largely worked alone for the dog-lab operations. On operating day, Ralph would lay out everything he needed. Once started, he could not walk away to fetch something. He would give the dog an intravenous line, then put the dog under. The young surgeon would prep the dog's chest, scrub his hands, and commit. At the initial operation, a model of esophageal atresia was created by opening the dog's chest and resecting a portion of the esophagus. The ends of the resected esophagus were each carefully closed in layers of suture. The dog's survival was essential. Once the model of the problem was created and the dog was recovered, a second operation was planned where the developing surgical repair would be tested.

Ralph liked that Dr. Graham was a thinking man. As a surgeon, he was not just cutting and sewing; he had a scientific interest. Success with the second dog operation would hopefully lead to a breakthrough that could help a child born with atresia of the esophagus. Ralph worked diligently in the lab, reporting his problems and progress to Dr. Graham, keeping records of each dog and each operation.

In addition to the research lab, Dr. Berg worked with all the other Barnes Hospital and Washington University surgeons. He assisted them in the operating rooms and tended the postoperative needs of the surgical ward patients. Dr. Graham's chest service was a separate ward. Most of those patients had received thoracoplasty procedures for tuberculosis and lung abscess. Contagious and in isolation, the tuberculosis patients all had chest tubes with closed suction. The nurses were adept with obtaining chest X-rays and handling the glass chest-tube suction bottles, which sat on the floor. Managing the postsurgical care of these patients became routine. Ralph's self-sufficiency in the dog lab mirrored his work with patients on the wards.

Over the summer, surgeons whose careers had been put on hold for military service finally started to return. Dr. Eugene Bricker (1908–2000), who was responsible for the general surgery residents and the rotating medical students for Washington University, returned to run the surgery service at St. Louis City Hospital.

The first dog Dr. Berg operated on solo in the research lab developed severe gastric bloat and became sick after the initial resection of a piece of esophagus operation. This dog eventually died a few weeks later. Dr. Berg took the dog to the hospital morgue in the basement and performed an autopsy. He found a large gastric ulcer that had eroded into the dog's aorta. During the initial surgery, he had cut the vagus nerve at the resection site on the esophagus. This unintentionally hindered the vagus nerve's ability to regulate acid production and gastric motility. By summer's end, Dr. Berg understood that the esophagectomy had led to gastric outlet syndrome, or gastric bloat. So Berg excluded this nerve from each subsequent operation, both the initial model and then the atresia repair.

A preserved vagus nerve helped. The gastric-emptying problem was lessened. In addition, young Dr. Berg moved to prevent the situation. He added a gastric-emptying procedure to the esophagectomy. This worked, and his dog models became routine and successful. Almost all the dogs did well after the first operation to create the atresia model. This was appreciated by Dr. Graham. The second operation, to attempt to repair the missing section of esophagus, got started. This line of research would take time to achieve success in terms of recovery, observing the return to eating without a feeding tube, and future implementation on the children affected.

Mary returned to St. Louis by train in late August 1945 with Ralph's sister, Margaret, and the baby. Ralph, working long hours at Barnes

Hospital, was happy to see his family. Their plans to rent an apartment when Mary returned were soon changed; so many young people were returning to St. Louis that there were no apartments available.

They had saved the $3,000 from the sale of their home, so Mary quickly found another brick house about the same size and type as their first. She made the $7,000 purchase and arranged the mortgage. Mary, now a stay-at-home mom, busied herself with her baby and fixing up the new house. Margaret helped for several weeks before returning to Spokane.

Dr. Graham had initiated his chest surgery fellowship back in 1929. Chest surgeon Dr. Brian Blades (1906–1977) subsequently helped Dr. Graham formalize the chest program into a two-year thoracic surgery fellowship and then left St. Louis in 1942 for military duty. Although Dr. Graham was hopeful that Dr. Blades would return to Washington University after the war, the surgeon decided not to. So Graham's search for a chest surgeon with enough training and experience to take over the chest fellowship continued. A few months later, Dr. Thomas Burford, another of Dr. Graham's fellowship surgeons, returned from Africa and took up Dr. Blades's position. It was late in 1945, and the surgery department threw a winter party to welcome Dr. Burford. Everyone was pleased he was returning to St. Louis. His military experience and presence thrilled Dr. Graham. Correcting congenital blue babies was becoming the problem of the day, and he wanted to start this line of chest surgery work.

Ralph's work continued at the same pace, bringing more responsibility and more operations. Overall, Ralph and Mary had another quiet but productive year. It was arranged for Dr. Berg to continue his surgical training the next year at a different institution: the Portland Veterans Administration Medical Center in Oregon. His training there would also repay his military obligation.

On the chest service at Barnes, a blue baby presumed to have tetralogy of Fallot was to have a surgical shunt. It was Dr. Burford's case, and the Potts–Smith shunt was planned. The larger shunt between the thoracic aorta and pulmonary artery had advantages over the Blalock–Taussig–Thomas. Berg assisted Dr. Burford in the surgery room that day. After anesthesia, prep of the chest, and exposure of the mediastinum, the large aorta and pulmonary arteries were identified and circumferentially dissected, with tapes then placed around them. The pericardial sac remained intact. Next, they clamped each vessel using a side-biter clamp. Developed by Dr. Crafoord, these C-shaped longitudinal clamps pinch the vessel so flow continues opposite the vessel yet prevents flow within the "C" portion.

The two vessels were opened with a blade inside the occluded parts of the vessels, which were near each other. Dr. Burford began to sew the thoracic aorta lumen, or cavity, to the pulmonary artery lumen. The suture chosen was a running silk. The first pass went relatively well. With the next pass of the needle, the suture pulled through the vessel wall and out. The delicate tissue did not hold but instead separated as the braided suture was pulled up. There was some bleeding. A pack was quickly placed to control the blood. It went quiet in the room. The case was not going well.

Dr. Burford pulled the pack back, cut his suture, and removed the running silk. He would have to start the suture over. Then one of the clamps released unexpectedly. The case appeared futile with the amount of blood loss and difficulty getting the dislodged clamp back in place. Then the case was over; the child died with a rush of bleeding on the table.

Dr. Burford left the operating room, frustrated. Dr. Berg remained, closed the child's chest, cleaned the surgical site, and applied dressings. He carried the child, wrapped carefully in a soft blanket, to her anxious parents in the waiting room. After gently talking with them about the events in the operating room, he confirmed their permission to autopsy. He brought the child to the pathology department and assisted with the postmortem exam. There, he found tetralogy of Fallot heart defects, with the heart valve between the lower-pressure right chambers narrowed. There was a hole between the two big heart chambers, the ventricles, and a failed suture outside the child's heart.

Knowing Dr. Burford had done his best, Dr. Ralph Berg resolved to learn and improve and never give up. After that case, he never used a running suture. He always interrupted sutures. If one suture pulled out or broke, the others would still hold.

Death from heart disease had been the norm. To touch the heart was taboo for most people. But there was now a glimmer of hope. Ralph was calm and very quiet when he told Mary about this case. He resolved that he would not give up when it was his case. He knew he could do better. He would never let go.

CHAPTER 6

Thoracic Training

Together, Mary and Ralph planned his next step in surgical training, and as June 1946 approached, they were ready. Mary and their now one-year-old child would again return home to Spokane for the first part of Ralph's training. Mary had their second St. Louis house ready for sale, their belongings stored. She and their son left for Spokane on the train. Later, Dr. Berg drove himself to Portland, Oregon, and started work at the VA hospital there in early July. The medical personnel quarters comprised a series of Quonset huts.

This two-year block of time would pay back the government for Ralph's medical school tuition. The Veterans Department of Medicine and Surgery was new, as was the GI Bill. With this new government agency, veterans hospitals across the country were able to recruit and retain top medical personnel and collaborate with local university hospitals.

After arriving in Portland, Ralph almost immediately ran into Dr. Karl Poppe. It was a pleasant reunion, both of them Washington University Department of Surgery men trained by Dr. Evart Graham. Dr. Poppe, about ten years older than Ralph, was now a chest surgeon attending at the Portland VA Medical Center. He had moved from St. Louis earlier that year. Ralph recalled, "Poppe was Dr. Evart Graham's number two man" during the lean war years. Now Dr. Ralph Berg, assistant surgeon, was to work with Dr. Poppe in the capacity of a chest fellow.

The Portland veterans hospital had a busy chest service, and the VA had begun building a 155-bed hospital addition for tuberculosis patients. For the sick veterans with tuberculosis and related lung abscesses, the surgeons performed thoracotomies and thoracoplasty. Ralph called the tuberculosis work "a crush."

Meanwhile, Mary, in Spokane, suspected she was pregnant again. Toward the end of the summer, she realized she was leaking some type of fluid. She was feeling ill and went to the doctor. It turned out she was leaking amniotic fluid. With rest, it stopped. Mary got to Portland in late September. Ralph was overjoyed to see her and pleased she was with child. She found a small apartment in Vanport, Oregon, while they waited for their St. Louis house to sell.

Vanport, a 650-acre complex of public housing, the largest in the country, was built to be a temporary community and had sprung up on the floodplain in response to the huge influx of workers to the Portland shipyards during WWII. The railroad trestle ran along the river and acted as the levy. Mary found Vanport to be a horrible place. She and everyone who lived there were concerned that the river would flood. The city, however, was not worried. It reassured the residents that the dikes would hold.

Mary moved out of Vanport as soon as their house sold. She earned a large profit with this sale, $5,000, and with it bought a nice house close to the veterans hospital on Marquam Hill. Ralph moved in.

Their second child was born November 15, 1946, premature by about six weeks. He weighed only a few pounds, so he stayed in the hospital, feeding and growing. He had bilateral inguinal hernia repairs before Mary was able to take him home at six weeks of age. Their child returned for surgical umbilical hernia repair when he was ten weeks old. By then, the baby was thriving and came home the next day. Mary was able to fix up their third house. She was strong, physically and psychologically, and dedicated to Ralph and their family. Working tirelessly, she repaired windows, put in new fixtures, and sewed draperies and, of course, clothes for Dr. Berg, always the best-dressed doctor.

The closed-heart procedures for blue babies were evolving, and Dr. Berg felt the shunts to mitigate tetralogy of Fallot demanded a research lab. Without a dog lab, Dr. Berg could not continue the esophageal work, nor start any congenital heart work. Further limiting the closed-heart work was the lack of children at the veterans hospital. Not to be deterred by these limits, the two chest men, Berg and Poppe, remained focused on research and wrote up their clinical casework. Bronchogenic carcinoma—a lung cancer—and surgical resection of the part of the lung with the cancerous tumor was the topic of many shared clinical case studies. The tuberculosis work, entrenched in surgical thoracoplasty care, was another topic where Berg and Poppe had multiple cases to present. Hiatal hernia repairs via the chest were also common.

Dr. Berg wrote, published, and presented chest work with Dr. Poppe based on their cases in Portland and their work from St. Louis. They continued with a weekly chest conference. They were busy surgeons and enjoyed each other's company (R. D. Berg 1957).

The success of the Blalock–Taussig–Thomas shunt for tetralogy of Fallot in 1944 continued to drive demand for blue-baby repairs. Meanwhile, Dr. Robert Gross's work in patent ductus repair had been improved and garnered increased surgical results (Chaphin 2014). Fired in 1938 by Dr. Ladd after developing and successfully performing ligation of patent ductus, Dr. Gross was rehired in 1942. He was named the William E. Ladd Professor of Children's Surgery chair at Harvard Medical School in 1947. This was the first surgical chair in the nation.

Dr. Gross's development of a repair marks in many respects the point in time that children dying of congenital heart disease became a focus of successful and durable surgical innovative force.

A few patent ductus patients grew to become young adults before their symptoms were sufficient to prompt a diagnosis. With compromised health and an awareness of a repair, they sought out and were referred to the chest surgeons. Some of these patients were admitted to the chest service at the Portland VA hospital.

When it was Drs. Berg and Poppe's case, they would place the patient under anesthesia and open the chest via a left thoracotomy; they did not open the pericardial sac, as this was a closed-heart procedure. They circumferentially dissected the aorta to place two long tapes around it, then circumferentially removed all the fibrinous attachments from the pulmonary artery and placed two tapes around that. The tapes were on either side of the patent ductus. They then clamped both sides of the patent ductus, often using a side-biting vascular clamp, and cut it with a surgical blade. The resulting small luminal openings in each artery were closed with interrupted sutures. The result: Both the aorta and the pulmonary artery were closed securely and physically separated from each other. With each heartbeat, these arteries moved with their blood flow.

Dr. Poppe recognized the talent of Dr. Berg and gave positive feedback to his former chairman, Dr. Evarts Graham. This time and work eventually was counted toward Berg's chest surgery fellowship and thoracic surgery boards.

Time flew for Ralph and Mary. They were both enjoying themselves, their family, and Portland. The summer of 1947 was a joy, as they were finally together.

In late January 1948, Dr. Ralph Berg was annoyed. A new patient had been admitted to the chest ward. The patient was sick, and the concern upon initial evaluation was that he had a post-thoracotomy complication. This patient's case had been a difficult thoracotomy, and a blood transfusion had been given. After examination, Dr. Berg said the patient did not have a chest issue. He did not want this patient on the chest service. However, being three months post-thoracotomy was enough to get him there.

Within a day, this patient got sick with vomiting, then yellow skin from jaundice. Dr. Berg sent him for a gallbladder removal, and a common bile-duct stone was also identified and removed at surgery. The patient came back to the chest ward with tubes to drain his biliary tree into a glass bottle on the floor. On morning rounds, the apparatus fell over, glass bottles shattered, and bile spilled everywhere. Ralph could smell it.

It turned out that the patient was infectious. The two nurses caring for this patient came down with hepatitis. One nurse almost died. About a week later, Ralph and Karl went climbing and skiing on Mount Saint Helens. That day, Ralph became unusually exhausted and could not finish the climb. When he returned home, he found that he too was ill with hepatitis. Being that he was contagious, he was sent away to Madigan Army Hospital in Tacoma, Washington. It was early February 1948. At that time, hepatitis was known to have A and B classifications. Convalescence and recovery were slow. Ralph and Mary wrote letters to each other; occasionally they called and talked.

Mary, left alone in Portland with two young children, was pregnant for the third time. Her husband sick and in another state, she took care of herself and her children. Her friends and family helped. In May, she delivered her third child and third son.

It is worth noting at this point in the narrative that before the May 1948 meeting of thoracic academic surgeons, Dr. Graham, who initially remained opposed to separating thoracic surgery away from general surgery, changed his mind. With these difficult closed-heart surgical procedures emerging for treatment of blue babies, Dr. Graham now agreed to initiate a separate board certification and designation for thoracic surgery training. The training would be in addition to general surgery training, with a new board, the American Board of Thoracic Surgery (R. Berg 2006).

Shortly after Mary arrived home with her healthy baby, the railroad levy in Vanport gave way. The flood was massive and fast moving, and many lives were lost on Memorial Day 1948. When Mary heard the shocking news, she sat and held her three boys close to her. They all cried.

Meanwhile, in Tacoma, Ralph discovered that he had contracted a chronic active form of hepatitis B from his patient, who likely received hepatitis from the blood transfusions during chest surgery. Ralph was always extremely cautious about blood transfusions after this experience, and he took to heart his doctor's admonishment to not use alcohol. He also learned that his sister had married his best friend from Spokane, Al, upon Al's return from the war. Then a letter came from Dr. Graham, forwarded to Madigan by Mary, offering a surgical residency in orthopedics or urology in St. Louis. Ralph thanked Dr. Graham when he wrote back but told him he was interested only in thoracic surgery.

Almost three months hospitalized, Ralph read every article in his field and followed closely the developments in heart surgery. In February 1947, Dr. Russell Brock (1903–1980) in England had performed the first successful pulmonary valvulotomy for blue babies with tetralogy of Fallot. He used a direct approach to the stenosed pulmonary valve in that he opened the pericardial sac, and by palpating and positioning the beating heart, he was able to identify the hard pulmonary valve that empties the right ventricle by its harsh murmur and thrill from the abnormal flow of blood across it.

The technique was done through a small stab wound in the right ventricle to cut the dense adhesions going into the pulmonary valve and separate its leaflets that were stuck together. Bleeding was controlled with positioning of the heart with stay sutures on the ventricle. The specialized knife almost immediately provided relief of the stenotic valve, and blood flow improved. Dr. Brock made sure to give credit to his junior surgical colleagues, who continued the pursuit of blue-baby repairs and open-heart surgical repairs. His paper, published in June 1948, reported three successful cases.

That June, Dr. Charles Bailey (1910–1993) performed a digital/manual valve commissurotomy (a process explained in chapter 8) on the mitral valve between the left atrium and left ventricle. This patient developed dreaded arrhythmias and died on the operating room table. This was the fourth death for Dr. Bailey's new procedure. Undeterred, he then drove to a second hospital and performed the same operation later that day. This patient was not so ill and survived. Dr. Bailey, like Dr. Brock, did not take personal credit for this step forward in procedures for heart-valve stenoses (Johnson 1970). He too figured the time had come, and three excellent surgeons, Drs. Bailey, Harken, and Brock, had stumbled logically onto this valve-repair procedure, finally becoming successful in performing the procedure on both the pulmonary and mitral valves of the four heart valves.

Finally feeling adequate, Ralph decided to return to his work. The idea of opening the pericardial sac and the heart itself had taken hold. Developing a heart-lung machine that conceptually would allow such surgical work inside the heart was his goal.

The next letter from Dr. Evart Graham was the one Dr. Berg was waiting for. Mary was excited when Ralph called and told her of Dr. Graham's offer to train in chest surgery. Although it was a lot of work, she would sell their house in Portland and meet him back in St. Louis with the children. Ralph wrote ahead to Dr. Graham and accepted the position as chest fellow. But Dr. Berg now had a time constraint. He was expected for the start of the training year on July 1, 1948.

In late June 1948, yellow and weak, Ralph Berg drove himself to Barnes Hospital in St. Louis, Missouri, from Madigan Army Hospital in Tacoma, Washington. His bilirubin blood level was twenty and thankfully trending down. The normal bilirubin level is one.

On the morning Mary left Portland with her children and enough clothes for a short trip, their third son was three months old. Mary and the boys went by train to St. Louis and stayed with her relatives in Walnut Grove. When Mary finally met up with her husband, they went to Quake Lake and stayed overnight. It was a nice reunion. She had worried and missed Ralph. Glad to see him and glad he was getting back to his old self, she started looking for a place to live. Mary found a great house in Hanley Hills just outside of St. Louis.

Ralph was proud of his chest residency. Having been invited by Dr. Evarts Graham was exciting. He loved his mentor, and so did Mary. Berg called Graham a "thinking doctor." The young couple was invited to visit his home on a beautiful spot where the Mississippi and Missouri Rivers came together called Windy Rise, and the Grahams were lovely people. Mary felt that Dr. Graham did not easily connect with people, but he did connect with Ralph. That evening, not wanting to overstay the invitation, Mary commented, "I think we should go." But Dr. Graham said, "Oh no, I am enjoying the conversation." They stayed and chatted into the night, sitting out on the porch overlooking the water.

The chest residency at Barnes Hospital was evolving, and Dr. Berg felt fortunate about this step in his career. Chest surgeons were pushing to find new technologies for huge problems: congenital heart defects, lung cancer, large esophageal procedures, and tuberculosis procedures. Closed-heart procedures were being done, and the thoracic surgery boards were approved that fall; Ralph still called them chest boards. Dr. Graham came to be known as the father of chest surgery.

The chest surgeons at Barnes were successfully ligating patent ductus. These surgeons, with limited diagnostics, were also doing three closed-heart shunts: the Potts–Smith aortopulmonary shunt, the Blalock–Taussig–Thomas subclavian pulmonary shunt, and the Glenn cavopulmonary shunt. Operative risks were high. The Potts shunt offered superior long-term palliation over the Blalock–Taussig shunt, which had received much press and public adoration with the hope of blue-baby repairs. The drive for technology to allow chest surgeons to operate inside the heart mirrored the chest surgeons' "make it work" attitude.

Evarts Graham and Ralph Berg worked well together. But Dr. Berg soon learned he was not popular with some general surgeons who had been called to wartime service and then returned to St. Louis wanting a coveted chest residency spot. One became assistant surgeon, a teaching position at Barnes Hospital. The pyramid system of filling training spots, the changes with chest boards separating thoracic surgery from general surgery, and the emergent heart procedures all clashed. This one general surgeon expressed his irritation that this young upstart, Berg, had been invited for chest training ahead of him.

Having stepped up and performed as a surgeon in an impressive way during the extreme shortage of surgeons during the war years, Berg had little tolerance for this behavior. Years later, while Ralph and I were collaborating on this story, he revealed that this assistant general surgeon became the thoracic resident following Dr. Berg, commenting, "He was a class-A shit."

One week per year was Dr. Berg's vacation schedule. Mary enjoyed the new house, tended to the children, and occasionally helped at the university surgery office.

After his thoracic fellow year, Berg did his general surgery training. Starting July 1949, Dr. Ralph Berg became assistant resident in general surgery. He continued to work the chest service, participate in chest conferences, and assist with chest surgical cases and the dog research lab.

Berg enjoyed his plastic surgery rotation. He had two sessions on the service, and both plastic surgeons, Dr. James Barrett Brown (1899–1971) and Dr. Vilray Blair (1871–1955), influenced young Dr. Berg to apply plastic surgery principles to his work. "The only thing patients remember about you is their scar" was Ralph's enduring advice to me decades later. The final detail of closing after any surgical procedure, an excellent scar was his style.

Meanwhile, Dr. Burford, not passionate about the congenital

hearts, made his career in esophagus work. The esophageal atresia congenital defect had been surpassed in numbers by chemical burning and scarring of the esophagus in children who had inadvertently eaten lye. The need for a repair was thus intensified, and Burford finished and wrote up the repair of these children. This work, the repair on these sick children, was dependent on the dog-lab model of esophageal resection and drainage-model creations. This was Ralph's first encounter with certain lapses in academics: Ralph Berg's name was not on the paper. Not being acknowledged hurt. Berg's work during his surgical intern year, where he discovered the gastric ulcers that eroded into the dog aorta, and his subsequent advances to the dog model had allowed this work to progress (R. Berg 1956).

Intriguing news arrived in 1950. Dr. Wilfred Bigelow (1913–2005), a Canadian surgeon with a well-developed research team, reported his research on hypothermia to the American Surgical Association. The dogs were cooled to a range between sixty-eight and seventy-five degrees, under anesthesia and monitoring. Then cardiac arrest was induced, and for fifteen minutes, the circulation was stopped. And then restarted. With hypothermia, mortality was 50 percent; still, this work was a huge advance. Dr. Berg brought this report to chest conference. Seeking intracardiac time with the heart stopped to provide a bloodless field to work within was the premise for a heart-lung machine. Hypothermia might allow more time for their current procedures and shunts. Berg, a thinking surgeon, took note. Of course, this was news from the dog lab, not yet advanced to a human or a blue baby (Oransky 2005).

Ralph's training was being continually modified and added onto as the field evolved. Another year added to the timeline set him off, and in July 1950, Ralph told Mary, "I've had it. Let's just quit."

Mary said, "No, we have put so much time and effort into this training."

Logic won, and Ralph stayed for his last year. Dr. Graham helped him apply for chief of chest surgery positions. Ralph also applied for his medical license in the state of Washington.

The following July, Mary was put in the hospital with ascending paralysis involving her legs. With three little boys at home, her husband busy at work, and she eight months pregnant, the experience was terrifying. Polio was diagnosed, and Dr. Graham paid her an immediate visit. He said, "Give her plasma."

They did. She suffered all night long with anxiety and discomfort, unable to lie still and unable to pass her urine. A nurse had to put in a bladder catheter. Soon Mary was asleep. Because of the immunoglobulins from the plasma, she quickly got better. Dr. Graham, always thinking, hired a babysitter for the three children at home. Mary was in the hospital for nine days before walking out with some relatively minor post-polio weakness. The children were glad to see their mother healthy, and both Mary and Ralph would always remember how supportive and caring Evarts Graham was with them.

The Washington medical license arrived in the mail in early August. When Mary delivered in late August, her obstetrician was Dr. Ralph Harsh (1913–1986), and everything went well. She had a healthy girl. Dr. Harsh and his wife, Louise, eventually moved to Spokane to practice.

Dr. Berg, trained under Dr. Graham and his new thoracic surgery fellowship, with his general surgery training at an institution that was performing cutting-edge chest surgery, was offered the position of chief of surgery at the veterans hospital in Boise, Idaho. He accepted.

CHAPTER 7

The Road to Spokane, 1952

After the delivery in August 1951, both Ralph and Mary were thankful for a healthy baby girl. Mary had some weakness in her upper legs from her brush with polio, but she was particularly thankful to Dr. Evarts Graham for her plasma treatment. She was busy and excited to be done with the surgical training experience.

Mary sold their house in Hanley Hills, her fourth home sale, and landed a profit significantly larger than the last. They were headed to Boise, Idaho. With a rented flatbed truck, they planned to haul all their belongings and the entire family together, new baby and three little boys. Mary felt comfortable making a home purchase ahead of their arrival, avoiding a temporary apartment and another move for the family. She bought a nice house in Boise near the hospital.

No sooner had they pulled into Boise, anticipating settling into their new house, than things changed. Ralph got word that the academic jobs had been switched. Instead of Boise, he was to start right away in Portland. They knew Portland and that hospital. It was certainly an advantage. However, the young couple had no money and had not planned for this dramatic switch. All their assets were in the Boise home. The planning and the hope for a smooth transition went out the window. Without a break, they turned around and headed off to Portland, Oregon. Mary would work with the realtor to sell the Boise house.

Ralph dealt swiftly with the first flat tire. He pulled safely off the road and fixed it. He was annoyed. With the second flat tire, Ralph exploded and started throwing rocks at the old flatbed truck, cursing in his style. He was upset, the truck was junk, and they were now behind schedule. On a tight budget and a tight timeline, her husband frustrated and throwing rocks, Mary, initially not sure what to do, was soon laughing. She calmly walked with the baby and the boys down the road to the off-ramp. They strolled into the first inn, and the pleasant owner listened to her story and was helpful. He got Ralph and the flatbed to the roadside inn. The family stayed the night and left refreshed the next morning, tires fixed.

They arrived in time for the start of Ralph's new job, chief of thoracic surgery at the Portland veterans hospital. The family settled into an apartment. Within a few weeks, Mary was able to sell the Boise house and purchase a new house in Portland. They moved in, and her two oldest boys started their grade-school education at the local school.

Dr. Berg tried to make the transition into academic surgery. He had the academic training. The promise for a research lab was important, and he was eager to set up. An academically trained Mayo Clinic chest surgeon was the chief of surgery at the hospital. After several weeks of meetings and discussions, Dr. Berg learned there would be no compensation for the move from St. Louis via Boise to Portland. Shortly after, he learned there would be no research lab. Ralph felt betrayed.

Dr. Berg sat for the oral exam, the American Board of Surgery, and passed September 24, 1951. He was pleased with this result. In November 1951, Dr. Berg was appointed clinical instructor in surgery at the University of Oregon School of Medicine. Dr. Berg's independence and fierce loyalty to his care and attention toward his patients was appreciated by the rotating medical students.

There was no longer a weekly chest conference at the Portland VA hospital; however, Ralph and many of the surgeons traveled and attended chest conferences at other institutions. Intracardiac issues were being shared. Dr. Charles Bailey and Dr. Dwight Harken had a bit of a feud over who was first with blind digital mitral valve commissurotomies. Their feud made the conferences interesting, and the surgeons who attended were invited to visit and watch a mitral commissurotomy at the two surgeons' respective institutions.

The surgeons often focused on how future valve-replacement materials would behave over time when implanted inside human patients. The replacement materials obviously needed to perform over a lifetime. They discussed a "fatigue" machine to test the durability of different materials. The concept of a heart-lung machine was always part of the discussion.

A chest surgeon in private practice and a consultant at the veterans hospital performed ligation of patent ductus on a blue baby who had grown into a young man. The diagnosis was made by stethoscope exam. At surgery, this surgeon confirmed the ductus had remained patent and was shunting blood left to right.

Dr. Berg learned of this closed-heart case in the middle of the night, when an urgent phone call came in. He rushed to the hospital and got the patient into the operating room for an attempt to save his life. When Berg opened the chest incision, he found only ligatures, no sutures to close each large vessel securely. With nothing to anchor either ligature, the pulmonary artery ligature had simply rolled off. The bleeding from the pulmonary artery into the chest had caused the surgical emergency. This patient died.

Dr. Berg did not like this complication, a death. He talked with the chief of surgery, who was not able to help other than to encourage Dr. Berg to educate this surgeon. So, Dr. Berg delivered to this surgeon the published research papers detailing the new, safer technique for ligation of a patent ductus. He offered to help him in surgery with the newer technique to clamp both the aorta and the pulmonary artery with the side-biter clamps, cut the ductus, and sew both sides closed with interrupted sutures.

When it happened again to another young adult veteran, the patient was salvaged because Berg was called in before the case was completed. This time, the surgeon had placed a large clamp on the aorta and tied a ligature across the ductus on the pulmonary artery side, followed by cutting the ductus and placing a single stitch on the aortic side. This was a quickie procedure full of risk, in Dr. Berg's opinion. Luckily, the patient was saved. Berg quickly performed circumferential dissection of both arteries and closed both sides of the ligated ductus with interrupted sutures.

Dr. Berg was incensed as the surgeon closed the chest. This surgeon's poor judgment and techniques could not be excused. The title of chief of thoracic surgery and its responsibility fell to Dr. Berg, yet he had no authority to teach, edit, limit privileges, or train this surgeon.

Sharing of surgical technique was encouraged, yet the politics—trading off patients to others with a perceived lack of direct responsibility, the stealing of ideas, the jockeying for position and labels—that he briefly experienced in academics was not Berg's style. Discussing ideas was a way for more established surgeons to steal ideas without credit to the original thinker. Berg attempted to convey his disappointment about these issues, only to be misunderstood. He found it difficult to understand or to protect himself from this moral affront in an academic environment. The Portland VA appointment was ending in December. Ralph did not attempt to renew it.

Mary summed up their half year in surgical academics thus: "We came back to Spokane, and Ralph went into practice alone on January 1, 1952. Our good luck continued." Dr. Ralph Berg returned to his hometown, leaving academic surgery for all the right reasons (M. Berg 2011).

CHAPTER 8

Dog Lab and Hypothermia, 1952

Ralph and Mary arrived in Spokane in January 1952 with their young family, the oldest eight, the youngest eighteen months. On the way to Spokane, they ran out of money. Fortunately, the house in Portland sold quickly, and Mary found a nice brick house on a quiet street, close to two hospitals. They moved in and were happy to discover that the neighbors across the street were Ralph's cousin Andy Berg Jr. and his wife, Alice.

Thoralf and his two brothers, Olaf and Andy, were running the North Hill bakery. Time seemed to have moved slowly in Spokane, while for Ralph and Mary, so much had changed since they left Spokane just eleven years earlier. Ralph, about to turn thirty, was now a trained chest surgeon with cutting-edge experience on closed-heart and emerging intracardiac procedures. His eagerness for technology, a pump, to allow surgical time inside an open heart sent him to the research lab.

Over the years, Dr. Ralph Berg would say about private practice, "We were beholden to no one." The freedom in private practice was great. "We were unencumbered by chiefs of surgery and academic life." The disappointment with not being able to set up a research lab at his first academic appointment was easily remedied in private practice.

He set up an office and solo practice as a thoracic surgeon at the downtown Paulsen Medical and Dental Building, suite 770. He applied for active-staff status and surgical privileges at all three local hospitals: Sacred Heart, St. Luke's, and Deaconess. He quickly received privileges to operate in the chest and abdomen and became a member of each hospital's medical staff. He joined the Spokane County Medical Society.

The medical training program based in Seattle at the new University of Washington School of Medicine, with outposts in Portland, Alaska, and Spokane, was run by an established internist. A new chest surgeon was an excellent addition to his teaching program. He met and helped Dr. Berg with advice and patient referrals. Dr. Berg soon developed a surgical team and became a well-established part of this teaching network.

Shortly, a general practitioner called up Dr. Berg. The doctor had a patient, a young lady who had developed rheumatic fever as a child and then suffered her whole life with a weakened heart. He explained to Berg about her mitral valve. He could tell it was abnormal, with calcifications seen on her chest radiograph. She had a loud heart murmur by stethoscope. The two doctors talked about whether her case was operable due to potential for complications such as atheroembolic stroke, where pieces of the hardened, scarred mitral valve could flake off during the procedure to travel out of the heart toward the arteries carrying blood flow to the brain and hemorrhage or cause a dreaded pulmonary embolism and death. This doctor told Berg about a similar patient he had recently sent to San Francisco, California, looking for cardiac surgery for the same problem.

When Dr. Berg saw the young lady, she described her nagging cough and shortness of breath, both of which were getting worse. The young lady explained, "I can't climb stairs." Her mother was with her and wanted something done. Her daughter was fading.

Dr. Berg recommended an intracardiac procedure, a manual commissurotomy of the mitral valve. This was a routine procedure at Washington University in St. Louis. It was brand new in Spokane, Washington. This twenty-six-year-old was still healthy, not yet a cardiac cripple, and Dr. Berg felt optimistic. "It was being done other places," he explained in retrospect. "It just hadn't been done here." She signed up for this procedure with Dr. Berg.

During surgery in the Deaconess Hospital, Dr. Berg performed the first manual commissurotomy in Spokane, a procedure inside the heart, using swift surgical technique.

Swift technique was how Berg operated. Simply put, he learned from each and every mistake, he incorporated what he learned into his subsequent cases, he sought as much preoperative information as possible, and he anticipated and moved smoothly through each step of the operation. Frequently this involved using a second glove to hold his retractable knife blade securely against his finger. He would insert his finger and palpate, finding his landmarks, and position his finger. He would release the blade and cut the stenotic leaflet, then retract the blade and safely remove the knife. Interrupted sutures were also a crucial part of his process.

The patient was placed under general anesthesia. Dr. Berg opened her chest on the left side. He carefully held that lung out of his field with retractors. The pericardium was opened. Then Dr. Berg placed a purse-string suture around the left atrium appendage. The appendage, an elbow of tissue where the blood flowing through the atrium forms an eddy of diminished flow, held the suture as a running line that could be pulled up to close the opening. With a secure purse string and positioning of the heart so the purse string and left atrial appendage were at the highest point, thus using gravity to delay the spilling of blood, Dr. Berg could control blood from escaping. He placed his gloved finger through it, pulled the purse string taut, and worked inside her heart.

He gently pried apart the calcium scarring the leaflets of her mitral valve together. The calcium made the valve into a dam, a stenosis preventing blood from flowing through the valve into the left ventricle.

It was also a drain on her life, forcing her heart to pump hard against the calcium blockade. This commissurotomy restored the valve's mobility so it opened for flow between the chambers when the heart contracted and then closed with each heartbeat, preventing retrograde flow back into her left atrium when her heart relaxed. Dr. Berg, satisfied that the valve was working, closed all the layers and then her skin. The case lasted about two hours, and the intracardiac work took about three minutes. When she awakened from anesthesia, she could breathe comfortably. It was such a relief. She felt wonderful.

Once home, Ralph walked across the street and told Andy, cousin to cousin, all about this first. He told Andy how it felt to put his finger into the calcified valve, how it felt to touch and identify the leaflets and gently crunch them free of the adhesions holding them together. Never sure how a surgical procedure would work out, and ever vigilant during the case, Ralph had been successful. The valve was no longer stuck together. The patient would be fine. He was pleased to report the patient also avoided a risky trip to San Francisco. Andy and his wife were impressed. Later they all learned that the general practitioner's other patient in San Francisco had died on the operating table. Dr. Berg was grateful his first intracardiac case went so well.

The hospital administrator at Deaconess Hospital had several surgeons doing chest work and was not interested in making accommodations for another one. From Dr. Berg's view, the established surgical group was favored. Competition from a new young surgeon seemed like a pointless uphill endeavor. The operating rooms were also small at Deaconess Hospital, so Dr. Ralph Berg stopped operating there except for an occasional emergency case. He was happy to work at Sacred Heart hospital just a few blocks away, where he had an advantage: Two older general surgeons who performed thoracic work were both retiring. Soon Dr. Berg would be the only chest surgeon at that hospital.

Berg immediately started making waves. The first shift occurred when the senior anesthesiologist at Sacred Heart, who preferred short, less demanding cases over the big chest and heart cases, complained about Dr. Berg's longer cases. The Sisters of Providence advised this Dr. Small to talk to Dr. Berg directly, so he pulled Berg aside one day and told Berg he could have anesthesia services from this group in the afternoon. The morning slots were for shorter cases. Dr. Berg's long, tedious chest cases were not remunerative for them.

Ralph Berg understood that Dr. Small wanted his group to make money and was not passionate about the new heart work enveloping the country. Berg knew he could not persuade Small to be part of his heart team and did not bother trying. He walked away. Dr. Small was content that he had limited Dr. Berg to the afternoons.

Dr. Berg never discussed this small disappointment. Instead, he went to the nurse anesthetist service provided by the hospital. In a formal meeting, these anesthesia providers were more than agreeable. They were both appreciative and passionate about hearts. From that day forward, Dr. Berg worked exclusively with the certified registered nurse anesthetists (CRNAs), and he never looked back. They gave superior service to his patients. Dr. Evarts Graham also used nurse anesthetists.

Another aspect where Dr. Berg set himself apart from other doctors concerned fee splitting. The main doctor would send a large bill for all the professional services on the case, collect the funds, and split them with the other doctors. Ralph felt strongly this was not ethical, as did his mentor, Dr. Graham. It brought money into the relationship with his referring doctors, it was difficult to account for the funds, and it further complicated the relationship with patients. The American College of Surgeons was against fee splitting. Dr. Berg therefore sent out his own bills for his services to each of his patients.

The most valuable part of the experience working at Sacred Heart was the dog lab. Ralph always credited the nurses and nuns who ran the hospital for providing space in the first-floor nursing quarters for the research lab. A $25,000 grant from the Eagles helped offset costs. With this first grant, Dr. Berg maintained a research fund his entire career.

Ralph swiftly set up a lab. Heart work was advancing fast, and research and time to establish the details and the pitfalls of each new procedure were crucial. The research lab followed the same concept as the dog lab in St. Louis—a small surgical suite outfitted with the same instruments and care as a standard operating room, with the patient being the dog.

The dogs were obtained from the local dog pound, and Berg became the owner of each animal. After a lab, a nurse or nurse student took the patient dog home and cared for it, reporting back to Dr. Berg how the dog was doing. The dogs did well. Dr. Berg detailed his most difficult cases and new procedures in the dog lab. The same team was used in the lab as in the main operating room, following the same standards of success.

A stickler for operative technique and acknowledgment of ideas and contributions, Dr. Berg always believed each team member was essential to the success. Without this synergy, failure was common. In 1952, Dr. John Lewis (1916–1993), working with a team at the University of Minnesota under the direction of Dr. Owen Wangensteen, reported the first successful case of an intracardiac repair of a ventricular septal defect—a hole between the lower heart chambers—using hypothermia with inflow occlusion. This significant step forward in the pursuit of intracardiac time was being done post-dog-lab on blue babies. After sixty successful cases, Dr. Lewis left Minneapolis for Northwestern University in Chicago, Illinois, where he was unable to continue intracardiac repairs with hypothermia successfully. Dr. Lewis ended up frustrated and retired from surgery early (Shumway 1996). Perhaps the dog lab, the heart team, the anesthesia team, or another critical component to success were not available.

One such crucial component, a well-trained nurse, appeared in September 1952. Donna Larson, a Sacred Heart nursing school graduate, landed her first job as circulating nurse, also scrubbing cases in the operating room. She had observed many of Dr. Berg's surgeries while in nursing school, so she was prepared for his diligence. During cases with Dr. Berg, she was graceful with his instruments, diligent, attentive, and smart. When Dr. Berg operated, regardless of the case, he was always demanding and precise. Many of the OR nurses found him difficult to work with; he consistently "let one know when he was not pleased and why," explained Nurse Donna.

Dr. Berg was quick and cool with his swift technique. The medical interns and residents were always pleased to assist or attend at Berg's operations because of his excellent technique, knowledge, and teaching skills. Nurse Donna enjoyed the challenge of difficult cases and soon began scrubbing on most of Dr. Berg's cases. This worked well for Dr. Berg. She was someone he could rely on for consistency and precision. After several weeks, he hired Donna as his personal scrub nurse. This job also entailed working in his Paulsen Building office; scheduling electrocardiograms and cardiac catheters at the hospital; helping with patient physical exams and new patients; keeping records; and being on call for emergency surgeries.

Dr. Berg was picky, meticulous, and focused on every minor defect, and he expected success. During his first year in private practice, 1952, he performed all manner of pneumonectomy, diaphragmatic and hiatal hernia repairs, closed-heart shunts for blue babies, patent ductus ligations, and open-heart digital valve commissurotomies (Larson 2011). Depending on the case, Donna would position the operating table and instrument stand to accommodate and give Dr. Berg advantage. She would place his instruments on the stand in perfect order so she could efficiently hand them to him as needed. She maintained organization and communication with him and the hospital and the operating room.

Dr. Berg also did smaller cases, such as bronchoscopes, foreign body removal, and cardiac catheters. The cardiac catheters were relatively quick procedures. However, analyzing the data took days. The data included pressure readings from inside each chamber of the heart and a tracing called a waveform. From analyzing the pressures, waveforms, and the dilutions after administration of the cardiogreen dye, Dr. Berg could determine whether a shunt existed, between which chambers, and the general size of the shunt.

Dr. Berg was the only doctor in a large territory—the Inland Northwest—doing bronchoscopes in 1952. The children who came in with chicken bones, candies, and other foreign bodies stuck in the throat were emergencies. An obstructed airway could take a life in minutes, and a child in distress was harrowing. At the time, this team would be flown in a small airplane to care for emergency foreign body cases in remote rural locations. With a quick bronchoscope, Dr. Berg could find the foreign body, sometimes in the lung, the esophagus, or trachea. Once removed, the child would restore spontaneous respirations, to everyone's relief. The team was efficient, fast, and successful.

A large part of Dr. Berg's chest training in St. Louis dealt with tuberculosis patients and patients with lung abscesses, who were not allowed in regular hospitals in Spokane because of contagious spread. Spokane's Edgecliff Tuberculosis Sanitarium housed and isolated tuberculosis patients receiving open-air therapy. Tuberculosis was a killer and a scourge dating back to medieval times. If open-air therapy failed, the old surgical therapy was to fill the chest with Ping-Pong balls, the idea being to permanently collapse the lung where the infection was brewing. The lack of oxygen was a benefit in fighting the persistent organism. However, an inadvertent partial collapse would lead to lung abscess.

From the moment he saw the sanitarium, a beautiful complex of redbrick buildings at the edge of a pine forest, Ralph liked it. The operating room was basic but well maintained. He obtained privileges there. A nurse and an anesthetist would come with him to operate. A definitive surgical collapse of the damaged lung, with controlled reshaping of the ribs that prevented any reexpansion, was performed. The abscess rate was much lower with this newer surgical procedure. Helping many TB patients, Dr. Berg spoke fondly of these rib-collapsing thoracoplasty procedures. It was all that was available for advanced TB patients, who were often treated poorly, like lepers, due to fear of spreading infection.

When new medications became available, this surgical procedure thankfully became obsolete.

Dr. Berg's cases were always interesting. Most of the ORs had basic instrument sets, but the necessary chest instruments were not available at the hospitals. He was operating at five facilities: Fairchild Air Force Base Hospital, St. Luke's Hospital, Edgecliff Tuberculosis Sanitarium, Deaconess Hospital, and Sacred Heart Hospital. He personally purchased the chest instruments. Nurse Donna brought them to the hospital where he was operating. She would select instruments from the hospital set and from his set, then sterilize them to make a complete set for Dr. Berg's case. At the end of the case, his specialty instruments were separated out, and both sets were cleaned and packed away.

At the downtown hospitals, Dr. Berg was making history with difficult and technical heart surgery. His results were excellent. He was open to all the different and interesting cases that came with chest surgery.

For instance, to increase blood flow into the heart muscle in order to alleviate angina, the theory of the day was to irritate the outside lining of the heart, the epicardium. The irritation would bring more blood flow to the heart muscle. Nurse Donna purchased commercial asbestos and sterilized it. In the dog laboratory, the first modeling surgery comprised placement of a coronary artery constrictor to create angina in the dog. One or two weeks later, asbestos was inserted into the pericardial sac. The procedure was technically successful, but it was impossible to tell whether the dog was any better in regard to angina (Larson 2011).

Once a week, there was an early-morning meeting held to present and discuss difficult and interesting cases. This case conference was basically Dr. Evarts Graham's chest conference reproduced in Spokane. Cardiologists, radiologists, pathologists, surgeons, anesthetists, and doctors in training attended. When it was pointed out that talc was safer than asbestos, Dr. Berg switched from asbestos to talc in short order. Talc got the job done. Asbestos was left behind.

Patients with murmurs and valve disease were more difficult. To improve on the manual commissurotomy, long instruments were being developed to be used inside the heart, accessed through the atrial appendage with a purse string. The Hufnagel valve came on the market in 1952. It was the first prosthetic valve—a plastic ball inside a plastic cage that, placed downstream from the failing aortic valve, only allowed forward flow, replacing the native valve that was failing from backward flow or regurgitation. Berg's team had their highest mortality with these patients. The Hufnagel valve was too big for a dog, so before the team attempted to use the valve on a struggling patient, Donna went with Dr. Berg to a funeral home. With written permission, Dr. Berg placed this valve in a cadaver (Larson 2011).

Children with intracardiac septal defects—defects in the wall of the heart separating it into its four chambers—were the most challenging. If the septal defect was large, the blue baby often died. These patients were still called doomed. They stayed on the list, getting some growth with medical therapy, such as digoxin, which slowed the heart rate, and living a limited lifestyle. It was felt these youngsters would benefit the most from the heart-lung machine. The concept: a machine that would perform the work of the child's heart and lungs while the heart surgeon stopped the blue-baby heart and performed the repair.

Dr. Berg was planning to use hypothermia to gain precious time in repairing an intracardiac defect. Dr. Bigelow, who had published his dog-lab results with hypothermia in 1950, and Berg were having breakfast together at the annual thoracic meeting that May and discussed details of Dr. Bigelow's hypothermia setup, techniques, and supplies. In Bigelow's experiment, the dog was given anesthesia and then lowered into an ice pool until the temperature dropped.

Stay sutures were used to angle the heart to minimize blood loss and facilitate the creation of the model. At the second operation, the repair of the septal defect was done.

In preparation, Dr. Berg had Donna purchase several sizes of curved needles at an upholstery shop. These were sterilized and used for the septal repairs. Dr. Berg would choose the size he needed, put one finger in the defect, and use the needle to make a purse string around the opening. The long, curved, specialized needle removed the need to place a needle-holding instrument inside the small cardiac chamber due to its ability to hold the upper thread. The "bobbin" or internal thread was controlled by Berg's finger acting as the footer and the shuttle hook. The tension could be controlled smoothly during and after the thread was set in place, thus avoiding pulling through the septal tissue. An advantage in the small space (Larson 2011). For a child with a larger defect, Berg planned to use a cellophane patch that he called "the Crafoord technique," as Crafoord had developed this patch to bridge the larger septal defects.

On March 25, 1953, Ralph earned the first chest boards certification in the area and number 235 of all certificates from the American Board of Thoracic Surgery. When he, at the front edge of this significant change, took the written exam and then sat for the oral exam, he "knew a lot more" than his examiner.

Later in 1953, a child patient growing slowly due to a congenital heart condition was referred to Dr. Berg. At the office exam, Dr. Berg determined by stethoscope that the P2 (pulmonary valve closure 2) heart sound was louder than the A2 (aortic valve closure 2) sound. At surgery, it was confirmed the ductus had remained patent and was shunting blood left to right. This flow was forcing the heart to work much too hard, robbing the child of peripheral flow needed for growth.

The surgical technique Dr. Berg used was familiar; it was the revised technique first developed by Dr. Robert Gross. With the youngster under anesthesia and both vessels dissected circumferentially away from the adherent connective tissue, he clamped both great vessels—the aorta and the pulmonary artery—with side-biting vascular clamps. He cut the patent ductus. Dr. Berg carefully sewed both sides of the ductus and closed both vessels with interrupted sutures. With his vascular clamps off the vessels, his surgical field clean and free from bleeders, the chest was closed, and the dressings were applied. The child was four years old. He did well in recovery and went home improved.

On May 6, 1953, a new report caught Dr. Berg's attention. Dr. John Gibbon (mentioned in "Historical Note 3") at Harvard's Massachusetts General Hospital had performed an open-heart case using his heart-lung machine successfully in a human. Gibbon's heart-lung machine was eighteen years in concept and development, then dog-lab research. His open-heart case outside of the research lab was an atrial septal defect (ASD)—a hole between the upper heart chambers—in an eighteen-year-old girl. However, after Dr. Gibbon's first success, he had three on-table deaths with his machine. Unable to move forward, Dr. Gibbon gave up heart surgery altogether. His heart-lung machine was subsequently purchased by IBM (L. H. Cohn 2003).

A physical exam, stethoscope auscultation, and patient history were adequate for diagnosing a patent ductus blue-baby defect; however, more information was desired and needed for the intracardiac septal defects. In preparation for the use of hypothermia for intracardiac septal defect repairs, Dr. Berg would use cardiac catheterization to obtain information. The heart catheters were performed in the radiology department. Nurse Donna set up the instruments in a sterile field and assisted Dr. Berg for these procedures. The catheters, ordered by Dr. Berg, were sterilized by boiling them in water on a Bunsen burner in the radiology room.

During the procedure, Dr. Berg would first decide whether the lesion was between the upper or lower chambers. To do this, he inserted the catheter via the femoral vein, using a small surgical procedure to expose the vessel at the groin. Through the catheter, an EKG lead wire was placed and manipulated into the right atrium. Donna ran the EKG machine; it was as big as a window and recorded pressures and waveforms. Berg gave an injection of green dye. A laboratory technician would then collect and run blood samples for oxygen content from each atrial chamber. Dr. Berg would analyze the data over the next few days, map out the results, and determine the location and size of the intracardiac defect. He made his surgical decisions based on this information.

The use of hypothermia continued to develop. At the American Medical Association meeting in June 1953, Dr. Henry Swan (1913–1996) at the University of Colorado in Denver reported a series of thirteen patients where his team used hypothermia to repair intracardiac septal defects, with one death. Dr. Swan rewarmed his patients by warming the fluids going into the heart, as well as with external sources of heat. This landmark paper established hypothermia as an effective tool for intracardiac repairs. This was validating for Dr. Berg and his plans to do the same (Swan n.d.).

As 1953 neared its end, Ralph and Mary were anticipating another child. Their family was well. The children were into sports, and skiing in the mountains was an activity the whole family enjoyed.

In one episode of note, Dr. Berg was set to operate and repair a hiatal hernia in the mother of his private scrub nurse. Nurse Donna was in the family waiting room, and the hospital scrub nurse assigned to the case was nervous. Dr. Berg reassured her, but the nurse fainted as he was making the chest incision. They called, and Nurse Donna scrubbed. The case went well.

In April 1954, Dr. C. Walton Lillehei (1918–1999) reported his successful intracardiac repair of a ventricular septal defect (VSD) on a four-year-old at the University of Minnesota using hypothermia, cardiac arrest, and cross-circulation from the parent. The blue baby's parent was effectively a heart-lung machine. Dr. Lillehei also considered his first case, performed on March 26, a success. There he had repaired a VSD on a one-year-old child, who died of pneumonia on the eleventh day after surgery. Within a year, Dr. Lillehei had performed forty-five open-heart operations with 33 percent mortality, which were reported (David K. C. Cooper 2010; Miller 2000).

Meanwhile, in Seattle, Dr. K. Alvin Merendino (1914–2011), chief of thoracic surgery at the new University of Washington School of Medicine and associate professor of surgery, was also interested in open-heart. As the only academic thoracic surgeon in the state of Washington, his work was followed by Dr. Berg. Merendino knew Walt Lillehei. They had both trained at the University of Minnesota with Dr. Wangensteen, though Lillehei was several years younger than Merendino. Open-heart was a bold concept. Lillehei's open-heart technique of cross-circulation, potentially lethal to both parent and child, seemed risky to Dr. Merendino. His team instead prepared a monkey as the biologic pump and lung oxygenator (Merendino 2011).

Back in Spokane, the class of 1954 graduating from the Sacred Heart nursing school admired and appreciated Dr. Berg's advances. They invited him to speak at the ceremony, and he prepared an eminently practical ten-minute speech for them:

> Members of the class of 1954 and guests, I am pleased to have the opportunity to speak to such a fine group. Congratulations and welcome. Rather than deliver a formal speech, I wish you would indulge me in covering a variety of topics which I believe may help you in your future in nursing. . . . Rewards of

nursing are many. Yours is a noble profession, more rewarding in personal satisfaction than in worldly goods. Remain aloof as you perform your duties. Remain grounded in the dignity, honor, and integrity of your profession. Do not become emotionally involved as you protect your patients' rights and care of them. Check and share responsibility with the doctor. If there is no correlation with the order to the patient condition, do not administer the medication. Avoid self-medication. If an order is confusing, ask the doctor to write it. Particularly with blood transfusions, take extra care. These good habits can protect you when fatigued and rushed. Thank you for the honor and privilege of welcoming you to clinical work in nursing.

Weeks later, in July 1954, Dr. Augie Senning (1915–2000) in Sweden successfully used his heart-lung machine to repair a mitral valve stenosis and remove a myxomatous mass from the right atrium. A myxoma, a noncancerous tumor, can break off in small pieces, travel in the flow of blood, and potentially cause a stroke. This was the start of Senning's first group of patients, which resulted in a 35 percent mortality. Dr. Senning used hypothermia and ventricular fibrillation to arrest the heart. His heart-lung machine was a drum fitted with rotating cylinders to pump and oxygenate the blood (Wettrell 2023). A young pediatric cardiology fellow who would become very important to Dr. Berg, Dr. Henry Lang from Harvard, was working in Sweden with this team. Ralph took note of this advance.

In the office on October 23, 1954, Dr. Berg saw a young girl named Linda and her parents for the first time. She was small for her age, and her pediatrician had picked up a heart murmur. He believed Linda had a hole in her heart. Dr. Berg examined the youngster with the assistance of her mother. He found a defect over her left chest. As he ran his hand over the lump, it was familiar, a precordial bulge with a palpable cardiac shock; no thrill, hammer, or shock pulse indicates no flow, an obstruction, whereas a thrill indicates flow with a stenosis. He heard an intense grade-3 to grade-4 systolic murmur, loudest in the pulmonic area and transmitted into the child's neck and back, by stethoscope, and the P2 sound was accentuated. By palpation of the abdomen, he found that young Linda's liver was enlarged. Both her hands and feet were cool to touch. The hole was robbing her of her blood flow to her extremities, and her heart was working too hard.

Dr. Berg warned the parents that Linda would continue to be sick. She might get pneumonia and even die. Until her heart was fixed, she was not allowed to play outside. Linda was a feisty little girl who would not cooperate with getting an office EKG, so she was scheduled to get an EKG and a heart catheterization to further define the suspected defect between her upper heart chambers at the hospital. On November 4, her EKG showed strain. Linda was started on digitalis, a medication to slow down her heart. The cost estimates were $100 for the cardiac catheter and $350 for the operation to repair her heart (Childs 2011). Her parents scheduled the surgery.

In the interim, a patient who had presumed coronary disease, his life and activities limited by angina, called the office. Dr. Berg had placed asbestos into his pericardium at surgery. This procedure had helped him become more functional. However, his chest pain returned. At the visit, Berg determined it had been about eighteen months since the asbestos procedure. He put Mr. George Caruso back on the list for heart surgery, this time with talc. Mr. Caruso stayed with Dr. Berg as a patient for the next thirty years.

A week later, Dr. Berg's office got a call. Linda's family had had a tragedy, a death. Linda's maternal grandfather had passed away. Linda's mother was upset. She was so upset that the thought of losing her daughter as well would not fade. Dr. Berg agreed to cancel, and they rescheduled surgery for six months away. The family thought Linda was going to die, as so many children with congenital heart conditions did. Her care and surgery were a real hardship for Linda's parents. Her other set of grandparents had declined to help pay for or loan money for Linda's condition.

At her six-month office visit, in the summer of 1955, young Linda was holding her own. She was still small for her age, but she had grown and remained out of the hospital. Dr. Berg told the family they could again wait for several months. He wanted to see Linda in January 1956.

Meanwhile, over in Seattle, Dr. Merendino's first chest fellow, Dr. George Thomas (1925–2021), started July 1955. A graduate of Johns Hopkins School of Medicine, Dr. Thomas had avoided repeating two years of general surgery residency by visiting with the chairman of surgery at the University of Washington. Dr. Henry Harkins (1905–1967) hired him inside of five minutes as a second-year general surgery resident (G. Thomas 2010).

In October 1955, Dr. John Kirklin (1917–2004) at the Mayo Clinic in Rochester, Minnesota, reported his series of eight patients undergoing intracardiac repairs with 50 percent mortality. Kirklin started with the IBM heart-lung machine, and modifications were made in the research lab. The first case of this series had been performed in the spring of 1954 (J. W. Kirklin 1955; Johnson 1970). Berg felt Dr. John Kirklin was onto something and followed his work closely.

What pioneer Spokane heart surgeon Ralph Berg Jr. was about to do the morning of December 27, 1955, dared the incredible. No one in the surgery made one unnecessary noise. His remarkable feat of operating inside a little girl's heart by "feel" alone was reprinted throughout the nation, transmitted by the Associated Press and published on page 1 of the *Minneapolis Tribune* and the Chicago Sun-Times, and by the New Orleans Times-Picayune, Amarillo Globe-Times, The Oregonian, Seattle Post-Intelligencer, and Seattle Times. The Associated Press commended the article in its log.

Excerpt from the Spokane Newspaper article "Deep Inside Her Heart," by Dorothy Powers (1921–2014), published December 27, 1955:

> Deep inside her heart, little Wileen Taylor was not like the other children. The games they played left her exhausted. A mild try at skipping rope left her gasping for air. Now 9 years old, she weighed a scant 50 pounds. Her face was pale, her bony chest abnormally enlarged. Wileen was the victim of a strange contraction. Her heart was severely overworked, yet she was starving for oxygenated blood. The words the doctor told her mother sounded funny. Wileen could not understand them.
>
> "Pulmonary valvular stenosis," he said, "with an interatrial septal defect." Translated, the big words meant that a tiny valve inside Wileen's heart was blocked almost completely. The dangerous stumbling block lay directly in the blood's vital pathway to the lungs for oxygen, damming the passageway between the right ventricle and the pulmonary artery. Blood barely squeezed through the malformed valve. The right side of Wileen's heart had to pump 5.8 liters of blood per minute, more than twice the normal amount.
>
> Without surgery, Wileen's case was hopeless. She did not know all this. She only knew that her parents, Mr. and Mrs. William E. Taylor, Spokane, took her to the doctor. From then on, science took over.
>
> A pediatrician made a diagnosis of congenital heart disease and referred Wileen to a team of doctors. The team catheterized her heart by running a slender length of plastic tube all the way from a vein in her groin through her heart and even out into her upper arm. Long before she entered the hospital, the surgeon knew exactly where the hidden blocked valve and the hole in her heart wall lay. He had to

know because once he sank his knife into the inner vessels of the child's heart, its blade would be buried from his sight. He would be operating by "feel" alone. Under the brilliant lights of the surgery, Wileen was strapped on her back. A surgeon, aided by a nine-man team, was about to cut straight into her heart. Moving briskly about the room were four nurses, three anesthetists, the surgeon, his assisting surgeon, and intern. Wileen was given injections and lost consciousness.

"Let's start," the surgeon said quietly. The heart did everything it could to hide. It forced the surgeon to split the child's breastbone in two for access to the vital organ. Hemostats, looking like cuticle scissors with crimped ends, clamped off the bleeding. In the entire room, the only sound was the sharp "slap" of instruments as the nurse clapped them smartly into the surgeon's hand.

Then, "Pericardial sac," he explained as he punctured the membrane encasing the heart. The surgeon was exactly where he should be. There, completely exposed, was the right ventricle of Wileen's heart. Its labored pulsing, clearly visible to the naked eye, brought a look of solemn awe to the ring of faces around the table.

Instead of containing three "cloverleaf" cusps which opened and closed, the malformed valve in Wileen's heart had only a "pinhole" opening. Blood barely squeezed through the tiny aperture into the pulmonary artery, begging to get to the lungs for oxygen. The second ailment, the septal defect, was a direct result of the first. "Backed up" blood behind the closed valve created terrific pressures in the right ventricle and indirectly forced open a hole which should have closed at birth between the right and left atriums (auricles).

Through the inch-wide hole, already-oxygenated blood mistakenly detoured from the left atrium to the right instead of carrying its oxygen load throughout the body. This burdened the right atrium with a double pumping load, badly overtaxing the right side of the heart. Working swiftly, the surgeon sewed a series of stitches in a circle on the surface of the defect. This "drawstring" stitch was designed to control the flow through the defect.

What happened looked impossible. The surgeon took a special knife and stabbed it straight into the heart. He withdrew it, leaving a small wound that a pen knife might have made. Into that, he inserted a pencil-like instrument called a valvulotome. Its end was perfectly round, its blade completely sheathed so there would be no useless cutting as it made its way to the danger spot, the blocked valve. Nobody breathed as skillful fingers guided the steel shaft on its journey through the heart. The surgeon piloted it entirely by "feel." The penetrating end was well beyond his view, hidden in the heart's interior. "There it is," he said tensely. His fingers pressed the protruding end of the instrument. A spring released the sheathed blade. Deep inside the heart, the blade struck.

The "miracle" was over for the moment. A surgeon had operated blind within a human heart on an obstruction he never saw. At the sudden rush of blood through its now-open gate, the heart valves leaped visibly. The eyes of the anesthetist, worried until now, suddenly met those of the surgeon over their masks. She nodded thankfully, satisfied at the sudden upsurge in her patient's pulse and pressure.

The surgeon re-sheathed his blade and withdrew the instrument from the heart. Gently, he then inserted another, a dilator to enlarge the valve still more. One thing remained: he had to explore the purse-strung hole in the little heart. He did it the simplest way. For an instant, he stood there, his gloved finger actually inside the child's heart. Then he straightened, after securing the purse string. "We'll close now. It'll be all right."

Layer after layer, the surgeon closed the covering about

Wileen's heart. Tiny holes were drilled down each length of the severed breast bone. Fine wires, laced from one side to the other, brought the bone into perfect alignment for knitting.

Finally, the tired surgeon dropped his gauze mask and rubbed a hand across his brow. Looking down at Wileen, he grinned. "Nice job," he told his team. And Wileen was getting well. (Powers, "Deep Inside Her Heart" 1955)

Dr. Berg was pleasantly surprised by the attention the team and hospital received after this article. The entire process was, for Berg, nothing more than swift surgical technique. Both defects were successfully repaired.

CHAPTER 9

Sister Mary Bede and the Transition to a Heart-Lung Machine

Dr. Henry Lang got Dr. Berg's phone number after reading the Dorothy Powers newspaper article. He wanted to talk to this chest surgeon in private practice across the state in Spokane who was using swift surgical technique with hypothermia and had successfully repaired an intracardiac atrial septal defect and a pulmonary valve stenosis in a blue baby, with a reporter watching.

Dr. Lang attended Princeton University for his undergraduate degree, earning his medical degree in 1947 from the University of Rochester, New York School of Medicine, then interning in pathology at Barnes Hospital in St. Louis. The postmortem exam was the main technique for diagnosing and understanding the various blue-baby defects, which held his interest. Dr. Lang went on to pediatrics at Children's Hospital in Boston. As a resident, he met and married his wife, Pauline, a college student at Radcliffe. Henry stayed on at Children's Hospital after his pediatric residency for a fellowship in pediatric cardiology with Dr. Alexander Sandor Nadas (1913–2000), a pediatric cardiologist known internationally for his care of children with heart disease (R. Berg 2006).

At Harvard and Children's Hospital, Dr. Nadas worked closely with chest surgeon Dr. Gross—a formidable team. Dr. Nadas typically sent his fellows to Europe, a tradition that had been disrupted by WWII for all but a few institutions. Henry spent a year at the pediatric department of the new Karolinska University Institute in Stockholm, Sweden. There, Drs. Crafoord, Bjork, and Senning's heart-lung machine had its first success on July 16, 1954. That team repaired a defect between the upper heart chambers and removed a mass inside one of the chambers. Dr. Lang was inspired.

A year later, in pursuit of a heart-lung machine and procedures to help blue babies, Dr. Lang landed an academic position at the University of Washington School of Medicine, starting June 1955. Teaching cardiology and cardiac physiology to the medical students, he also saw patients in the cardiology clinic. His work centered on cardiovascular physiology, especially congenital heart disease. And so it was that one day early in 1956, Dr. Lang called Dr. Berg.

Dr. Lang learned that Ralph Berg had an established dog lab separate from his private practice. The animal laboratory at the university in Seattle was a multianimal hospital consuming the entire top floor of the medical school, with an annual budget that was over four times the annual earnings of this private surgeon. Yet Dr. Lang told Ralph he wanted to come over and work with him in Spokane. Ralph said, "Yes, come on over," and was happy to have him. Henry took the risk. He left his academic position to establish a private practice where Dr. Berg was located. Dr. Henry Lang would become his pediatric cardiologist (R. Berg 2006).

Linda's mother sat and cried while watching home movies of Linda for days preceding her hospital admission in February 1956. Knowing the heart catheter had gone well did not help her. Her husband had just lost his job. Linda, now six years old, could not be outside, nor play with kids. She was kept inside to avoid stressing her congenital heart defect. She was sickly, blue, and could no longer wait for repair.

On February 1, 1956, the hospital called Dr. Berg's office. Linda and her family were being refused admission, a matter of the bill. Dr. Berg settled the issue by arranging a loan agreement for the $2,000 with the hospital. Young Linda, aware of the financial stress for her parents, was impressed by how easily Dr. Berg solved the problem. It made her feel better. Dr. Berg would take care of her (Childs 2011).

The heart catheter had revealed the defect between Linda's upper chambers and a duplicate of the vena cava. A second cardiac angiogram done in the operating room showed pressures higher on the right side of the heart. Dr. Berg felt the distortion of her left chest would not help him if he approached from the left.

At surgery two days later, Dr. Berg made a right anterior thoracotomy. Linda's pediatrician assisted. After the lung was retracted, a T-shaped incision was made in the pericardium, and the duplicate vena cava was circumferentially dissected out and encircled on umbilical tapes. Great care was taken to avoid the phrenic nerve, which controls the diaphragm. The purse string was laid around the right auricular tip after dissecting the interauricular groove, and then Berg inserted his finger.

He found a large defect, a hole in the atrial septum of the secundum type and an enormous orifice to the coronary sinus, which drains oxygenated blood to the right atrium. The heart was tilted, so he placed the atrial purse string at the highest point to minimize bleeding by gravity assist. Then he repaired the septal defect using a large, curved upholstery needle to place the single #5 braided silk around the circumference of the defect, with each bite of the needle also catching the Crafoord cellophane patch. The closure of the auricular tip was routine. The duplicate vena cava and the large coronary sinus did not need repair. The pericardium was loosely closed after cleaning it of all blood.

Linda's father had been pacing the halls for the seven hours since being separated from his daughter in the preoperative holding room. He knew he might lose his child. It was a hardship on every level. When Dr. Berg came out and told him and his wife how well Linda was doing, well, it was hard to believe—hard to let go of the fear. Berg informed them that Linda would spend several weeks recovering in the hospital. Both parents continued to worry she was going to die early, no matter the open-heart surgery outcome (Childs 2011).

Over Valentine's Day, the Catholic children on the ward received small presents from the hospital. Linda, in her bed when presents were handed out, was passed over. Her upset father quickly reassured Linda, left, and returned with letters and presents. It turns out he had gone to her first-grade class. The letters and presents from her classmates kept coming over the following days. In the playroom down the hall, Linda met another young girl, Judy, recovering from congenital heart surgery. They both had Dr. Berg as their heart surgeon and became recovery mates. Her friend, Judy, had ligation of patent ductus. Judy's mother was single, and Dr. Berg had made arrangements to cover the expense. Soon the girls were racing each other in wheelchairs up and down the halls. On one run, they ended up hitting the nurses' station desk. They were released from hospital the next morning (VanVoorhis 2011).

When Linda walked into her first-grade class, the kids were surprised at how good she looked. She grew normally and rapidly after her heart was fixed. These two young girls met again, by chance, in their college religion class when their professor asked his students to learn something about the person sitting next to them. Linda and Judy became healthy and are lifelong friends.

The Langs arrived in Spokane in March 1956, welcomed by the medical community and the medical auxiliary. They bought a house and set up an office where Dr. Lang could walk to both hospitals. He worked several other jobs to supplement his income.

Drs. Lang and Berg both felt Dr. Kirklin and his Mayo team were true pioneers. After IBM bought Dr. Gibbon's original heart-lung machine in 1953, Dr. Kirklin's Mayo team further modified and used it, reporting a mortality rate of 50 percent in October 1955 for intracardiac repairs. It was now available for purchase. Although the Scandinavian team had success a year earlier with lower mortality, their machine was not for sale. Both Berg and Lang wanted to purchase the Mayo Clinic heart-lung machine, and they well understood the need to raise moneys and be frugal with the funds for this pursuit.

In Seattle, Dr. Merendino and his chest fellow, Dr. Thomas, moved from monkeys to dogs for their biologic oxygenators. The lung preparation was based on Dr. Lillehei's cross-circulation with several modifications. They did not expect the dog to survive. They ran blood from the blood bank through the dog's lungs. It would oxygenate the human blood. They had achieved success in their research lab, and they respected the sacrifice of each dog.

As Merendino's team was preparing to use a Great Dane's lungs as the oxygenator for their first human case, one final step remained. He asked the superintendent of King County Hospital whether they could bring a dog into the operating room. The answer was yes from the superintendent, but they would have to use the back stairway. It was March 1956. With a preoperative diagnosis of blue baby, they anticipated a tetralogy of Fallot anomaly. However, when the pericardial sac was opened, a much more complex defect was found: transposition of the great vessels.

"It was sobering to visualize," so Dr. Merendino decided to close the child's chest rather than attempt the case. Despite this sound judgment, the child died on the table (Merendino 2011).

Finding more complex defects and the need for more precise preoperative diagnoses was a problem for all the pioneering open-heart surgeons. The diagnostics were emerging, as were the heart-lung machines. After this case, Dr. Merendino decided that monkey or dog, a biologic lung oxygenator was not the way forward. He switched to a commercially available Lucite bubble oxygenator and went back to the research lab. Congenital hearts and specifically transposition of the great vessels became his career focus.

Henry worked well with Ralph at all levels. Ralph welcomed his colleague's expertise, especially in the operating room with his most difficult cases. Henry would monitor the case and assist all the team members as they cared for the blue patient under anesthesia. The bond of friendship, camaraderie, and respect between these two doctors became sacred. Dr. Lang admired Berg's dog lab. It was a simple setup, successful, and led to excellent surgical results. The Sisters of Providence, supportive of the pursuit of better health for the blue babies, maintained a hands-off approach regarding the dog lab.

Dr. Lang set up a fundraising talk with the local branch of the American Heart Association. At the fundraiser, Dr. Lang explained the rapid advances in both Sweden and the Mayo Clinic in developing technology for intracardiac surgical repairs. He revealed the plans to bring this open-heart technology and surgical procedures to Spokane. Upgrading the research laboratory was the first step. Mrs. Jewett, a board member of the northeast branch of the Washington State Heart Association, was interested.

"What piece of equipment?"

Upon hearing "A heart-lung machine," Mrs. Jewett stood and said, "I think this is great. If our northeast branch of the Washington State Heart Association raises five thousand dollars, I will match it!" The branch voted and agreed to the challenge and the match.

She made a personal contribution of $1,000 toward this open-heart pursuit that night, which stunned the heart team. Dr. Ralph Berg was able to get commitments from pharmaceutical companies to provide supplies needed in the lab. The same supplies would be needed in the main operating room when the team took an open-heart bypass machine to patients. Besides helping the most vulnerable of patients, there was a frugal financial reality and an expectation of financial return with this major advance. Drs. Berg and Lang estimated it would take over a year of experimental dog-lab work before they could use the heart-lung machine with patients.

Sister Mary Bede came to Spokane to visit the town and the Sisters of Providence hospital and its staff ahead of her expected arrival in

Spokane by the fall to administrate Sacred Heart. She had a genuine willingness to work with the team for the blue babies. She took note of Dr. Ralph Berg. He was talented and right minded about the care and future of these most vulnerable children.

Dr. Ralph Berg, a thinking surgeon driven by the surgical principles of the blue-baby repairs, especially credited Sister Mary Bede for helping him with his research despite the somewhat controversial nature of the dog lab. Often referred to as the research lab, the dog lab was the enduring foundation for the scientific and clinical success of the Spokane heart team. For Ralph Berg, Sister Mary Bede's influence and support was the seminal fortuitous event of his career. His service to his patients, to the blue babies, was his work. The dogs were cared for as he would care for human patients. He respected all life.

Drs. Berg and Lang were planning to modify the hypothermia method with the hope of allowing repairs on some of the larger blue-baby children on the list who were at the next level of complexity. The list of pediatric congenital heart patients was critically reviewed, and every attempt to do small procedures, gain diagnostic knowledge of the blue child's heart, and hold until the child had grown was made. When a child remained on the list or became too ill or sick to wait, they became the next patient. Drs. Berg and Lang chose this approach understanding that new surgical procedures and the heart-lung machines were advancing rapidly. These methods offered hope against the certainty of death.

This line of risk versus benefit was difficult—when to wait, when to get a cardiac catheter, and when to operate. These children returned to the heart team for evaluation at regular intervals. Both cardiologist and heart surgeon gave particular attention and hope to these blue babies' mothers. They knew if the mother was fearful or lost hope, these children were doomed.

Marty, three years old, was sickly and blue and on the list. He could wait no longer. His heart catheter procedure showed a complex shunt between the atrial chambers. Lang and Berg both determined he needed to be next as his condition was worsening. There was no more benefit to waiting. The operation was scheduled for April 1956. A single working mom whose husband had abandoned her and her unborn child, his mother understood that her son was dying, and she was grateful when Dr. Ralph Berg told her not to worry about the bill for the operation.

In the operating room, the child was put to sleep by the anesthetist. After the monitoring lines were placed, the team carefully lowered the child's body temperature in a tub of water chilled with ice cubes. Next, the child was placed on the operating table. Dr. Berg began with a left chest incision. Dr. Henry Lang monitored the readings from the cardiogram. Once the pericardium was opened, the heart was exposed. An atrial septal defect was repaired, and then things began to go wrong. First an arrhythmia; then, despite all efforts, the child was lost.

Young Marty's mother waited nervously. When Dr. Berg came out, he was very kind in informing her of her child's death. She was in shock with grief. He asked her to consent for an autopsy, which was important. She consented. She went home and cried. The autopsy showed additional congenital anomalies. Marty's mother specifically remembered there was a blockage between her child's kidney and bladder: "The child was doomed." She felt blessed to have received Dr. Ralph Berg's compassion and concern (Patient of Dr. Berg 2010).

The irreplaceable Nebraska Stephens (1931–2022) arrived in Spokane later that April 1956, a trained OR technician from Fairchild Air Force Base Hospital. Several surgeons from Spokane were consultants at this military hospital, and Nebraska first met Dr. Ralph Berg when a surgical consult led to an operation. Nebraska found Berg to be regal, focused, controlled, and technically precise. A few weeks after this operation, Nebraska took a second job working nights at Sacred Heart. He was one of the three members of the military hospital's daytime

OR team that made up the night OR team at Sacred Heart, on the 11 p.m. to 7 a.m. shift.

One night, close to midnight, the front desk phone rang at Sacred Heart's operating room. Calls this time of night usually meant an urgent case. Nebraska answered, expecting a stressed surgeon to be on the other end of the line. It was Berg. Cool and authoritative, he told Nebraska to go check on a dog in the lab, located by the nursing student living quarters. Nebraska was not sure if he could or should do this task.

"Call me if the dog is alive. Don't if he died," Berg said. Nebraska did not have a lot of time to be away from his post, and he did not know what a dog lab was. Still, he went to the location and found the lab, as instructed. In a large, open kennel lay a dog. Nebraska did not need to call Dr. Berg. He was shaken yet curious. Later he learned the dog-lab cases went on once or twice a week (Stephens 2011).

As summer rolled in, the big expansion of the research lab was underway. Sister Mary Bede had arranged to purchase the first heart-lung machine. It arrived in June. The open-heart team would use the machine in experiments, working out all the details before transitioning to the main operating room for the benefit of the blue babies. Nurse Donna had trained her replacement before stepping out for maternity leave with plans to start a part-time job in the new lab that fall. She had been hired by Sister Mary Bede.

Vascular surgeons, whose special interest is blood flow and procedures to repair arterial aneurysms and create procedures to bring more arterial flow to downstream blockages, were logically interested in the bypass heart-lung machine. Dr. Richard Kleaveland (1926–2018) had chosen Spokane as the location in which to investigate this development. He and his wife arrived in August 1956 after driving across the country with their kids, stopping in Rochester, Minnesota, to visit family. Money was tight. Dr. Kleaveland's resident-in-training salary of $25 per month at Massachusetts General Hospital had left them with no savings. During those lean years, his family came to eat with him weekly at the hospital-sponsored meal. His wife made sacrifices to support the family during his training. Financial stability was important to Dr. Kleaveland.

His training at Harvard was excellent. He was ready to practice and knew his surgical skill was sound. "Precision is the main thing, repetitively precise. Speed follows precision," Kleaveland reported.

Dr. Robert Linton, the vascular surgeon teaching him at the end of his training at Mass General Hospital, said, "Well, I can see you are not going to send me a lot of cases," acknowledging his mentee's skill with a difficult vascular case. In fact, Kleaveland wanted to be far from any academic institution so cases would not be pulled out by doctors referring to academic surgeons. Spokane fit all his criteria. It was a medium-size town surrounded by a huge territory, with two hospitals and beautiful neighborhoods minutes away. There were many medical practices with doctors who could refer, and the only medical school was new and across the state.

Almost immediately upon arriving in Spokane, Dr. Kleaveland ran into Henry Lang at the hospital. They had skied together during the winter of 1953, when Henry had a car and long, white government-issue skis. They were both Harvard men who had trained at Boston Children's Hospital, Dr. Kleaveland on a pediatric surgery rotation with Dr. Robert Gross and Dr. Henry Lang as the pediatric fellow. A pleasant reunion for both. Henry informed his friend and colleague of Ralph Berg, the open-heart dog-lab team, and their purpose to develop a heart-lung machine. This was the big technology push of the time. During Dr. Kleaveland's surgical training from 1951 to 1956, Dr. Churchill was the surgery chairman at Massachusetts General Hospital, and chest surgery was still a part of general surgery training. Closed cardiac surgery procedures were a further subset of chest surgery.

"Only Mayo Clinic and University of Minnesota had crossed over into intracardiac procedures with a heart-lung machine," explained Dr. Kleaveland. This was experimental technology, and chest surgery was still in its fledgling state in Massachusetts, with Dr. Gordon Scanlon, the chest surgery fellow when Kleaveland was the vascular surgery resident, mostly self-trained under Dr. Churchill. Kleaveland went on to explain, "Vascular procedures were farther along than open-heart techniques. Stick your finger in the heart and fracture the mitral plaque was the cutting-edge, inside-the-heart procedure at the time." He was pleased with what he found in Spokane (Kleaveland 2011). He fit in with Drs. Berg and Lang—three well-trained doctors in pursuit of a heart-lung machine and all manner of excellent surgical skill and procedures around this machine.

The Kleavelands bought a house close to the hospitals. He set up a private office and began working with vascular patients. He did not wait for an invitation from the open-heart team and was welcomed, as he had a lot to offer. In fact, he helped with every detail of the expansion, including new surgical lights and plumbing. His attention to details, vascular training, instrumentation, and techniques were appreciated. However, it was his additional knowledge of veterinarian medicine that most impressed Ralph Berg. Kleaveland, an escapee from his family of veterinarians, made improvements for the dogs. Kleaveland contacted a local vet with a clinic not too far from the hospital. The vet agreed to support the dog lab. This care and support were big advantages to the dogs in terms of medications, diet, and being able to take them to the veterinary clinic after a surgery to recover before going home with the nurses. Dr. Berg greatly appreciated this advance (R. Berg 2006).

On August 6, 1956, Dr. K. Alvin Merendino and chest fellow Dr. Thomas successfully used their heart-lung machine on a six-year-old boy with a blue-baby defect and performed an intracardiac repair. The preoperative diagnosis was "congenital heart." The postoperative diagnosis, due to the intraoperative findings, was "pulmonary artery stenosis." The valve stenosis was successfully excised and repaired. The child did well.

Dr. Merendino took credit for being the first at the University of Washington and on the West Coast to use a heart-lung machine. An academic chest surgeon in San Francisco claimed he did the first heart-lung-machine intracardiac repair on the West Coast, then later retracted the claim (Merendino 2011; G. Thomas 2010).

Dr. Berg, not interested in accolades, stayed focused on outcomes and low mortality.

When Nurse Donna returned to work in late August 1956, the new lab was ready. The schedule was blocked out for experimental lab work on Wednesday and Saturday mornings. The team got to work. The purpose of the first experiments was to refine and develop the pump's use. They practiced cannulation, volumes, lines, pressures, and the status of the dog going "on" and coming "off pump." The surgical procedures were not technical at first (Larson 2011).

In November, Sister Mary Bede arrived in Spokane. First a schoolteacher teaching algebra, then a nurse, and then a nurse educator, she transcended to Sister of Providence late in life. In her service of the mission, she came to Spokane, where she became Mother Superior, running the entire Catholic hospital system. A talented woman with vision, her service to the mission was solid. She saw the talent in young Dr. Ralph Berg and his team. She knew well the difficulties with these doomed blue babies. She also recognized the talents of Drs. Lang and Kleaveland and was pleased that Dr. Berg had partners in this pursuit. Sister Mary Bede was equally pleased that the first heart-lung machine was being put to good use. Her involvement, despite the negatives of a dog lab, was insightful and deeply appreciated (R. Berg 2006). An experimental research laboratory was the best way to safely bring these children into the clinical operating room. Make all the mistakes in the lab first.

One evening, Dr. Berg was operating late with Nebraska, OR technician. Sterile, scrubbed, and gowned, Nebraska handed Dr. Berg the first instrument, a scalpel. The surgeon tried to cut the skin for his incision and only left a red line without opening the skin. Dr. Berg was upset. It was late in the day, and obviously this reusable blade had not been sharpened. So, Dr. Berg called for Sister Mary Bede to come into the operating room. The nuns lived in the hospital and were always close by. She came in.

Dr. Berg showed the Sister the red line and for her benefit tried again to make his incision, without success. He said to the Sister, "I want to cut your heart out with this scalpel." She turned bright red at his dark humor, a dull knife, and a challenge. It was her job to have the blades sharpened. She often did the sharpening herself; it was cost effective.

Ralph said, "I want a new blade for each case." Sister Mary Bede acquiesced and laughed with Ralph. The hospital made the transition to disposable blades, a new blade for each surgical case (R. Berg 2006; Stephens 2011).

Ralph's next concern: the pumps were perhaps part of the problem. Emerging reports from hospitals using heart-lung machines were concerning, showing long stays in hospital, tracheotomies to come off the ventilator, and difficult recovery after simple single intracardiac repairs in the patients who survived. The mortality started at 50 percent with Dr. Kirklin's first series. It remained high. This was both an exciting time and a time of caution, particularly for Dr. Berg. In the same intracardiac repairs without a heart-lung machine, his mortality was below 5 percent with swift surgical technique and hypothermia; but rapid advances in the pumps and techniques of each repair were being pioneered and shared. Dr. Lang particularly wanted lower mortality and felt *1* percent mortality was the goal.

The Mayo pump retained the Gibbon membrane oxygenator, contained in a glass cylinder that sat on top of the pump. "It was a visual, a red cascade," said Dr. Kleaveland, describing the blood running down over a stack of membranes of increasing size. The technology had advanced to bubble oxygenators; most heart teams had also abandoned the biologic oxygenators: human, monkey, then dog.

Needing a large surface area, the first bubble oxygenator used by the Spokane team was constructed of two sheets of thin, flexible, white plastic sheets measuring three by four feet. Sealed at the edges and along the interior to create a flow channel, the sealed sheets were rolled and placed in a containment cylinder. Oxygen from the pressurized tank bubbled between the sheets from vents along the top edge of the device. The blood flowing through the channel was exposed to the oxygen bubbles and exchanged gases, dropping carbon dioxide and oxygenating. The blood, depleted when it entered the device base, found its way back to the opposite side of the base, exiting fully oxygenated at the output port, then heading back into the pump for travel through the patient's circulation. They tried this first bubble oxygenator and rejected it after a few experiments (Kleaveland 2011).

A commercial Lucite bubble oxygenator of the type Dr. Merendino was using was brought in. Dr. Berg, never interested in the biologic oxygenator, was not convinced the bubble oxygenator was better than the cascading membrane. None of these oxygenators with pump were close to hypothermia in terms of efficacy. Dr. Berg considered his congenital heart work "the jewel in the crown of heart disease." Getting more time inside the heart for the repair was the goal. With hypothermia and swift surgical technique, Dr. Berg was able to achieve intracardiac times of ten to fifteen minutes. The field not free of blood, the heart still beating, he successfully made these repairs.

The dog would be brought into the lab early in the morning. The lab, set up like an operating room, was ready. Dr. Henry Lang determined the pump circuitry volume based on the size of the dog. He would prime the pump with that calculated volume. They used blood that came from the veterinarian, six to eight units per research case to prime the pump. Placing the first intravenous required help to hold the feisty dog. The drug to relax the dog was quickly delivered. The dog was put under exactly as done in the main operating room—general anesthesia with an endotracheal tube, Ambu bag ventilation, and monitoring lines. Dr. Lang monitored the volume, pressures, and waveforms via these lines.

Dr. Berg would open the dog's chest, exposing the pericardium within the mediastinum, and Dr. Kleaveland the groin, exposing the femoral vessels. They placed the dog on the bypass pump in a coordinated cannulation. The venous return cannula was placed into the femoral artery at the groin, which took the blood to the pump for a run through the oxygenator. The inflow cannula bringing blood from the oxygenator went into the aorta. Nebraska ran the pump, and Dr. Lang managed circulation arrest and every detail that came up. If all went well, they would venture into the heart and create a hole between the upper chambers.

They did flow studies, alternating oxygenated arterial inflow at the aortic versus the groin location; same for venous return routes. Eventually they chose gravity flow for the venous return, and Berg preferred to keep this cannula at the groin site. Gravity venous return from the patient back to the pump was the least toxic to the dog. They tested different-size tubing as well. They used a cold and heat exchanger and could decrease the dog's temperature in twelve minutes. Dr. Lang also used "Fox Green" (indocyanine green) dye injections prior to collecting multiple sequential blood samples. After the research lab to create the dog model of an ASD, he calculated the green dye dilution curves to estimate the size of the shunt they created as a model in relation to cardiac output.

Then they would come off the pump. This was the most harrowing part of the experiment—slowly and methodically waiting for the dog's heart to pick up a rhythm and then sequentially removing the pump and then the lines and closing the chest and groin. They awakened the dog, and after recovery overnight with the veterinarian clinic, someone would take the dog home. Most of the procedures were successful. After the research case, they would drain the blood from the pump. Nurse Donna occasionally used this old blood to feed her houseplants—perhaps morbid, but the overarching intent was to never waste or misuse blood products. This heart team respected all living entities and were attempting to save and prolong life. Together, they were able to create dog models that survived and weeks later became ready for the repair experiment.

Running, setting up, and cleaning the pump was time consuming. Dr. Kleaveland kept a book and critiqued each case, noting how they could do better. He developed a small cannula to perfuse the coronary arteries while the heart was shut down. The simple but elegant design was a malleable aluminum tube through which a green nasal oxygen tube passed and fit into a soft, graduated rubber gasket. The soft gasket fit snugly into any-size coronary opening, making perfusion to the heart muscle, the myocardium, much easier and more reliable.

Determining lengths of Tygon tubing based on the dog's size and setting up the mayo stand, Nurse Donna measured, cut, cleaned, and sterilized every product they used. Engrossed in the details of the pump, she was often on hands and knees, watching the lines and tubing as she and Dr. Lang prepared and ran the pump. One research day, the lab was ready for Drs. Berg and Kleaveland when, with no warning, the dog woke up, struggled, and pulled the breathing tube out. The dog jumped off the operating table right onto Nurse Donna's sterile stand full of perfectly positioned instruments. It was a fiasco. As the dog attempted to escape, the lab was pelted with flying instruments. That lab session was largely spent cleaning the pump and the instruments. Cleaning the pump with all the interchangeable components was a precise, daunting task (Larson 2011).

With several successful dogs modeled and then repaired using this pump, still Dr. Berg held back the decision to move forward into the main OR. The dogs took a while to wake up and a long time to recover. It was a problem. With hypothermia and swift surgical technique, neither the dogs nor the patients had this problem. The dogs did follow commands post-pump, but they were slow. Drs. Lang and Berg became concerned that the pump itself was the cause of this suboptimal recovery.

Ralph continued his phone calls and visits to the other chest surgeons using a heart-lung machine or in pursuit of intracardiac repairs. It was a small group of surgeons who were doing experimental work in preparation to go open-heart. It was an even smaller group of pioneers who were already on pump. Drs. Berg, Lang, and Kleaveland were not interested in being first. They wanted safety for the patients.

Dr. Kleaveland's father-in-law was a physiologist in Rochester, Minnesota. On a family visit, he ended up watching Dr. John Kirklin do intracardiac cases at the Mayo Clinic. Dr. Kirklin's advice was "Don't close the pericardium, weigh the patient before and after pump, and transfuse extra volume until good cardiovascular dynamics emerge." Dr. Kirklin gave the blood used to prime and run the pump back to the patient in an amount greater than 10 percent of body weight. In Dr. Kirklin's cases, this was delivered by the right atrial venous return catheter at the end of the pump run.

When Dr. Kleaveland relayed this information, Dr. Berg accepted the advice and found it helpful. Over the years, this rule was modified to Berg's rule: "Give two times the amount back in transfusion as what is lost in the chest drains" during the early postoperative period. For Dr. Henry Lang, this evolved into "Boost the child." They went to the annual thoracic meeting in May 1957. Much was shared, and invitations and plans to visit were made.

Reporter Dorothy Powers, whose article the year before had been picked up by the Associated Press, came into the office one day and talked to Dr. Berg. She wanted to update the public and report on the pump.

The current heart-lung machines were part of the problem, and Dr. Berg was not going to make the transition with the current pump, but he needed more moneys for the experimental lab to advance the design. Fundraising required the public to participate, but Berg did not want the public to learn of the dog lab. The information that the pump itself was hurting the dogs was critical to his decision to delay and hard to explain to the public. There was a professional dilemma.

Dorothy understood and reassured Dr. Berg of her intent to share their work accurately and respectfully with her readers. Ralph and

Henry chose a case where she could film the procedure and report to her public. The bypass pump stories would have to wait.

The team set up for a hypothermia case. The hypothermia room was half the size of the regular operating rooms. The night before, Nebraska brought in the large stainless-steel tub from the gynecologic room to use for the ice tub. It was covered with a soft blow-up swimming pool. The child had been on the list, and his was a most complicated set of multiple blue-baby cardiac defects. Dorothy agreed to limits; she was allowed to film into the OR using mirrors from her position outside the room. On June 4, 1957, Dorothy Powers published an article about this case in the *Spokane Review*.

> The boy on the table, everybody in the room knows, has no chance to live without the corrective surgery they are about to attempt. Already, in his ten short years, Patrick has leaned heavily on his supply of "borrowed time." Since birth, Patrick has been starving for oxygen. Total pulmonary venous anomaly plus an atrial septal defect and pulmonary valvular stenosis were the words the doctors had used. The big words meant simply that all veins carrying oxygenated blood from both Patrick's lungs emptied their supply into the right atrium of the heart via an anomalous channel—where it short-circuited uselessly back into the lungs again.
>
> Normally, the veins should carry oxygenated blood from the lungs to the left atrium (rather than the right), where it would be pumped via the left ventricle and aorta to all parts of the body. The vicious short-circuit robs Patrick of oxygenated blood on which to exist. Only a strange combination of defects, the doctors explained, has kept him alive even this long. Nature has made her mistakes in a weirdly kind manner.
>
> His second error, an atrial septal defect or abnormal "hole" between the atriums, allows a small bit of oxygenated blood from the lungs to find its way from the right to the left atrium

and out into Patrick's systemic circulation. And her third mistake—pulmonary valvular stenosis or partial blockage of the pulmonary heart valve—has protected his lungs from excessive circulation. In a strange combination of errors, then, Patrick has parlayed his brief years to ten.

Shortly now the cardiac surgeon will enter the pericardial sac, slit the tip end of the left atrium of the heart, and sew it to the common venous pool (juncture of veins from the lungs). Modern surgery will try to give Patrick what nature did not—a connection for oxygenated blood from his lungs to the left atrium of his heart. In the quiet of the surgery, an anesthetist moves briskly around Pat's ankles, inserting narrow, transparent tubing which will carry the anesthetic, Pentothal. Throughout the operation it will be given with Anectine, a muscle relaxant. Pat is still awake.

"You'll be all right, Pat," the anesthetist tells him. "You'll go to sleep soon, and when you first wake up, I want you to promise me to breathe as deeply as you can." It's necessary to prevent lung congestion. The boy nods soberly. Other tubes supply him with sugar solution and blood intravenously to nourish body cells during surgery and keep body fluids in correct balance. In one corner, nurses ready the ice bath which will "deep freeze" Pat. An electric rectal thermometer will record his slightest temperature change during the "freeze" and throughout the entire operation.

"We're ready," the surgeon says briskly.

Carefully they lift the boy's now sleep-saturated body, tubing and all, and submerge it in the bath of ice cubes and water, at 32 degrees Fahrenheit. A nurse begins systematically pouring basins of ice and water over the still form draped in heavy toweling. Twenty-two minutes tick slowly past, every one of them marked by a slowing of Pat's body processes . . . until his temperature is 91 degrees Fahrenheit. "Take him out now," the surgeon directs. "He'll drift about 7 degrees lower, to about 84. We don't dare risk his going much lower." Below 82 degrees, there could be damage from ventricular fibrillation (a fatal arrhythmia).

Surgery begins. With Pat turned on his side, the surgeon makes his initial incision, between the fifth and sixth ribs. The incision is carried into the lung cavity, the boy opened almost halfway through his chest. Intently, the operating team concentrates on one small area in the big room—the boy on the table. To one side, the pediatric cardiologist constantly monitors an electro-cardiograph of Pat's heartbeat and an electro manometer which registers the pressure in various chambers of the heart. A second surgeon assists the cardiac surgeon.

The surgeon is well inside the chest cavity now. He reaches for a tong-like instrument, attaches it to the bright pink lungs, and hands it to an assisting nurse. "Keep these lungs well out of my way," he instructs her, "but be gentle. Don't exert the slightest strain on them."

"Pericardial sac," he reports—and in an instant Patrick's heart lies exposed, bulging and laboring toward the surgeon with every beat. With intricate care and almost imperceptible strokes, the surgeon begins to slit the tip of the heart's left atrium. The cardiologist reports quietly from his machine: "We're getting an auricular flutter; better take care of it." A small amount of digitalis is administered, to slow the fluttering beat of the atrium into rhythm with the other chambers of the heart.

The cutting continues. "His temperature has dropped to 82 ½ degrees," the anesthetist warns. "He's too cold!" Mild rewarming is carried out via several hot water bottles. Everything about the boy, in his refrigerated state, feels cold. His face is cold to the touch. The surgeon remarks that heart and lungs are cool to handle. Finally, the connection is ready to be made. Gently the surgeon pulls a section of the pulmonary venous chamber toward him, clamps it off. "Stitch!" he says brusquely. The heart tissue so delicate it looks as though it will tear at every touch, he begins to sew the slit tip of the left atrium to the venous chamber. The rest of the room scarcely breathes. Finally, he raises his head. The connection is made. Patrick now has a direct route for oxygenated blood to reach all parts of his body.

One problem remains: What to do with the old "mistake" channel which had carried Patrick's blood wrongly. Tied off completely, the channel would cause such high pressure in the heretofore-left atrium that the patient would die. The surgeon's challenge is to restrict the channel as much as possible, yet not cause too high a pressure in the atrium.

"Cellophane!" he calls next.

A nurse hands him a strip of the transparent material, dulled on one side by chemicals which will cause formation of scar tissue. With deft fingers he sews it around the offending channel, tightens it a bit.

"How's that?" he asks the cardiologist.

The cardiologist checks his electro manometer, immediately reports the pressure the restricted channel causes in the various chambers of the heart. Again and again, they try, until the tightness of the cellophane knot produces exactly the right pressure the heart chambers can tolerate. He ties it then. In time, formation of scar tissue will restrict the channel still further. By then, the heart chambers will be able to adjust to higher pressures.

The closure begins. Once the pericardial sac is closed, the surgeon gently lays Pat's lungs across its top, tucks them in like so much fluffy pink foam rubber. Five hours have elapsed since the start of surgery, two hours of which were spent within the boy's chest. The cardiologist, free now to leave his post at the electro-cardiograph, glances at the clock. "I think," he says, lowering his mask, "I'll go say a word to the parents." Another hour is required to bring Pat's temperature back to 98.6 by placing him this time in warm water, in the same pool in which he was "deep frozen." He goes from there to a recovery room.

Downstairs, for Patrick's parents the hours have gone slowly. Time after time, as the elevator clangs, the mother rushes to the door, stares down at the face of the child on the surgery wagon. At 6 p.m., ten hours after she took up her vigil, the right face stares back. "Hi, Mom. Hi, Dad," Patrick whispers softly. "Gee, it only took a few minutes, didn't it?" (Powers, "Cool Heart" 1957)

This case was another successful intracardiac repair using hypothermia, excellent preoperative heart catheter diagnostics, and swift surgical technique. Berg's suspicion of the heart-lung machine itself being part of the high mortality experienced by a few pioneering heart surgeons for the same work was further solidified. Berg used inflow occlusion and avoided cardiac arrest. He did not want to add a heart-lung machine unless it would benefit above what they were already capable of. The team was pleased with the Dorothy Powers article.

That July 1957, Mary Berg threw a baby shower for Pauline Lang. The Bergs' new house was on Melinda Lane in a quiet neighborhood just across the street from a large and beautiful park with a swimming pool. The open-heart team members and many friends came and enjoyed the party. The families were close. Together the wives had a monthly potluck dinner. The couples would get babysitters and get together at one of the homes, enjoy each other's company, and share their best recipes.

A Bird ventilator came into the research lab in the late summer. It could mechanically take over the previous hand bag ventilating technique. With hand bagging, the anesthetist delivered each breath to the patient with a squeeze of the Ambu bag. On long research cases, this was exhausting. With the new technology of the respirator, the volume of each breath and the rate of delivery could be set, and the respirator would do the work. The anesthetist was able to set up a medication line to keep the dog sedated. With the new ventilator and the drip of medication, a long pump run was now possible.

The team had an experiment all set up. They kept the dog on the heart-lung machine for almost two hours, then monitored the dog late into the evening hours while sedated on the ventilator. The blood foamed so much that foamy blood ran under the door at night during these "time on pump" experiments.

Doing longer times on the heart-lung machine with a recovery on the ventilator quickly showed that the pump was not benign. The dogs survived the longer pump runs, but they were not right. They did not respond to commands. They were blank emotionally. Some came around and were able to walk and eat. Some passed on a few days later. Ralph knew the bubble oxygenator was the problem; it was "hard on the blood" and not yet safe for humans.

The new chairman of thoracic surgery for the University of Oregon, Dr. Al Starr (b. 1926), arrived in Portland that August. Dr. Ralph Berg called him to welcome this third pioneer into the Pacific Northwest, pick his brain, and make a connection. Starr had been to Minneapolis and Rochester, Minnesota, and spent four weeks with the two teams there, learning how to use his new pump. Trained at John Hopkins, Dr. Starr expected to be out of the dog lab and on pump performing open-heart procedures within a year.

On February 21, 1958, the new president of the Northeast branch of the Washington State Heart Association gave an interview that was published in Spokane's newspapers. He reviewed prior contributions to the Spokane open-heart team—the first heart-lung machine, matching funds from the American Heart Association, and the pharmaceutical companies' donations. He reported plans for the upcoming year that included more testing in the research lab, going "live" in about a year, and earmarked money to train hospital personnel for the transition to patients. The president requested public donations to support the Heart Association. Later that month, Dorothy Powers's follow-up article on Patrick also helped with fundraising.

Drs. Berg and Lang were pleased with the results of Patrick's repair. The extra cardiac connection between the venous pool and the left atrium was working well, and the endless recirculating had been stopped. The intracardiac work to partially close the large ASD, assisted by the pressure monitoring to get a balance in the two chambers, had worked. Patrick did not have arrhythmias or high pressures. His heart size was almost normal now, and it had gained strength. Patrick was well. Dr. Lang said, "There's no cyanosis [bluing of the skin] anymore. There's also less clubbing, or bulging, of his fingertips. His chest deformity—formerly a bulging which showed over the heart—disappeared. Pat's pulmonary arteries—swollen by previous excessive circulation on the right side of the heart—are returning to normal size" (Powers, "Nine Months Later" 1958).).

In April 1958, Dr. Starr and his team at the University of Oregon did their first successful intracardiac repair with his heart-lung pump. There was media and a front-page article in the Portland newspaper. Dr. Starr wanted the attention; he wanted Oregon's blue-baby cases to stay in Oregon; previously, they were being referred to the two Minnesota teams.

At the annual thoracic meeting in May, Dr. Berg and his team were invited by Dr. Al Starr to see his lab and study his transition to human operations. The pump aspect of a heart-lung machine was either a finger pump involving sequential tabs—or "fingers"—that milked the blood forward in the tubing or rollers that moved the blood forward via a rotating occlusion. Dr. Starr was using an advancement of the finger pump originated by Dr. Lillehei's Minnesota team, who had found theirs at a local farm, where it was used to milk cows. Berg was also invited for a visit by Lillehei during the meeting.

All three doctors on the Sacred Heart open-heart team traveled to Portland after the meeting. They drove down from Spokane in Henry Lang's new convertible and watched Dr. Starr in the lab and in the operating room. Dr. Starr was ahead of the Spokane team. It was an enjoyable road trip with lots of discussions, learning, and fun.

Dr. Berg and some of the Spokane team then went to visit Dr. Walt Lillehei at the University of Minnesota. Ralph and Walt became friends. Dr. Berg preferred the roller pumps used by the Karolinska team and in Texas by Dr. Denton Cooley, former intern to Dr. Alfred Blalock. The rollers had fewer moving parts, were easy to switch out if one failed, and were easy to repair. Dr. Berg shared with Lillehei that his team's present method of oxygenating the blood, the Lucite bubbling oxygenator, was being replaced by a process of "filming" the oxygen on rotating disks. Other refinements had also been added, including sterilization for all parts of the new machine, which was not possible with the older machine. From what Berg and the Spokane team members learned, a new pump had been ordered with the disc oxygenator. The new heart-lung machine was expected in a week or two and would be delivered to the open-heart lab for testing first.

The new pump arrived in early July 1958, again purchased by the Sisters of Providence with Sister Mary Bede's vision guiding. The open-heart team was able to use many parts from the old pump, including the roller pumps and the base with the sigma motor pump. Tuffy sponges and detergent were used to clean all pump parts. The new pump had a hand crank attached to the base; in case of an electrical failure, they could still pump. This was an important advance. The old plastic bubble oxygenator was replaced by rotating discs that dipped into the blood and were gently covered with a film of blood. There was no foam. The rotating discs were on a rod, and the oxygen was delivered into the hollow rod and discs. This was housed in a separate compartment, a cylinder on top of the rollers in the base. The only criticism was that the discs tended to stick to each other on the rod.

Testing in the open-heart lab continued. They set up for a time-on-pump experiment with the new upgraded disc oxygenator in the lab. Dr. Ralph Berg called Nebraska at midnight and sent him to the lab to check on the dog. Nebraska had to call Dr. Berg—a first! Nebraska recalled that this phone call was an event. He woke up Dr. Berg. The dog was alive, sedated on the ventilator after a long pump run.

With this huge improvement, Berg started to plan the next step. The new oxygenator was time consuming to clean. The heart-lung machine comprised a multitude of parts: cylinders, nuts, bolts, rods, discs, and Tygon tubing. The stainless-steel discs were cleaned individually and loaded onto a long metal rod. Gaskets were used to close the loaded rod into the cylinder. To keep the discs from sticking together so that they could rotate freely on the rod, they would rub silicone on the discs. After each case, Donna and Nebraska would scrub the entire pump, a lengthy cleaning process. They had to clean each disc, dry them, and bake them to get the silicone off. Then they applied silicone spray to each one before the next case.

To save time, Donna would bring the clean discs home, bake them in her oven, and take them back to work in the morning. She would set up the pump again, assembling the disc oxygenator, and autoclave it inside a large metal box for an hour. The lab was a learning process for everyone.

On October 14, 1958, a baby was born to welcoming parents in a small town not too far from Spokane. At three days old, he was circumcised. Baby Greg's color changed to blue, induced by intense crying. The doctor at the nursery looked him over closely and discovered he had a major heart murmur and was in heart failure. Greg's mother, Lyta, took him home on digitalis drops and instructions not to let him cry. Lyta worried that her job—holding babies for fluoroscopy—might have contributed to the defect. When she took her new blue baby to see her husband's parents, it was a moment of reckoning. The grandparents' family had experience with three blue babies who died shortly after birth. They were appalled that Lyta was breastfeeding her new blue baby, as working at breastfeeding had preceded the blue-baby deaths in their family. Baby Greg had trouble nursing and would spit up the digitalis. It was a nightmare for Lyta.

She found hope when the baby was referred to Spokane. They saw the new pediatric cardiologist, Dr. Henry Lang, and baby Greg was directly admitted to the hospital. Dr. Lang arranged a cardiac catheter with Dr. Berg. The procedure was done the next day. Dr. Lang and Dr. Berg used local anesthesia, a sedative, and a sugared nipple to perform a heart catheter. The procedure took ninety minutes. They entered at the groin and collected pressures and waveforms. They injected a green dye and took blood samples at time intervals after the dye. Both doctors came out and talked to the family.

Baby Greg had a major ventricular septum defect. They were not able to do open-heart surgery on such a small person. But Dr. Berg had read in a journal about a procedure where they could partially tie off the pulmonary artery so the ventricular pressures would be more equal and the blood would not endlessly recirculate through the lungs. The recirculating from the abnormal pressures would dilate the chambers dangerously. The family was advised of the need for this first surgery, followed later by a second surgery to repair the VSD. The family was also given more detailed instructions about the digitalis and breastfeeding. The digitalis was typically given by gavage and, because a symptom of cardiac stress is vomiting, not before or soon after breastfeeding.

The surgery was set for early December. Baby Greg was sent home with supplemental formula via a bottle. At the next dog lab, there was a new urgency. They had one dog ready with the VSD model. The plan was for a series of experiments involving banding the pulmonary artery with the VSD modeled dog. There was no discussion of baby Greg in the open-heart lab; they focused on the work directly in front of them (Soehren 2011).

That Saturday, the VSD model dog, which was moving slowly

but following commands, was brought into the lab from the home of a team member. When the dog was on bypass, Dr. Berg did not have to reopen the pericardium. The pulmonary artery work was a closed procedure. Dr. Berg was able to isolate the pulmonary artery and its two branches. He constructed a band out of pericardium and laced umbilical tape to secure it. The dog was awakened after a pretty short case. This dog was to be brought back for a third lab a few weeks later. The self-adjusting pulmonary band was evaluated. There was little to no damage to the banded pulmonary artery, and the outflow constriction was maintained. The VSD did not increase in size.

Heart catheterization evolved rapidly in October 1958 when Dr. Mason Sones (1918–1985), a pediatric cardiologist working at the University of Cleveland in Ohio, made a major advance. Previously, either the right or the left heart chambers would be interrogated. During a left heart catheterization on a pediatric patient, while his patient was tilted on his side to shoot the lateral image, a minor malposition allowed the catheter tip to slip inadvertently into the origin of the right coronary artery. Contrast dye injection was given through the catheter when its tip was at the origin of the aorta but not across the aortic valve. Dr. Sones expected to see contrast within the left ventricle and back to the left atria. Instead, the right coronary artery and its branches imaged.

Stunned, and knowing both coronary arteries originate at the base of this great vessel, the aorta, Dr. Sones understood this advance. Now both the right and left heart chambers *and the coronary arteries could be imaged* (Legget 2009). Dr. Sones, credited for developing coronary artery imaging, subsequently developed catheters that helped the cardiologist drop into either coronary ostium when at the aortic root. These catheters eventually became available commercially; however, the time for this advance to disseminate was longer than the Blalock–Taussig–Thomas shunt.

Also in October 1958, National Heart Month, Dr. Lang gave a talk to a Valley Service Club for further fundraising. He outlined the heart-lung machine project, the eight-person team, and the need for $8,000 before the machine could be used on human patients. The successful use of hypothermia resulting in repair of multiple combinations of heart defects with low mortality and the expectations of a heart-lung machine were discussed. The national push was to get more than ten minutes inside the heart in a dry field without serious complications. Dr. Lang reported that the wait list for his practice was six to eighteen months. Dr. Lang also commented on the decrease in mortality that had occurred over the prior three years, from 50 percent to less than 20 percent nationally—though still nowhere close to the 1 percent he sought.

When baby Greg was just nine and half weeks old, in early December, he was readmitted to the hospital with Dr. Henry Lang. The closed-heart procedure was performed the next day. Dr. Lang was in the operating room with Dr. Berg. After placing the intravenous, the anesthetist put the baby to sleep. Dr. Berg opened the chest with a right anterior thoracotomy. The pulmonary artery was already large, bulging from the excessive flow recirculating through the large VSD. Dr. Berg dissected the pulmonary artery. The wall was thin. He constructed and laced the pericardial band that would retard the expansion of this vital vessel. Then he snugged down the band. The overcirculation was not totally corrected, but it was slowed, and the ventricle and pulmonary artery were protected from ever-expanding pressure and flow.

Dr. Henry Lang watched, pleased, as the chest was closed. Baby Greg woke right up and did well. The adjusted band limiting the excessive pulmonary artery blood flow was a temporary repair, reducing the chances of congestive heart failure by minimizing left-to-right shunting. The hope was that it would allow the baby to grow, and then a staged repair would be possible when the blue baby was larger and older. The digitalis slowed the heart, and Greg was sent home on this medication to grow and gain weight. Drs. Lang and Berg had boosted the child, buying time for him to grow as a step toward a more definitive repair (Soehren 2011).

Drs. Berg and Kleaveland went to a surgery meeting in Boston. At the meeting, Dr. Gross invited them to come to his lab and see the new disc oxygenator; it was better engineered, and the discs were convoluted. This oxygenator had been designed by heart surgeon Dr. Kay Cross, influenced by the Karolinska team and heart surgeons Augie Senning and Bjorn Bork. Berg liked the convoluted shape of the discs, which was less traumatic on the blood as it filmed. In Dr. Gross's research lab, they were still using a finger pump to propel the blood through the tubing. They watched Dr. Gross operate in a dog experiment. When the tubing connections came loose from the finger pump and blood sprayed all over the place, there was chaos.

Dr. Kleaveland, unimpressed by these events, stated these connection problems were one thing; the response and cleanup were another, and were substandard compared to what they were doing in Spokane. Still, the Spokane team purchased this new commercially available disc oxygenator from Cleveland's Case Western University. Dr. Berg knew there were no more funds to purchase this oxygenator, so they came up with a "buy-in" plan for this last advance. The doctors would own the pump used for their human patients (Kleaveland 2011).

The buy-in for the latest bypass pump was a lot of money and a big decision for the Kleavelands. Still new in his private practice, Dr. Kleaveland planned to use the bypass machine for his vascular work as well as Dr. Berg's open-heart cases. Dr. Kleaveland approached several local banks to finance his part of this large purchase. He was turned down by several; so was Dr. Berg. But on December 23, 1958, the new oxygenator arrived in Spokane, purchased by the three doctors who planned to use the machine on their patients.

After testing, Dr. Berg noted the thin convoluted discs did not stick together like the flat discs did. When the discs stuck together, the overall surface area was decreased, which defeated the purpose of maximum surface area. With these discs, the pump was easy on the blood. Dr. Berg noted the dogs awoke from anesthesia and were not "goofy."

The media was eager to get a story on the transition to open-heart repair on a human with this new pump. On a Friday night in early January 1959, the long pump cylinder for an adult patient was set up. The cylinder held fifteen stainless-steel convoluted discs on a rotating rod. After it was loaded, the rod was inserted onto two plates. The plates were set onto the cylinder with a gasket. Both ends were tightened loosely, and the cylinder was set in a box of steel, ready for a one-hour autoclave run the next morning.

Nebraska knew this painstaking process signified that the first case in the human OR would occur the next morning. He also knew this cleaning and setup process would limit the number of open-heart cases that could be done in the future. The Tygon tubing, with three different diameters, came in rolls from which exact lengths needed to be cut and sterilized for every case. All parts were sterilized separately and then assembled under sterile conditions. Not to mention the cleanup: After each case, these discs had to be individually scrubbed, baked to remove excess silicone, and resprayed with silicone for the next case.

Early the next morning, the young lady was brought into the operating room. Reporter Dorothy Powers was there, but no film crew.

The patient was a cardiac cripple with a large hole between the atrial chambers of her heart. She was an adult, and her life was limited to rest. She had been on the list for years, and now she was ready and willing to take on this role as the first patient. The new bypass pump was in the operating room, and all the components had been tested and sterilized. It had gravity venous return. Donna and Nebraska primed the pump with saline solution to check for leaks and to rinse the circuit. The convoluted disc oxygenator sat elevated on a table.

Next, they primed the circuit with four units of banked blood. This machine had roller pumps, a hand crank, a built-in pacemaker, the ability to cool the patient, and pressure recorder device, specifically added for Dr. Henry Lang.

The patient was put under anesthesia. This machine had a heated cylindrical unit. The heated blood entered the pool where the convoluted discs would rotate like records in a jukebox stacked sideways and pick up the blood as a film. The surface area, about 1,000 square feet per minute as the discs rotated at 90 to 100 revolutions per minute, facilitated the exchange of oxygen and carbon dioxide on the disc surface. Dr. Lang was pleased.

Drs. Berg and Kleaveland worked simultaneously, opening the patient's sternum for exposure to the pericardium and her groin for exposure to the femoral vessels. Once Dr. Berg had the superior and inferior vena cava exposed, he did a test clamp. The patient tolerated the test. Next, he applied the clamps and moved swiftly to place tubes securely into each of those veins. With a "Y" connector, both tubes joined a common tube that delivered the patient's blood into the machine. The clamps were removed. Dr. Kleaveland securely inserted the single venous return cannula at the femoral artery. A coronary sinus sucker was hooked up on the other side of the machine to deal with the small circuit perfusing the now isolated heart.

They were set. It was a moment.

Dr. Lang said in his calm voice, "Okay, we're ready."

They clamped the venous return, opened the pump circuit, and then opened the femoral return by removing Dr. Kleaveland's clamps. They were on pump. The heart was exposed and then stopped. Dr. Lang anticipated and corrected every detail. Dr. Berg opened the atrium. The defect was big, almost two inches. He worked quickly using a standard needle driver and was amazed at how much easier it was without blood and frequent breaks to clear the field. The doctors prodded each other, of course; they were from different areas—pediatric cardiology, chest surgery, and vascular surgery.

Because this defect was so big and she had back-and-forth flow through it, the pressures on either side of her heart were about equal. Once the repair was tested and secure, they closed the heart. Coming off pump—the most agonizing process in the research lab—was initiated. With the heart beating again, they slowly and sequentially stopped half the flow to the pump with the removal of the inferior vena cava tube. Then the superior vena cava tube was shut down.

They gave the "boost" of 10 percent of the pump-primed blood. When Dr. Lang was happy with the hemodynamic and pressure volume recordings, they shut down the femoral line. Everyone relaxed, and closing began. It was done. It was a success. But it was quiet that Saturday morning. They were cautious, and the patient was cared for in the operating room for several hours. When she was taken to the ward much later by her anesthetist, she was off the breathing tube and smiling.

This accomplishment, after the trying months, over fifty dog experiments, and three heart-lung machines, each progressively better, was almost anticlimactic. It went so well, so smoothly. The pump was as "nontoxic" as they could make it. Their first human repair of an intracardiac defect using the heart-lung machine was a success.

There was a champagne celebration at Dr. Henry Lang's house later that evening. It was an understated, classy affair. The team brought family. They all talked about the case. They discussed the research done in preparation and how smoothly the transition and work in the main OR had occurred. Everyone was elated.

Reporter Dorothy Powers delayed until all was well and the patient was comfortable with the story being published. "Gowned, masked and observant of the sterile field, it was the privilege of this reporter to stand within inches of the patient on the table at Sacred Heart Hospital," she wrote. "The result is the first eyewitness account of use of the heart-lung machine in the history of Spokane medicine." Her article was published January 28, 1959 (Powers, "Open Heart" 1959).

CHAPTER 10

Using the Heart-Lung Machine

The year 1959 opened on this great success of crossing into open-heart procedures with heart-lung technology. The accomplishment was well received in Spokane. Dr. Berg's surgical practice was growing. The additional time with the heart stopped and a surgical field free of blood allowed for more complex repairs. Dr. Berg was grateful to retire the upholstery needles for standard needle drivers and interrupted sutures. The team looked ahead.

Ralph found balance from the intensity of his work by leaving his work. His hobbies and sports showed a common thread of precision and focus. He liked to hunt, shoot, travel, work outdoors, and golf. The president of the exclusive Duck Club invited Ralph to join. The duck hunting was superb. The club members were business owners and community stalwarts. Ralph accepted the invitation and became friends with the president.

Together they marveled at the disregard for human life in the name of all manner of religion. Influenced by his grandfather Anders and his father, Thoralf, Ralph Berg held respect for life and hard work in high regard. While hunting, both men noted there was little to honor the lives and work of doomed people. Corsica—the island off Southern France where, during the Middle Ages, despite the pope and religious guidance, people lost their land and lives to more powerful neighbors—was a frequent topic of these discussions.

Across the state in Seattle, in reviewing his cases where single intracardiac defects were repaired with the heart-lung machine, Dr.

Merendino found the mortality was trending down but still above 10 percent. And he again decided a new oxygenator would help him advance and lower mortality. The Lucite bubble oxygenator had too many limitations.

Dr. Merendino further explained, "The work was demanding. The congenital lesions of blue babies were being identified in adults. The spectrum of patients needing open-heart procedures was expanding. Many of the established heart surgeons who had developed and performed closed-heart procedures did not make the transition to open-heart." Merendino got a new membrane oxygenator and continued to care for his wait list of blue patients. One of his private patients was at the Virginia Mason Hospital in downtown Seattle. Dr. Merendino and his partner, Dr. Henry Harkins, had offices in King County Hospital, so they developed the "Have pump, will travel" method. For the patient, they would travel downtown with the heart-lung machine in the back of Merendino's truck. This problem resolved when the new University of Washington Hospital opened in 1959 (Merendino 2011).

Dr. Ralph Berg found the heart-lung machine fit well with hypothermia and swift surgical technique, and more challenging cases were scheduled. During the repair of a child with tetralogy of Fallot, Berg needed more than cellophane to bridge the large intracardiac ventricular septal defect. He used a piece of the child's pericardium instead. The decision, made in the heat of the moment, was the logical extension from leaving the pericardium open to allow swelling after surgery and prior use of the pericardium for pulmonary artery banding. Removing some of the pericardium to use in the repair was reasonable. "It worked swell," Dr. Berg said. "It was superior."

Depending on patient needs, up to thirty of the convoluted discs would be loaded onto the rod; in the dog lab, they rarely used more than twenty. Dr. Lang took care of volumes, how much blood was used to prime the pump, flows during surgery, and pressures and assisted Dr. Berg with drug management as he operated on his human patients.

The similarities to the dog lab always pleased Dr. Ralph Berg.

Although the main purpose of the dog lab had been achieved, this heart team did not close it down. The experimental focus simply shifted from pump safety and congenital intracardiac surgical repairs to heart valves and a special interest of Dr. Berg's: chamber wall aneurysms. Berg had noted aneurysmal dilations of the left ventricle wall in the blue babies. Berg wanted to repair the wall aneurysmal defect, which was typically small and focal. So, the team created a model, which was done with a coronary artery constrictor to achieve a lower-chamber-wall aneurysm in the lab. Then they removed the constrictor and plicated the lower chamber wall, inverting the thinned aneurysmal defect and placing several vertical sutures to hold the inverted tissue. These sutures had to be strong, and permanent. They had some success, and these wall aneurysms remained a focus for Dr. Ralph Berg.

Installation of valve-replacement devices was a frustrating line of investigation in the lab. They developed and tested new clamps to assist with each intracardiac or valve repair. Thoracic aneurysm repairs were stalled due to the need for a replacement for the diseased aorta. Both chest and vascular surgeons were focused on this problem; Dr. Kleaveland was developing aortic grafts. At autopsy, Dr. Kleaveland would occasionally be able to harvest a normal aorta, which he would pack in ice prep and send to Seattle.

At the University of Washington, a new process brought about the beginning of Washington's state organ bank. The process—lyophilization—took the water out of the aortic tissue and freeze-dried it to achieve product stability and shelf-life. It could subsequently be used as a replacement graft for aortic aneurysm repairs. These grafts were so precious that a research-lab experiment was not done. There was a reluctance to send a freeze-dried aortic graft back to Spokane. The university did not want the community hospitals doing big vascular cases, but Dr. Kleaveland would find a way.

Dr. Kleaveland took one of his thoracic aneurysm patients to Houston, where surgeons were using heart-lung machines for thoracic aneurysm repairs. Dr. Stan Crawford, who used the heart-lung pump to do this case, had trained with Dr. Kleaveland at Harvard and was now at Baylor with pioneering open-heart surgeon Dr. Cooley and vascular surgeon Dr. Michael DeBakey (1908–2008). The patient had Marfan syndrome, a congenital disorder that is associated with aortic aneurysms at a young age. Dr. Kleaveland watched the case as a visiting surgeon. In Spokane, the volume of these cases was small and remained small (Kleaveland 2011).

Back at Sacred Heart Hospital, a research council was formed in late 1959. Everyone agreed that Sister Mary Bede was the de facto leader. Under her understated and steady leadership, all the departments at the hospital had been upgraded, including the accounting department to accommodate the research funds and the needs of the families with blue babies. She was supportive of the heart team's efforts. She had formal architecture plans—albeit no funds—for a new hospital tower to sit along the ridge above downtown. She found funds to begin the remodel of the front entrance to the hospital to accommodate cars driving up to drop off and pick up and remove the imposing stone stairway (Locati 2012).

By the early 1960s, heart-lung machines had become even more commercially available, and the John A. Hartford Foundation Inc. offered substantial grants to university and private hospitals all over the country to help with the costs of developing an open-heart program. A private hospital in Seattle sent Dr. George Thomas, Merendino's first chest fellow, who had been in private practice a few years, to the foundation to apply. Hartford awarded a $344,312 grant on January 22, 1960, and the Heart Center in Seattle opened September 24, 1960 (G. Thomas 2010). Medical schools and training programs sent chest surgeons who were coming out of their chest residencies with knowledge of open-heart procedures and the heart-lung machine.

Meanwhile, Henry Lang and Ralph Berg reviewed their first pump cases, their outcomes. Centers currently publishing outcomes and mortality data were large and academic. Berg and Lang decided to not publish their first series of patients treated with open-heart surgery—for the simple fact that they were at the top of the list for outcomes, with a mortality below 2 percent. They did not want accolades, nor did they want naysayers.

For the Spokane heart team and the rest of the pioneering heart surgeons who had crossed into open-heart procedures, valve disease was becoming a priority. The Hufnagel valve, in use since 1952 and now produced in smaller sizes, was not durable in the research lab. At home with a team member, several weeks to months after insertion, the dogs failed when the Hufnagel device traveled and shut down arterial flow to the legs. Like aortic grafts to replace aneurysmal aortic segments, heart-valve replacements were a difficult line of research.

One of Dr. Berg's patients who had undergone a closed aortic-valve commissurotomy was back in Dr. Berg's office in early 1960 with the same symptoms. He was short of breath and avoiding stairs. The evaluation revealed that his aortic valve was once again stenosed, symptomatic, and in need of repair. Berg and team performed an open aortic-valve repair with the heart-lung machine. More precisely, Dr. Berg removed the calcifications and repaired the holes in the leaflets of the valves with the superior field. Berg hoped the valve would not restenose.

At the May 1960 thoracic meeting, Dr. Berg recalled, there was not much choice when it came to the heart valves. Berg was using the Braunwald–Cutter valve—the first and only mechanical heart valve available commercially. He admired the accomplishments of Dr. Nina Braunwald, likewise the first and only (at that time) female chest surgeon. She worked at the National Heart Institute, and her husband was a cardiologist. However, Dr. Berg preferred to repair the heart valves. Even with the heart-lung machine, the valve repairs were a technically demanding and tedious operation; but once repaired, the valves performed well and quietly.

However, one patient's situation pushed Dr. Berg to seek a better alternative. Within six months, a twice-repaired aortic valve was failing for the third time. This time it was failing with insufficiency, which meant Berg's patient was on borrowed time; heart failure and death loomed without a third aortic-valve procedure.

Jean, a nurse anesthetist who had completed her training in Spokane, had moved to Portland and was working with Dr. Al Starr at the University of Oregon. Miles Edwards, a mechanical engineer, was helping design the cage-and-ball metal device for heart-valve replacement. They were testing the Starr–Edwards valve in their research lab, and it looked promising. Dr. Starr was ready to transition to human patients with his mechanical valve. Hearing about this from Jean, Dr. Berg wanted to know more. He admired Dr. Starr's work.

Jean drew Ralph's attention to Dr. Starr's first thoracic fellow, a Dr. Kendall, who had worked in the research lab for a couple of years in the testing phase of the mechanical valve. A few months earlier, in the spring of 1960, Drs. Starr and Kendall had implanted the Starr–Edwards mechanical valve on the first patient. The case went well. However, as they rolled the patient for the X-ray plate, an air embolism moved out of her heart and into her brain. She died immediately. The valve went back into the lab phase, and they were close to coming back out with a second patient.

Berg called Dr. Starr. After talking, arrangements were made to get Dr. Berg's patient to Portland. In September 1960, Dr. Starr assembled the same team. Dr. Bob Kendall (1927–2019), now in private practice, was willing to assist. He had graduated from Stanford University in 1949 and attended the University of Oregon School of Medicine, finishing in 1953. He took a general surgery residency at the Portland Veterans Administration Medical Center, then a thoracic residency with Dr. Albert Starr that morphed into a cardiothoracic residency at

Oregon Health & Science, finishing July 1960.

The case went smoothly, and the Spokane man did fine, though Dr. Ralph Berg recalled that his patient complained about the loud click with his new mechanical valve upon returning to Spokane and with each follow-up appointment over the years.

Describing it later, Dr. Kendall said simply, "Dr. Starr asked, I agreed. It was the first successful Starr–Edwards valve done in the world."

Open-heart procedures continued to gain acceptance, and more programs were emerging going into 1961. At Deaconess Hospital, seven blocks west of Sacred Heart Hospital, a new wing opened. Its new administrator wasted no time when he arrived. The wing had larger operating suites, an open-heart room equipped with a commercial heart-lung machine, and a research lab in the basement, not far from the morgue. A local private practice chest surgeon started doing open-heart pump cases. He too used a pediatric cardiologist as the pump doctor.

In April, Dr. Robert Gross was the visiting guest professor at the Spokane Surgical Society meeting. Dr. Berg presented his paper "Experiences in the Treatment of Aortic Valvular Disease by the Open Method Utilizing Cardiopulmonary Bypass." The paper was delivered with precision and supporting slides.

Since arriving in Spokane in January 1952, Berg had operated on thirty-eight patients with aortic-valve stenotic lesions. The first group of fifteen patients received a modified manual commissurotomy with the Lebsche knife. This early surgical technique for commissurotomy was blind. The surgeon operated by feel, with his retracted blade ready. Because of the higher pressures on the arterial left side of the heart, a digital commissurotomy was not safe. Since going "live" with the heart-lung machine in January 1959, Berg had operated on an additional twenty-three patients using the open-heart technique. Now, with a heart-lung machine, more could be done to repair the aortic valve.

In an interview, Berg described seven patients in the second on-pump group with congenital lesions of the aortic valve who had two instead of three leaflets on their aortic valve. The rest of his patients had "acquired" lesions on their valves. All his patients had angina, fainting, shortness of breath, and harsh murmurs. Berg reported the results of the preoperative cardiac catheter results, the gradient of pressure across the valve (max 150mm Hg), the calculated valve orifice size, and the mean systolic injection pressures. He showed a slide of the heart-lung machine, noting it was built by the PEMCO Company with modifications—the DeBakey roller pump heads, arterial filter inspired by Dr. Gross, a bubble trap, venous reservoir and setting chamber, the modified Kay Cross disc oxygenator with convoluted discs, and a heat exchanger to provide hypothermia and normothermic phases.

During operations, Berg focused on the most efficient way to reduce the gradient across the valve. He opened the aorta with a corkscrew incision above the valve, placed a Potts dilator through the valve, and pulled the valve up into the operative field. Berg would preserve and repair the resulting rents and perforations in the valve leaflets after the calcific masses were removed. He used pieces of the patient's pericardium to do patch repairs of these holes. He would reef up the commissures so the valve leaflets would meet smoothly. Sometimes this repair of the valve ring would include resuturing an old aortic dissection and damaged aortic wall. The goal was to get the gradient below fifty. Berg would close the aortic opening, come off pump, and close the chest.

He reported five patients died before they could get into the cardiac cath lab, and four died after the diagnostic cath but before the operating room. Of the twenty-three patients Berg operated on, three died with the operation, and four had "late" deaths (R. Berg 2006).

He was therefore immensely pleased that a mechnical valve was now available to end this line of operations.

Ralph also shared a funny story. A car enthusiast, he had a favorite auto mechanic, Doug, who liked to tease Ralph about how his engine repair techniques were like the repairs Berg performed on the heart, which Doug had read about in the newspaper. One day, when Ralph came in to pick up his car, they again started talking repairs and hearts. The mechanic outlined each step done to the engine and how it was like heart surgery. Ralph listened, nodding, and then said, "Okay, Doug, now turn the engine on and do the repair at 80 rpm." They both smiled and laughed.

The heart-lung machine support and penetration into community hospitals seeking open-heart surgery was slow to become standard for all heart specialists—even those cardiologists who had recently finished training. Enter newly trained Montana cardiologist Dr. Paul Shields, who was on the hunt for a practice that was ready for open-heart surgery in 1961. "Entering the heart with a knife, a finger or a catheter was still far from accepted, certainly not standard, and in many places considered extremely dangerous," he explained.

After graduating with the fifth class of the University of Washington School of Medicine in 1954, Dr. Shields went to Indianapolis General Hospital for his internship and medical residency and became fascinated with the heart. He subsequently landed a cardiology fellow year with his mentor, cardiologist Dr. Charles Fisch, and together they set up a heart catheter lab for the hospital. Shields and Fisch made equipment decisions about catheters, transducers, X-ray equipment, monitoring equipment, printouts of data collected, red goggles, and lead aprons.

"It took six months to get it all together," said Dr. Shields. The next year, he worked as a cardiac and research fellow. Commissioned into the Air Force, he then served his country for two and a half years in his field, cardiology. He wanted another year in cardiology fellowship, but his search found only two-year programs, and repeating a year was too painful. Spokane, he learned, had cardiac research labs, heart catheter labs, and chest surgeons at both hospitals performing open-heart cases. There were emergency rooms with phone operators who could call in the teams at a moment's notice. Deaconess Hospital's new administrator was welcoming, and further introductions led to arrangements for Dr. Shields to share office space with the Deaconess heart team. He arrived in Spokane in late spring, 1961 (P. Shields 2011).

Dr. Shields assisted the busy pediatric cardiologist with heart catheters. At Deaconess, heart caths were done under standard fluoroscopy in the radiology department, wearing those red glasses and lead aprons as protection against the imaging radiation. Dr. Shields placed a left radial artery needle for the sole purpose of blood draws and blood gas analysis. There was a lot of guessing in getting images of the right heart that were clinically useful. It was considered taboo to enter an artery with a catheter, so Dr. Shields used the veins to pass his wires and catheters into the right heart. Shields changed the X-ray plates by hand, adding to the guesswork. Dr. Shields remembered that an image intensifier, a device that changed the X-ray film plates, twelve plates in twelve seconds, was installed before his first two years were over. During those first two years of his practice, he noticed the chest surgeons did not venture too far from their teams or their hospitals.

Elsewhere in Spokane, Andy Berg Jr. and his wife, Alice, had their cousin Mike Berg's family over to their new house on Twenty-Seventh Avenue. Mike and his wife, Virginia, who had spent the summer of 1961 in Spokane with Mike and Ralph's parents, Thoralf and Leila, up on North Hill, brought their baby boy, who was a few weeks younger than Alice and Andy's baby girl. Pregnant again and due in November with me, Virginia planned to continue with college at Washington State University and was signed up for the fall semester. As the babies cooed at each other on the floor in the living room, Alice wondered how Virginia could handle the burden of two babies and college. Andy took a Polaroid of Mike for his early-decision application to the University of Washington School of Medicine. Dr. Herb Eastlick was advising Mike and recalled advising his older brother, Ralph, back in 1940 (A. Berg 2010).

Later, in 1962, Mike and Virginia would move to Seattle to start medical school at the University of Washington.

During Dr. Kendall and Jean's honeymoon to Austria in February 1962, the newlyweds met up with Ralph and Mary Berg for a week, renting a Volkswagen bug to go between ski resorts. Soon they talked about working together in Spokane. Kendall was invited and agreed to come look at Dr. Berg's practice. When Dr. Kendall visited and operated with Dr. Berg in the early spring, he was more than pleased with the open-heart team. He returned to Portland with plans to close his private practice and move to Spokane within a year.

Back in Spokane, Julie Spores, a young registered nurse, got interested in working with the open-heart team while training to become a nurse anesthetist at Sacred Heart. Julie hung around the open-heart room, coming in early to help the senior anesthetist set up the case. Upon returning from vacation in March 1962, the senior nurse anesthetist welcomed Julie onto the team as backup.

Each team member was vigilant of how interconnected they were in the care of these patients. They searched for and trained their replacements and fellow team members. Julie, determined to be a part of this amazing team, had freelanced in Spokane until she landed her CRNA job at Sacred Heart. Shortly after she joined the team, the lead anesthetist had a personal tragedy and took an extended leave.

The team was shocked but carried on. Julie settled in and was able to pick up the demanding work with ease. She came in early and set up the operating room, including reels of music on the stereo and a homemade, themed, and decorated cake on a small table in the operating room. The surgeons would come in, perform the case, and then eat cake—in the operating room! Carboholics, all of them!

Heart repairs weren't the only advances being made around this time. In August 1962, the inoculation for polio became available, and Dr. Henry Lang was at the forefront of bringing it to the public in Spokane.

That fall, the seventy-third annual convention of the Washington State Medical Association was held in Spokane at the Davenport Hotel. On the last day of the weeklong convention, an open-heart surgical procedure was featured for the audience of doctors to view on live closed-circuit television. The local Spokane TV station, KHQ, provided the televised coverage from the operating room at Sacred Heart Hospital, where Drs. Berg, Kleaveland and Lang were set to repair a ventricular septal defect on a five-year-old boy.

This was bold. Even in the best, most experienced surgical hands, these congenital defect cases were difficult. Recently, a noted academic open-heart surgeon had a child patient die during a televised open-heart procedure. All hoped for the best.

This situation put the Berg heart team under pressure. Their audience was made up of the public and doctors who wanted to learn and refer their patients for surgical repairs. A second room at the hospital was set up for the panel of four doctors moderating the events of the case. Experienced with open-heart procedures, the panel explained each step of the procedure and answered live questions from the doctors in the audience. Dr. Walt Lillehei, professor of surgery at the University of Minnesota, was the featured guest and first panel member. Well known as the first in the world who had undertaken cross-circulation using a parent as his heart-lung machine back in 1954, Dr. Lillehei was also friends with Dr. Berg. The open-heart surgeon from Deaconess—a Seattle Heart Center surgeon who went "live" with pump cases in December 1959—and Seattle cardiologist Dr. Gordon Logan made up the rest of the four-man panel.

On September 19, 1962, inside operating room 10, the team was left undisturbed by the audience and had little ability to communicate with the panel. However, they knew they were being observed live via the camera.

The case went well. The youngster did well. He went home the next week, pink and feeling well. The local newspapers reported the event a week after it occurred. It was positive media coverage for the team. The names of the surgeons, Berg and Kleaveland, were not revealed (Stephens 2011).

Nebraska left Spokane shortly after this media event, following honorable discharge from the military. He was anxious to return to his hometown of Philadelphia; Spokane was not his kind of place with its blue laws. He never expected to return.

Nebraska's replacement noted that the open-heart patients stayed in the OR after each case. The nurse anesthetist cared for every aspect of the patients' recovery and intensive care, influenced by Dr. Henry Lang, who set this standard of monitoring. Dr. Lang would frequently come into the room and get an update, making minor changes. This all-day, all-night care by the team predated cardiac anesthesia, standard recovery room, and intensive care units of today.

Nebraska wasn't the only loss on the heart team. Sister Mary Bede was called up to the Provincial Council in 1962 to help run the system of Catholic hospitals in the Northwest. This exceptional teacher, nurse, administrator, and supporter of the open-heart team left Spokane to attend her next higher calling. Her farewell party was understated. Her presence and her vision were never doubted. She left with little fanfare and the fervent hope that her influence would live on (R. Berg 2006).

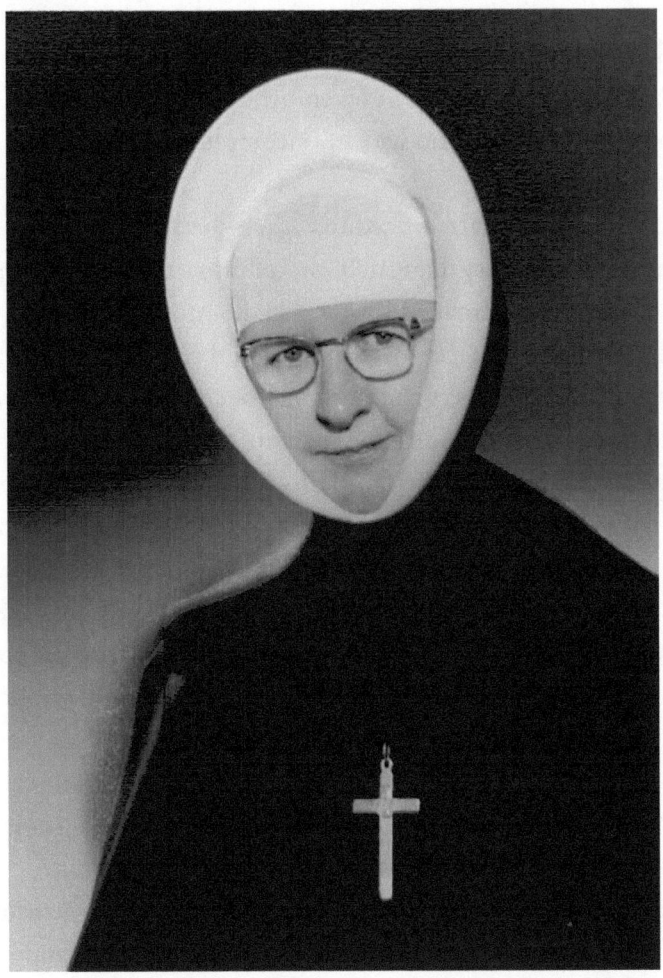

Photo of Sister Mary Bede (Providence Archives 1960).

By November 1962, baby Greg, now four, was large enough for the open-heart machine. The family returned to Spokane to have Dr. Berg do the open-heart surgery after years of agony and vigilance for Greg's mother. The pulmonary artery banding performed at nine weeks of age had prevented the dreaded massive expansion of his right ventricle, limiting the flow like a governor limiting gasoline flow on an engine. Baby Greg did well with the pulmonary artery band, the digoxin, and the monitoring. On Thursday, November 29, 1962, young Greg went into operating room 10 and had an uncomplicated VSD repair using a pericardial patch.

After his open-heart procedure, Greg developed a heart block arrhythmia. Dr. Henry Lang felt the pacemaker node on the left ventricle had been damaged by the repair. After all, it was a huge VSD. Dr. Berg thought the arrhythmia would clear up. In fact, he was sure it would clear up, as it had never happened before to a patient of his. "He acted like it wouldn't dare persist," described Greg's mother.

When the family left the hospital with their son's heart repaired, the arrhythmia did not clear. Sometimes, when Greg was sleeping, his pulse would drop to the midtwenties, and when he ran a temperature, his pulse might get up to forty. The next year, Greg had his first pacemaker placed to ameliorate the problem. The pacemaker box was large, and Greg was still small. The box was placed on his abdomen, below his waist. Greg had problems with broken wires over the years. The leads, which had originally been sewn onto his heart muscle using an anterior thoracotomy for access, were never removed. A new box under the skin was the procedure used when the leads broke.

Greg's mother was not overly fond of Dr. Berg but "trusted his ability." She remembers waiting in Dr. Berg's waiting room and "seeing so many sick children, so much sicker than Greg. Somehow, that never made it any easier for us." Greg named his pacemaker "the alarm clock."

"If Dr. Berg had not been willing to try a new procedure, the pulmonary banding, Greg would not have lived long. We are so grateful for his ability to do this for our son," she remarked during a later interview. Also, while there were some hurts connected with the continuing arrhythmia problem after the open-heart surgery, she understood the risk. She said, "I am sure this block would have happened whoever had done the surgery. There was just something about Berg's attitude when he talked to me the last morning in the hospital that upset me quite a bit. I think I was so disappointed with the block, expecting everything would be fixed with the second operation, that I probably was hypersensitive" (Soehren 2011).

The small, incremental steps and staged procedures that Drs. Berg and Lang used to buy time for their sickly blue babies were successful. The question of how best to care for the complicated congenital defects remained unanswered.

Across the state at the University of Washington, Dr. Merendino stayed focused on transposition of the great vessels. "These were truly doomed blue babies," he said. "Transposition, lethal without additional defects to allow the two circulations to mix, is so much more complicated than a single or several defects between the upper or lower chambers. Most of these blue babies did not survive their first year," he explained.

Merendino developed a modification to the transatrial switch. The original technique of atrial switch had been presented by Dr. Augie Senning in 1958. Technically challenging, it required long suture lines to switch the atria inflows via moving the intracardiac atrial septa and not the wall of the atria. His modified operation used permanent Invalon sutures and a long strip of mesh to reinforce the inverted suture line, mostly along the atria wall. Merendino's team achieved success in the research lab with the new method. When Dr. Merendino took his atrial switch from the lab to the clinical arena, a four-year-old child was his first patient. At surgery, the case was difficult. The parents were able to see their child postoperatively. Briefly she was pink, the blue gone. But the sutures did not hold. She passed in her parents' arms.

Dr. Merendino continued working in the lab, determined to capture a mold of the intra-atrial defect with compressed Styrofoam. Eventually, with the assistance of a dental technician, Dr. Merendino got the atrial mold to a point where they were ready to go clinically to a child. The mold was taken intraoperatively and then developed and would guide the atrial switch procedure. The first case was the child of this dental technician, who had transposition of the great vessels. The intra-atrial switch procedure went well. The child's mother saw her child pink and was pleased. When the surgical resident put the child on the bed, she died (Merendino 2011).

The blue babies who lived with left-to-right intracardiac shunts subsequently developed peripheral resistance or hypertension. "These were tough cases, in balancing the risk of operating. The peripheral resistance stayed the same for a long time after the open-heart surgery ended the intracardiac shunt. Some patients died, and some survived with correction of the shunts or defects," explained Dr. Merendino. He told of a family where the sister asked the hard questions of Dr. Merendino about the chances of death for her brother, a young man of twenty. She decided to take her brother to Mayo Clinic for the surgery. She returned months later with a gift for Dr. Merendino, for his honesty and integrity in explaining to her the risk. Her brother had died with his repair.

An academic publication from the University of Sinead in Japan caught Dr. Merendino's attention. Intracardiac VSD was being closed with hypothermia, which allowed a limited twenty minutes of intracardiac time in blue babies. Dr. Merendino, who admitted he was not the fastest surgeon in the world, was intrigued. "This was an area where this new technology of bypass pump and surgical skill was still inadequate for the very small blue babies. The heart-lung machines did not adapt to small size," he explained.

Merendino took a different approach from Dr. Berg's small procedures to buy time for growth. He invited this Japanese surgeon to come to the University of Washington. Dr. Yerisano came and spent a year. Then Dr. Morhi came the next year from Japan. They worked in the research lab. Their goal was to achieve an hour of intracardiac time using deep hypothermia. It was felt that with sixty minutes of time, the surgeon could successfully repair a single or complex intracardiac defect (Merendino 2011).

With the New Year, 1963, the open-heart team at Sacred Heart was anticipating changes. Change was planned as much as possible, as the unexpected could rock the stability of these educated, intelligent, hypervigilant, and hypersensitive personalities.

Dr. Kleaveland had grown his vascular practice, and his team had been making their own aortic grafts in Spokane since the first time they had difficulty retrieving a freeze-dried aorta from Seattle. In Spokane, the cadaveric grafts came in a glass tube. The operating team would reconstitute the graft, and both Drs. Kleaveland and Berg would use it for aortic aneurysms.

Dr. Kleaveland repaired both abdominal and thoracic aneurysms. He also proved himself a valuable member of this open-heart team by developing specialty instruments for each need that arose. He performed the vascular femoral vessel exposure and cannulated the femoral artery to help place each patient on the heart-lung pump.

Plastic aortic grafts came on the market. At first the plastic grafts comprised braided nylon woven over a glass tube, which acted as a form stent. Sealed with formic acid at both ends, it would make a tube graft. They corrugated it to achieve flexibility. Shortly, Dr. Sterling Edwards (1920–2004) came out with a knitted tube graft. Dr. Edwards had been a couple years ahead of Dr. Kleaveland during training at Harvard and took an academic position in New Mexico, where he came up with the grafts. They were softer, more flexible, and easier to use.

Dr. Kleaveland was busy with aortic aneurysm repairs, which were remarkably successful and did not require the heart-lung machine. It was a bittersweet but organic and professional separation for surgeons Kleaveland and Berg when Kendall and his wife arrived in Spokane in the spring of 1963. For Kendall, closing his Portland surgical practice and settling into the Spokane medical community was a smooth transition, and he kept busy, performing groin access and assisting Dr.

Berg's pump cases while he developed his own referrals. Kendall, the first partner in the Berg Surgical Group, was impressed by the way Berg and Kleaveland, who had not formally associated their practices, continued to support each other. The pioneering open-heart work kept them close.

Dr. Berg remained passionate about the blue babies and always acknowledged the surgical skill of this vascular surgeon. Operating on humans and animals is a high calling. To take on responsibility for another's life, to help a patient overcome a life-threatening situation, leads to a confident and self-assured demeanor, which came naturally to Dr. Kleaveland. He had grown up with animal surgery and looked at it like carpentry, as a skill. He identified and fixed the problem. Solving problems surgically was an enduring challenge. To be done after the repair and move on was also attractive.

Dr. Berg's mindset was a bit more complex. A thinking man's surgeon, he believed surgeons are "more than fix-it people." He was comfortable forging ahead into the places of the heart where most were not willing to go. His artistry and independence were hard to appreciate, as he often set a difficult standard to follow. Dealing with the deaths of the blue babies had steeled Ralph Berg to perform his best and not look back.

Bob Kendall started his chest training after heart-lung machines were safe, missing the early work on blue babies. He took advantage of this luxury, focusing on valve disease. Kendall did not like working on the blue babies; but Dr. Lang more than made up for that deficit. On one occasion, a child on the blue-baby list who was taking digitalis came in sick to the emergency room with digitalis overdose, the treatment for which at that time was an emergent exchange transfusion. Dr. Lang, a universal blood donor, performed the transfusion in the hospital recovery room, himself the donor. Henry was fabulous with children. He could make that connection that gave comfort and security to the child because he was a child at heart himself. Henry rode a dirt bike to work, rode horses, and ate candy all the time—yet restricted his kids to candy only on the weekends.

Dr. Kendall recalled, "Henry Lang was always in the operating room, helping us." The intraoperative atmosphere was cordial, and when the case was going well, they all chatted about more personal issues. Henry would argue with Bob about how long it took to drive to Sun Valley from Spokane, eight versus ten hours. They were all skiers. Henry had his farm south of town and liked to jump fences on his horse. Ralph, an avid hunter, always took time off during duck season.

At the beginning of the Kendall–Berg partnership, there was one open-heart case a week. By the fall of 1963, they often performed two cases and sometimes more weekly. But that did not mean they were routine by any means. The void left in Nebraska's absence remained.

The lead CRNA, Julie Spores, left work one Friday in early spring, 1964, after a challenging case with Dr. Berg. She rode her motorcycle up to Bonners Ferry, Idaho, visiting her parents for the weekend. Late that evening, a nurse supervisor from the hospital called, awakening the entire family. Julie was needed immediately for an emergency open-heart case. The local police drove Julie back to Spokane, lights flashing.

The case was a take-back of a patient with aortic dissection after an aortic-valve replacement earlier that day. Emergency take-backs were rare but urgent in the extreme. That night, they were on pump in room 10 when the cooling system clogged. The temperatures rose dangerously. Without Donna or Nebraska, the fix was tense. They called for help. The nurse supervisor had to locate the janitor. First time in scrubs, first time in an operating room, this janitor remembered Dr. Ralph Berg's language was "salty" as he directed the janitor in what to do. "The base of the pump, a large metal box, was also acting as the roller pump cooler with a water bath. The drain, which emptied out in the operating room floor drain, was clogged," described the janitor. Fortunately, he was able to unclog it and drain the pump so the pump technician could refill with cool water—problem solved (Spores 2011).

Later that spring, Dr. Berg, typically cool and contained, was visibly upset, even tearful one evening at dinner with his family. Upon inquiring, the family learned a patient had been unable to come off the pump. Dr. Berg performed open cardiac massage for hours before they lost the patient, a man with a family. It was difficult, the grief overwhelming.

With a new partner and increasing volume of open-heart cases, a need arose to find and train a dedicated replacement to manage the heart-lung machine. A few of the OR circulating nurses volunteered to learn the pump, and the team struggled with this arrangement. Nebraska had the best understanding of the position. After consulting Berg and Lang, Donna started the process of getting Nebraska to come back to Spokane to run the pump. Eventually, the local community college developed a program to train pump technicians (Larson 2011).

Shields's neighbor called him on a Sunday morning, panicking. Her husband was on the ground, having passed out. It was most likely a heart attack, with the man showing a weak yet fast pulse. Shields immediately started chest compressions and gave mouth-to-mouth breaths. The neighbor regained consciousness, became combative, pushed Shields away, and relapsed into cardiovascular collapse. When the ambulance arrived and loaded the patient, Dr. Shields jumped in. His neighbor insisted on Sacred Heart Hospital, so the ambulance called ahead, and Dr. Shields performed chest compressions all the way to the emergency room.

At Deaconess, Dr. Shields had a mobile DC defibrillator stationed in the emergency department that could travel all over the facility as needed for patients, but this new defibrillator was not in the Sacred Heart ER when they arrived. Shields kept his neighbor alive for ninety minutes using the old AC defibrillator and closed-chest compressions. Then this neighbor died of his heart attack with ventricular fibrillation arrhythmia (P. Shields 2011).

Death from heart attack was prevalent. After more than a decade in research, Dr. Arthur Vineberg presented his work with humans at the annual thoracic meeting in 1964 (Katrapati 2008). In Montreal, Canada, he had developed a procedure to increase blood flow to the heart muscle. Ralph, intrigued, was able to have coffee and breakfast with Dr. Vineberg the morning after his presentation. He asked many technical questions about the mammary artery and how it was tunneled to allow blood to trickle into the open spaces around the heart muscle.

Heart muscle is different from skeletal muscle. Myocardium is a syncytium, meaning the borders between each cell are open, whereas in skeletal muscle, each cell is contained by a closed membrane, a border. Vineberg's concept—perfusing the open space with blood that could get to the cells of the heart muscle—would benefit a large area of this specialized muscle. This was appealing to Berg, who believed a sudden lack or decrease in the blood flow to the heart muscle from its coronary artery was the cause of a heart attack.

Dr. Berg wanted to perform the Vineberg procedure right away. His chronic angina patients were growing in number, significantly surpassing the blue-baby list. The asbestos powder had evolved to talc powder into the pericardium, but still these patients were crippled by their chest pain. In the research labs, the heart team in Spokane had a simple dog model to create angina. Next, they learned to dissect the internal mammary artery off the left chest wall, where it originated from the subclavian artery, swing it over to the heart, and, with the use of a special instrument, pull the prepared artery through a long myocardial tunnel. Once the clamp was removed from the internal mammary artery, the syncytium took up the blood flow, like a soaker hose lying across the grass. It worked so well in the research lab that the number of labs was small before the okay to transition to patients was given.

Mr. George Caruso, a longtime patient of Berg who had undergone the asbestos epicardium irritation and collateralization years earlier, then a talc procedure, was having worsening chest pain. He was one of the first patients to undergo a Vineberg internal mammary artery graft. His case was more technical, as his pericardium was scarred down onto his heart. Caruso did well with the procedure and became free of his angina, continuing to return annually to see Dr. Berg.

At the University of Washington, the hypothermia team was ready to transition from the lab to the OR in the late summer of 1964. Dr. Merendino had monitored their research work; pleased with the success, he did not perform the lab procedures. The Japanese surgeons deferred to Dr. Merendino regarding performing the procedure on a human in the main operating room. Plans were made, and the first pediatric blue baby was identified.

In the days before this big transition, Dr. Henry Harkins, the chief of surgery, unfortunately suffered a heart attack and died. Finding himself not only the new chief of surgery but also without his trusted surgical partner, Dr. Merendino faced a challenging situation. At this time of great achievement and grief, Merendino felt responsible for training the general surgery residents. He set the example, undertaking the biggest and most difficult cases in both general and chest surgery. But it seemed untenable to both perform as chief of surgery and focus on pioneering cardiac cases. The entire field of heart disease was rapidly advancing.

Merendino pushed ahead with the deep-hypothermia case for a blue baby too small for a standard heart-lung machine. He performed the case. The blue baby had an intracardiac defect. Merendino lost the patient on the operating room table. It was a blow.

Dr. Merendino made the best of the situation, putting the experienced Japanese surgeon who developed the deep-hypothermia setup together with the new chief of thoracic surgery, Dr. David Dillard (1923–1993). A medical student at the time, Mike Berg recalled that the blue-baby surgical deaths continued at the University of Washington and were upsetting to him; he chose a different field of surgery, ophthalmology.

Back in Spokane, Olaf Berg turned sixty-five in 1965, and another amazing benefit of the new country came: Social Security. He and Thoralf both sent away to the old country for their birth certificates, and both received Social Security. Olaf no longer needed the daily bakery work for his pay. Thoralf, pleased, closed the bakery and retired.

Olaf had worked his entire life in a Berg bakery. Thoralf had cared for Olaf since their mother died in childbirth with their younger brother, Andy, and he cared for Olaf into old age. Olaf moved into an apartment close to the bakery. His nieces and nephews visited frequently. Thoralf found retirement to be an amazing experience; he slowed down and got some real sleep. Many of his grandchildren said he mellowed nicely.

For Ralph Berg, well trained, well respected, and a leader in his field, life was going well at work and with his home life. Mary was, as Ralph explained, his "greatest asset." When she was gone on real estate trips or with the children, he counted the time until she returned. The team could tell when Mary came home because Ralph would become calm. His younger brother, Mike, graduated medical school and was off to train in a surgical field. Ralph and Mike Berg's families visited over the summer at the lake. Ralph and Mary's youngest, Rory, age nine, taught Mike's oldest, about to turn five, to swim.

Meanwhile, the medical community in Spokane was growing and performing at a level comparable with academic institutions. They had attracted excellent physicians. Ralph, with few limits, was content.

CHAPTER 11

Acquired Heart Disease Intrudes

Nebraska decided he did like Spokane and was pleased to come back after Donna called him twice. Sister Mary Bede sent him a personal letter; then the new administrator confirmed that Sacred Heart Hospital would like his services. His experience with the pump and the open-heart team was highly regarded. He was offered a job as a salaried perfusionist.

When he returned to Spokane in 1965, he found the team had done less than fifty pump cases since he left in October 1962. One planned case and occasionally a second urgent case were done in any given week. The cases needing open-heart were stacking up on the list. Nebraska described the response to his return: "I lit the house on fire." He got the team moving, doing more cases, better and faster.

During his time away in Philadelphia, Nebraska had worked at the university hospital as OR circulator for an academic open-heart surgeon. "They had a fancy heart-lung machine," he explained. They would match one patient to another in terms of blood type. After the first case of the day, they would cut the lines of the pump before the filters, place new screen filters, wash the outside of the pump, and start the second case, preprimed with the first patient's blood. They did more cases in Philadelphia than the Spokane team. Their steps shortened the time cleaning the pump and lowered the number of banked blood units needed to prime the pump.

Drs. Berg and Lang would not hear of implementing such techniques with blood. Since becoming sick with infectious hepatitis from a patient, Dr. Berg had always avoided unnecessarily mixing blood or any body fluids. However, they were all intrigued by the concept of decreasing pump cleaning time. The team wanted to be able to perform two elective cases a day, and cleaning was a major obstacle.

Nebraska noted the loss of Sister Mary Bede. However, her vision endured through the new administration, who sent Nebraska to visit academic institutions with open-heart programs. He was to observe their pump setups, learn, and report back to the heart team as well as to administration. Around the country, everyone wanted to advance the success of open-heart surgery. Nebraska ran into many pioneers, as they were frequently lecturing on the same circuit of institutions he was traveling to. First he listened to Dr. John Kirklin lecture about moving the patient's temperature probe. Monitoring temperature was critical, and avoiding high temperatures was more serious than low temperatures. Kirklin had abandoned rectal temperature probes, as they often fell out during the case. He moved to a probe attached to the catheter that drains the bladder. Drs. Berg and Lang implemented the temperature probe change (Stephens 2011).

Meanwhile, Drs. Berg and Lang realized that the blue patients did not tolerate the new intravenous dye injections. The new dye showed on X-ray film, in real time, which could be preserved for review as a cine and stored in the radiology department, and more precisely imaged the heart chambers, the congenital defects, and the valves. While significantly superior to the green dye that demanded hours of mathematical equations to get cardiac outputs and shunt flows, this new dye was potentially toxic. The small children developed concerning kidney problems after injections.

Some academic institutions were using specialized radiology equipment to accommodate the small size of these blue babies. The newer tables could rotate and move, so the same information could be obtained with a single dye injection. Drs. Berg and Lang gave two dye injections, as they had an old X-ray table, which perhaps is why they were some of the earliest doctors to note the toxicity.

Drs. Berg and Lang's combined work, typically enhancing each other's abilities with precision results, was occasionally dysfunctional. On one occasion, Dr. Lang performed a heart catheter and diagnosed a ventricular septal defect on a young patient with a heart murmur. With this diagnosis, Dr. Lang made a referral to Dr. Ralph Berg, who confirmed a heart murmur on his physical exam and recommended open-heart surgery to repair the defect. At surgery, Dr. Berg placed the patient onto the heart-lung machine, opened the patient's heart, and found it was normal. There was no VSD.

From the operating table he said, "Henry, I think you made a mistake." Henry looked up from the pump and immediately said, "He does." Meaning he felt he was correct in his diagnosis of a VSD. Henry then reviewed the patient's films and disagreed again, even in the face of the operative findings, that the youngster did not have a VSD. Ralph closed the heart and then the chest. He was upset and told Henry to go talk to the family.

The dilemma of accurate preoperative diagnosis was not new. In this case, the cardiologist overread the heart catheter. This patient recovered just fine.

After this case, Dr. Berg reviewed all his preoperative heart catheters regardless of which doctor performed the heart catheter procedure. Berg was aware of criticisms going around, especially from the bigger academic institutions, about how performing a heart catheter and then recommending and performing a cardiac surgery was a "self-referral"; but Dr. Berg cautiously continued with the diagnostic heart catheters. The procedures were evolving and becoming less difficult, just like the open-heart surgery. Berg was better than most at performing them both. His main concern was the safety and accuracy of the catheter procedure, especially in the blue babies. Accurate diagnostics made for better surgical results.

On Nebraska's next institutional visit, Nebraska headed to Palo Alto, California, and Stanford University Hospital. He met a woman of small stature, kind and friendly. She was scrubbing her hands at the scrub sink when Nebraska walked up. She was alone, so Nebraska assumed she was not a heart surgeon. They always had an entourage in his experience. This woman knew Dr. Berg and was happy to meet the famous doctor's perfusionist.

They entered the operating room. Nebraska was there to observe and talk to Dr. Norman Shumway's (1923–2006) perfusionist. This woman was showing Dr. Shumway an aortic valve that she had developed. She had to stand on a box in the OR to see. Nebraska assumed she was a professor at Stanford and her husband an engineer. During that case, Nebraska observed the use of disposables for the first time. This team used disposable components for the heart-lung machine and on the operating table. They used special pumps to control the flow of the intravenous fluids. Nebraska enjoyed the visit and their recognition of his surgeon, Dr. Ralph Berg (Stephens 2011).

It turned out he had just met Dr. Nina Braunwald, the pioneering heart surgeon herself. It was a defining moment for Nebraska. Nina was nice to him; she did not lord over him. After he finally realized she was in fact a surgeon, an open-heart surgeon, she invited him for coffee. Over coffee, she asked Nebraska all about Dr. Ralph Berg and his program. Of course, Berg used her valves, the Braunwald–Cutter aortic valve, that had come out commercially in 1963.

Back in Spokane, the upgrades from this visit included Travenol infusion pumps and the disposables on the OR table. Dr. Ralph Berg was first in Spokane to use the intravenous line pump to control the flow rate of any intravenous medication. He liked the more precise delivery of fluids to his patients. The nurse anesthetists embraced this advance. The pumps were attached to a standard intravenous pole. Previously they would jack an intravenous bag up the pole to get more gravity flow. Now the CRNA could even add a second or third pump if needed. And the disposables made the time between cases much shorter. A bunch of the sterile products used—patient drapes, towels, pads to collect lost blood, suction tubing, and gowns—could be tossed and replaced with a sterile disposable pack. The issue of disposables for the heart-lung machine was not settled.

Dr. Berg's first encounter with the new administrator was jarring. Sister Mary Bede had understood and envisioned that with great care and excellent results, the hospital would be full of patients. Dr. Berg set a time to question her replacement after several of the blue-baby children on the list had recently come back to their Northwest families in a pine box, deceased after surgical care provided far away.

"Why are some of the blue babies being referred to San Francisco instead of retaining them in Spokane?" he asked.

The new administrator answered without shame, "Because that open-heart surgeon has a federal grant for this work at the University of San Francisco. It is financially less risky to send the patients there."

It was sad and infuriating to hear this. Most of these blue children were from vulnerable families where funding was an issue. The new administrator would not lift a finger to promote the Spokane team, nor acknowledge their fundraising or success. This was the opposite of Sister Mary Bede and her vision. Together, Ralph and the Sister had shunned accolades and media, while for this administrator, accolades were important, even above a relationship with the care team and the doctors.

In her void, Dr. Berg appreciated Sister Mary Bede even more.

He also began looking for other opportunities to care for his patients. Then the open-heart surgeon in San Francisco lost the federal grant due to poor results, the local bank agreed to offer low-interest loans more formally to the blue-baby families, and Drs. Berg and Lang began educating their patients about these loans.

By 1966, the Deaconess Hospital team was also performing the Vineberg procedure successfully. Dr. Shields and his older partner had a wait list of chronic angina patients. Together they performed the heart catheters.

These two cardiologists agonized before referring to open-heart surgery for significant obstructive coronary arteries on heart cath. By selection, these patients were chronic or stable angina patients. Some of these chronic angina patients did well with the Vineberg artery implant. Occasionally Dr. Shields got a chance to inject into the mammary artery graft on a postprocedure patient—"You could see the blush of the myocardium." More acute patients, typically with chronic angina, sometimes developed a heart attack. These patients would often die or spend weeks in the hospital on bed rest. Many of the cardiologists' patients referred for open-heart Vineberg surgery did not recover.

In 1966, at the Children's Hospital of Philadelphia, cardiologist Dr. William Rashkind (1922–1986) developed his idea to more easily perform the difficult open surgical procedure of atrial septectomy. Credit goes to Vivien Thomas, who first developed the surgical atrial septostomy while working in Dr. Blalock's research lab to modify the known model for hypertension into the stable dog model with an atrial septal defect, which was then used to develop the famous shunt. The

Rashkind balloon was perhaps the first catheter intervention device. The balloon, inserted from the umbilical vein or other large vein and then positioned across the two atrial chambers, could create or enlarge an ASD with its cutting blade.

Dr. Berg and particularly Dr. Lang took note of this advance. The need to create an ASD was rare except in the transposition defect, where creating an ASD would be urgent and lifesaving (W. Boehm 2006).

Nebraska was sent to the University of Washington to observe a special blue-baby case, not a young child or young adult. The Spokane team was interested in the pump setup for a baby, as the pumps being too big was the dilemma Berg and Lang wanted to address. But at the university hospital, a nurse came out of the operating room and informed Nebraska that the case was "too difficult" and he was not allowed in that day. Nebraska's visit was finished.

Nebraska talked with the OR desk staff. He felt this academic team did more pacemaker placements and not as many open-heart pump cases as the Spokane team. When he returned home, Berg was upset that his perfusionist had not been allowed into the OR to see the blue-baby case. "A wasted visit," he commented. Berg was interested in how Dr. Merendino was approaching the blue babies and how it compared to the technique Drs. Berg and Lang were using in Spokane: staging with an initial closed-heart procedure followed by a definitive procedure when the child had grown enough to use the heart-lung machine.

Having watched and worked with many open-heart surgeons, Nebraska noted that Berg was unique: "He never rushed, always steady, methodical, and well prepared." Berg's swift technique led to the best surgical results in the shortest times (Stephens 2011).

Soon there was negative press about the hospital, a landowner's dispute with Sacred Heart administration over the value of a land parcel. This parcel was needed for the new hospital tower dreamed of and outlined by Sister Mary Bede, which had finally been funded, but administration had created an enemy out of the landowner of said parcel with multiple lowball offers, followed by filing legal action against the property owner. The press reported the court had sided with the property owner with prejudice; the administration and hospital lost the opportunity to purchase the land in the future. At significant legal expense on the hospital's part, much greater than the initial disputed amount, the landowner won.

Everyone on the heart team further appreciated Sister Mary Bede and her vision. Administration, now stuck, decided to build the tower jutting out from the hill instead of along the hillside with its associated beautiful views. There was further cost to do this, and extra cost for subsequent additions to the hospital complex, which is on a steep slope.

Planning and construction neared completion on the base of the tower. At monthly meetings that Nebraska called "fat cat" meetings, where the construction and plans to move the clinical services were discussed, Dr. Berg sat in a chair next to the administrator. Nebraska noted Berg occasionally did not make this meeting.

At Deaconess Hospital, the senior cardiologist broke both legs in a skiing accident. Dr. Shields was given his colleague's list of angina patients and brought a nurse from the OR into the cath lab to help. Able to perform the heart catheter procedures without an assistant doctor, he then independently referred his patients for the Vineberg implant open-heart procedure. Dr. Shields kept a list of surgical results. He soon became the main adult cardiologist at Deaconess Hospital.

Aware of the advance in imaging the coronary arteries, Dr. Shields shared in the increased interest and knowledge of coronary artery anatomy. Following this gain in knowledge was curiosity about the infarct syndrome, also known as an emerging heart attack. Dr. Shields contemplated going to the Cleveland Clinic to work with Dr. Mason Sones and learn his newer technique of coronary imaging. However, he moved on to direct coronary injections after obtaining Dr. Sones's commercially available catheters (P. Shields 2011).

In 1967, pulmonary embolisms were treated with an open-heart operation, a pulmonary artery thromboembolectomy. With the heart-lung machine and early surgical intervention, more of these patients survived compared to Dr. John Gibbon's era in 1930. One patient was a forty-two-year-old woman. She had just delivered a child when she developed chest pain and severe shortness of breath. A massive saddle pulmonary embolism was diagnosed on heart catheter. The doctors immediately consulted Dr. Berg, and he recommended urgent open-heart to remove the clot from the pulmonary artery.

They moved quickly into the operating room. After surgical sterile prep and opening the chest, Berg was on the heart-lung machine, cannulated at the femoral. "Real easy," as Dr. Berg described his time to get on pump. Everything seemed fine at first. Dr. Berg was intently working in the chest. Nebraska noted he had lost one of the three units of pump-priming blood. He reported to Dr. Berg, who did not want to hear about it. He did not like to be disrupted. Nebraska lost another unit and replaced them. He was worried. The patient became unstable, blood pressure dropping and anesthesia not able to maintain it. Dr. Berg pulled back the drapes, and she looked pregnant, with her belly full of blood. They lost her on the table.

The autopsy showed the femoral artery had split between the layers and dissected all the way up to the chest. After this case, Dr. Ralph Berg rethought femoral cannulation. He had previously not wanted the arterial pump line in his field, at the open chest. After searching the literature, he found a single paper reporting this problem of femoral artery dissection. From that day forward, Dr. Berg no longer cannulated at the groin. Instead, he cannulated at the aorta where the cannula was right in his field and any problems would be immediately obvious.

Nebraska acknowledged one of Dr. Ralph Berg's defining attributes. When they lost a patient, any patient but especially a child, it was very upsetting. But Dr. Berg was always calm and thoughtful. When asked, Dr. Ralph Berg explained, "Some are meant to die, some to live. Well, we did all we could." And he always did his best. Dr. Berg, intense, focused, did not walk away.

At the annual thoracic conference in May 1967, the valve-replacement and congenital-heart case discussions were replaced by discussions about heart attack patients. The Vineberg procedure was being criticized. Patients with angina needed something more. Chest surgeon Dr. René Favaloro (1923–2000), a new staff surgeon at Cleveland Clinic with Dr. Don Effler (1915–2004), was at this meeting. Ralph liked him. René was young, in his thirties, and he really enjoyed Dr. Berg. They became friends. Dr. Berg was invited and later went to Cleveland to visit with René.

Like Dr. Henry Lang, Dr. Mason Sones at Cleveland Clinic, a pediatric cardiologist by training, was always in attendance in the operating room. And Sones could more precisely image the coronary arteries than Dr. Berg had ever imagined. Sones had developed this coronary catheter procedure a few years earlier. He needed a heart surgeon to correct the artery blockages he was imaging and was working closely with Dr. Favaloro.

In the clinic's research lab, the doctors were working on a more direct way to increase flow to the heart muscle. Dr. Sones, always looking to get better results for his patients, felt the surgeons should have less mortality and the patients should have less angina. He had convinced Drs. Effler and Favaloro that the internal mammary implants, the Vineberg procedure, was not durable. The procedure was indirect. It brought arterial flow from the mammary artery into the heart muscle via a tunnel into the muscle, relying on the pulsatile arterial flow to absorb and distribute cell to cell via the open membrane syncytium. At Cleveland, the surgeons did not poke holes in the internal mammary artery nor leave all the side branches open—the soaker-hose configuration. Instead, the internal mammary artery, in a submyocardial tunnel, had only the most distal end open to flow. Constructed this way, the implant was not reliable from Ralph Berg's view. He noted that even with the soaker-hose method, the chronic angina recurred a year or two later (R. Berg 2006).

Heart attacks, a major cause of death, often affected men in the peak of their productive years. The traditional treatment for a heart attack at the time was bed rest for six weeks, and people who survived their first heart attack often died within one or two years with a second heart attack. The belief that a heart attack was related to occlusions, or plaque, acquired over time inside the coronary arteries seemed logical to many. These arteries brought blood flow to the heart muscle. A lack of flow would affect the heart muscle's ability to perform. The scientific proof, however, was lacking and daunting to even contemplate obtaining.

The Cleveland Clinic was working on using the saphenous vein and directly opening the coronary artery to remove a plaque. The greater saphenous vein, as the conduit, brought more flow compared to the Vineberg configuration. The flow was into the partially blocked coronary artery, which had multiple branches before the capillary system to more directly bring the oxygenated blood into the cells of the heart muscle. They used a peripheral vascular technique, performing a short segment jump graft around a focal coronary artery stenosis, which had been modeled in the lab.

In the dog model, with a single coronary artery, a constrictor caused a narrowed artery. This was easily fixed with endarterectomy at the second procedure. An endarterectomy would be limited in its use for humans with their three coronary arteries. It was not uncommon for all three coronaries to have at least partial blockages.

Dr. Berg enjoyed his time with Dr. Favaloro and looked forward to his results. When he returned to Spokane, Dr. Berg started to harvest saphenous vein in the lab and occasionally in patients.

Just after the operating rooms opened in the basement of the new Sacred Heart Hospital tower building, Nebraska went to Texas Heart to visit Dr. Denton Cooley. He was amazed that they were doing twenty open-heart pump cases per day. He noted how they used disposables in every aspect of the operating rooms. The insides of their heart-lung machines contained disposables. Cleaning the pump involved tossing and replacing disposables. They used a different kind of venous return and lactated ringers to prime the pumps, no banked blood. Dr. Cooley had a technician who made his instruments. Nebraska got this technician's name and number, anticipating that the Spokane team would continue to grow and need a third complete set of instruments. Nebraska found Dr. Cooley to be a nice, average guy, easy to talk with.

Nebraska debriefed administration and then Dr. Ralph Berg that Henry Lang was the main blockade to decreasing time to clean and prime the pump, as Dr. Lang was resistant to disposables. Disposable oxygenators and avoiding banked blood for the lactated ringers' solution would decrease turnaround time. Dr. Lang's monitoring and assistance was being taken over by the Travenol pump, the new monitors, and now disposables. Dr. Lang's continued control of the venous return reservoir occasionally upset Dr. Berg, as it led to blood backing up in the operative field. If they redid the venous return lines like the Denton Cooley team, it would be much easier to set up the pump and go (Stephens 2011).

Upon hearing about these advances, including cutting three feet of line out of the venous return so they could lower the operating table, Ralph wanted to advance with these products. Berg's attitude: "If Dr. Denton Cooley can do this, I can do this."

The Texas team's venous return was a disposable collapsible bag. Berg was not impressed with this device. But the difference in the filters was a different matter. Cooley and his chief perfusionist had been concerned the pump rollers were shearing off particulate matter from the tubing; the twenty-micron filter was too big to catch it, so they used a fifty-micron arterial filter. Lang and Berg both became concerned that their twenty-micron arterial filters were letting "air and aeroembolisms by." At Spokane, everyone watched the lines for bubbles; Nebraska was scared to death about bubbles. Patients might not wake up intact mentally, like the goofy dogs. When the Spokane team went to the smaller fifty-micron filters, the patients' benefit was immediate. The fifty-micron arterial filter was better and easy to add, catching the smallest bubbles and debris.

The new equipment, including disposables for the dump, were purchased and ready to go for a Monday case. As luck would have it, a twenty-two-year-old patient had come in over the weekend with a massive pulmonary embolism. The patient was driving long hours to Spokane and chain-smoking cigarettes. At this time, Dr. Berg wanted and had advised all his patients to quit smoking, as nicotine is a chemical vasoconstrictor.

The patient came in through the emergency department, collapsing. Pulmonary embolisms were diagnosed using a heart cath to visualize the clot inside the pulmonary artery. Dr. Berg was called in on a Sunday.

Nebraska primed the pump with two liters of sterile normal saline and installed the disposable bubble oxygenator. Without having to calculate the number of discs to use and then load the discs on the rod for the oxygenator, they were ready to start in a short time. The weekend on-call system had also notified Dr. Lang of the emergent case. Anticipating the team would be about ready to go on pump when he came in, instead Henry found they had already been on pump for twenty minutes, and Ralph was currently pulling large clots out of this patient's pulmonary vessels.

On Monday morning, Henry was mad at Nebraska. "So, the convoluted discs are out?" Dr. Lang had not been briefed on the new updates. He blocked the new disposable oxygenator for the next case, making Nebraska take it down and put in the convoluted discs, which Nebraska did. Then Dr. Berg was mad. Nebraska was stuck in the middle. That was when Dr. Berg took over as the open-heart team leader, calling all the shots.

Like Dr. Sone, Dr. Lang's skills pulled him into the cardiac care of adult patients, a most difficult transition. Caught between the more detailed needs of the congenital blue-baby cases and the demands to move quickly and precisely with the ever-increasing volume of adult patients needing open-heart procedures, Dr. Henry Lang was starting to be a hindrance in the operating room when they worked on an adult—a dilemma shared by every pediatric cardiologist in the country. Henry Lang loved working with children. He moved at a slower pace, addressing and attending the child's every need. However, the need for coronary artery imaging and cardiology care for the adult patients with angina was huge.

At the Cleveland Clinic, a Dr. Carroll Simpson started his three-year cardiology fellowship with Dr. Mason Sones in June 1967. The meteoric rise in acquired heart disease was intruding. Since 1958, Dr. Mason Sones had developed catheters to drop into the coronary ostia more easily at the aortic root. He taught his technique to his cardiology fellows. He traveled and lectured to every open-heart program that invited him. His catheters were available commercially. "Then basically he switched careers and became an adult cardiologist. He was brilliant," explained Simpson, who trained with him for adult cardiology. It felt like an honor, and Simpson was proud. However, others at the Cleveland Clinic did not appreciate Dr. Sones's move away from pediatric blue babies. "Dr. Sones was moved down to the basement. This was a punishment from the staff, not ready to allow adult coronary work into the hallowed halls of the radiology department where pediatric congenital heart work was being done," said Dr. Simpson (Simpson 2011).

Another young cardiologist was being lured to Spokane: Dr. Tom Mouser. An avid fly fisherman searching for a job that would accommodate this passion, he spotted an advertisement for a staff physician in the Northwest and applied at the Spokane Veterans Administration hospital. He graduated with the second class from West Virginia University School of Medicine in 1963. His class was paid to take the National Medical Board exam, and Tom ranked above the 98th percentile of the 3,000 medical students across the country that took the exam that year. The WVU medical faculty was largely from the University of Minnesota, including Dr. Herb Warden (1920–2002), a chest surgeon who was a part of Dr. Walt Lillehei's cross-circulation team back in 1954.

Dr. Mouser, board eligible and with a year of cardiology fellowship from WVU, got the job of staff internist at the Spokane VA hospital. So, he drove across the country with his son, Bill. They arrived July 25, 1967, his son's sixth birthday, and Dr. Mouser started work right away. His wife sold everything and hired a mover, paid for by the new job, and arrived in Spokane a few weeks later.

During Mouser's fellowship year, he had experienced the transition from cardio green dye to intravenous contrast dye. With the new heart catheters, rather than spending the day calculating dilution curves to obtain cardiac output and assess for a shunt and then its size, both the right and left ventricle were injected with intravenous contrast.

Images and cine films were obtained as the contrast dye showed on radiology film.

Prior to Mouser's arrival, the Spokane VA hospital only offered medical management of the cardiology patients. Patients who needed a heart cath or a pacemaker were sent downtown. Pacemakers required a chest surgeon and an operating room. The surgeon placed the pacer pocket holding the pacer box in the anterior abdominal wall, then sewed the leads into the heart. Sewing in the leads required access into the pericardium and the heart muscle. The chest surgeon had to perform a thoracotomy to place these leads for permanent pacemakers.

Leading up to 1967, urgent transvenous pacemakers were only temporary, used for dysrhythmias after open-heart surgery or in the emergency room. The stylet, a hook at the end of a pacer wire, was jabbed into the ventricle via the wire coming into the heart from the vein. If the patient did well, the patient would be referred for a permanent pacemaker. The limitations of the early stylet were the reason why these pacers were temporary. Over time, the stylet would release, and the wires fell off the myocardium.

The American and Irish medical device company Medtronic developed a permanent transvenous pacer wire with a better stylet. These new wires and stylets no longer needed to be sewn into the myocardium, nor did they need a pocket on the abdomen. Dr. Mouser was hesitant but well prepared from his fellowship and performed the first permanent transvenous pacemaker placement in Spokane—no chest surgeon, no operating room, and without a surgical backup. The patients did well.

Soon Mouser was routinely placing pacemakers in his patients in the operating room. With the patient appropriately positioned, anesthetist giving sedation, and Dr. Mouser giving local anesthesia into the area, the needle entered under the collarbone, then the vein, and a rush of dark blood came back. Next a wire was threaded through the needle. Dr. Mouser removed the needle but not the wire, then placed a sheath over the wire into the vein to secure access into this vein. He pulled his wire and placed the pacer wires via the sheath, confirming their position with fluoroscopy. A pocket was made on the left anterior chest wall where the pacer box, connected to the new wires, was positioned. He would close the pacer pocket incision, and the patient would stay overnight.

Many of his patients had had a heart attack, even a second heart attack. They had chronic angina and were on the verge of being cardiac cripples. This advance kept many patients from a large chest incision, saved lives, and reduced the number of treated arrhythmias.

In 1967, cardiac care as a specialized hospital ward or unit was an emerging concept. The heart-lung machine initially a concept to allow intracardiac time, its success was now driving every aspect of care for heart disease. The cardiac care unit (CCU) emerged in response to heart patients being treated successfully, gaining a chance for survival.

Dr. Mouser set up the Spokane VA hospital's CCU, first visiting the Deaconess and Sacred Heart care units for ideas and ways to solve problems. He educated the VA hospital nurses and assistants. At the time, nurses and ambulance drivers were not trained with the cardiac defibrillators, though the older AC defibrillators were in a little red box at every ward nurse station. Dr. Mouser was impressed with the DC defibrillator at the Deaconess CCU. Although it was big due to its large capacitor, it worked consistently. Eventually, the DC defibrillators were miniaturized (Mouser 2011).

Dr. Shields, a consultant with the VA hospital and avid EKG reader, came once a month and discussed the cardiac patients with Dr. Mouser. Shields appreciated Mouser's passion for reading EKGs, maybe 200 a day at the VA. With Dr. Sones's advance in imaging the blood supply to the heart muscle with coronary angiography, coronary angiogram cases for chest pain or angina patients were stacking up. By the fall, Dr. Mouser was content with his Spokane position.

Back at the Cleveland Clinic in Ohio, Dr. Favaloro's first human case to test the use of the saphenous vein was a stable angina patient with a right coronary artery blockage seen on coronary angiogram. Drs. Sones and Simpson, the cardiology fellow, were involved in every detail in the operating room that early fall 1967. Once the open-heart team was on pump, Dr. Favaloro harvested the saphenous vein and performed a saphenous interposition graft at the right coronary artery blockage. Dr. Favaloro opened the right coronary artery and sewed the proximal and then the distal anastomosis, a few centimeters away, onto the right coronary artery.

Dr. Simpson was so pleased that he reported, "René was a technical master." He continued, "To see the first direct coronary bypass with Dr. René Favaloro, well, it worked. The patient survived the procedure, and his chest pain resolved" (Simpson 2011). From there, the Cleveland team started using longer vein segments, moving the proximal vein connection up onto the aorta, as it was a more reliable source of high inflow. They also used an aortic punch with a side-biter clamp to make the proximal connection. The cases were successful. They anticipated publishing them.

Another line of research on acquired heart disease was occurring in Spokane. At the Spokane Surgical Society meeting in the fall of 1967, Drs. John Hershey and Manuel White presented their research results on transmyocardial punctures. The punctures into the ventricles' outside wall, done with a Titus needle, directly deliver blood into the syncytium of the myocardium, providing immediate revascularization of the myocardium.

The two doctors had a dog model with a progressing coronary artery constrictor that led to an acute ischemic event. The transmyocardial punctures were the second procedure to repair and recover the model's heart attack, an interesting and successful solution to acute ischemia, or lack of blood flow. Dr. Kendall, whose interest was cardiac valve disease and not coronary ischemia, was not impressed; Dr. Berg, however, was. The two dogs were healthy and hearty on leashes.

Dr. Hershey, a general surgeon, had come to Spokane in 1957 after training with Drs. Harkin and Merendino at the University of Washington. Hershey's father died of a massive heart attack in 1959; at the time, it was common knowledge that about half of all men died of heart attacks. When Holy Family Hospital opened in Spokane in 1967, Hershey joined the staff—as did Dr. Berg—and traveled less to do his surgical work.

Drs. Hershey and White's lab was located inside a veterinary hospital on Francis and Wall Streets near Dr. Hershey's northside private practice office building. They operated on forty modeled dogs, progressing from abrasion of the epicardium to skin grafts onto the heart and then to omental grafts, to assist collateralizing the coronaries. These were similar lines of research to the Spokane team's asbestos and talc experiments before going live with their custom-built pump. Dr. Berg gave them a grant from his research fund and recommended their work to the local chapter of the American Heart Association.

Combined, it was a $2,000 grant to continue this research. Drs. White and Hershey used the grant and took their laboratory-supported work to patients in 1969. After six successful transmyocardial puncture procedures were done at Deaconess Hospital, Dr. White, a technically excellent board-certified chest surgeon, left Spokane for another state. The transmyocardial puncture work ended in late 1969. Later it was shown that these punctures eventually led to significant and morbid cardiac arrhythmias (Hershey 2011).

With immune suppression breakthroughs introduced by pioneering surgical teams, the world was in position and waiting for a human heart transplant to occur. In Dr. Christiaan Barnard's (1922–2001) South

Africa research lab, he transplanted the heart and immunosuppressed about fifty dogs.

Dr. Barnard had a patient willing to undergo the procedure, a fifty-four-year-old grocer suffering from diabetes and heart disease. When a suitable donor came available, Dr. Barnard performed the world's first human heart transplant operation, assisted by his brother. The operation lasted nine hours on December 3, 1967. The patient survived eighteen days; the immune suppression was borrowed. Heart teams across the globe mostly ignored this advance (Cooper 2018). The success of organ replacements came with true immunosuppression through the diligent scientific work of the Stanford University team and Dr. Shumway.

Dr. Merendino noted that the South African surgeon's admirers were everywhere, though. Ten minutes into Merendino's presentation at the annual meeting of the American Heart Association in San Francisco on his series of patients with valve repairs and replacements using open-heart and a heart-lung machine, the chairman of the meeting stood and said, "Your time is up." This was to accommodate Dr. Barnard talking about his transplant. Concerned about Dr. Barnard's jumping ahead with a heart transplant, Dr. Merendino did not stand, nor did he stay for this presenter (Merendino 2011).

Dr. Francis Everhart trained at the University of Minnesota with Dr. Jesse Edwards (1911–2008), a world-renowned cardiac pathologist. The postmortem exam of the heart was still essential for learning and understanding cardiac anatomy, the blue-baby defects, and acquired heart disease. The hope of better imaging and better treatments hinged on detailed knowledge of the heart.

After finishing his cardiology training, Everhart worked with a private group for two years in Minneapolis. He was frustrated with the slow pace and resistance to incorporating the new coronary angiograms and catheters into their private practice. Francis knew about Dr. Berg's open-heart team in the Northwest, so when an ad appeared for an adult cardiologist proficient in the new coronary artery catheter procedure, he responded. After interviewing with Drs. Berg and Kendall, he arrived in Spokane in July 1968 with his family.

He soon found that Drs. Berg and Kendall were themselves performing heart catheterizations. The surgeons wanted to learn to manipulate the catheters for imaging of the coronary vessels and for planning the surgical procedures. Dr. Lang would provide the sedation medications and the monitoring when either surgeon did this procedure. Dr. Everhart had not expected heart surgeons to have any interest in performing heart catheters but quickly found out how closely the surgeons worked with Dr. Henry Lang. A surgeon would show up for all of Dr. Lang's heart catheters, both adult and pediatric patients. The surgeon would assist in the catheter case. Dr. Lang would then do the report and make any referrals.

In contrast, Dr. Francis Everhart worked alone in the cath lab at Sacred Heart, needing only a technical nurse to assist him. Dr. Everhart approached the heart from a simple needlestick at the groin. Heart patients came in by ambulance, referred by their doctor with chest pain. Sometimes the heart patients were sent in from a private office, sometimes from an emergency room at an outlying hospital. Mostly they came straight to the cath lab. Sometimes they went first to the emergency room.

The heart catheterization suite at Sacred Heart Hospital was under control of the radiology department. In the mornings, the radiologists preferred to use it for special procedures, cut film, and angiography. They allowed cardiac studies in the afternoon. Cardiac studies were performed using a catheter manipulator with mirror imaging off the fluorescent screen, and the cardiac angiography was recorded on sixteen-millimeter cine film at a low rate of frames per second due to the limited X-ray power. The official "hospital" interpretation of heart and coronary angiography was performed by the radiologists. However, the clinical decisions regarding medical or surgical implications of the study results were made by the attending cardiologist and chest surgeon.

Dr. Everhart made referrals after his procedure with coronary imaging and depending on the result. He tolerated the heart surgeons coming in for his procedures. He got to know them well. He resisted their doing much more than watch (F. Everhart 1975).

Dr. Lang continued to supervise the heart pump in the operating room. He also followed all of Berg and Kendall's open-heart patients in the postoperative period. Dr. Everhart once called up the perfusionist and asked him, "Are you independent in the operating room?" Nebraska jokingly replied, "Henry gets in my way." Once, when a case came up that Dr. Everhart referred to Dr. Berg, Dr. Lang was in the operating room, and Dr. Everhart came in to observe. Ralph looked at his perfusionist and winked. The tension was almost palpable, and Dr. Lang left the room. When the patient was safe on the heart-lung machine, Everhart also left the operating room.

Dr. Lang made the painful decision to separate and isolate the pediatric practice from the rapidly growing adult cardiology. The new pediatric cardiologist was to arrive in June 1969 and would not perform coronary angiograms for the simple fact that coronary artery disease was not seen in the blue babies. Henry planned to bring in another adult cardiologist the following year, knowing he would be further pulled into adult cardiology. It was the era of fast. An adult with acquired heart disease, coronary artery occlusions, and chest pain would be referred for a coronary angiogram, and it was expected to be completed within days if not hours of the referral. Meanwhile, the blue babies would wait months before being moved to a heart cath.

In the fall of 1968, a third open-heart surgeon came from the Mayo Clinic to work with Drs. Berg and Kendall in Spokane, bringing an electronic system for patient data entry.

Berg and Kendall's practice continued to grow. When Nebraska traveled to San Diego, California, to learn about the heart-lung machines and setup there, the visit went so well that he almost took a job there. When Ralph found out, he hired Nebraska, luring him away from Sacred Heart Hospital by matching the salary offered in San Diego. Nebraska stayed in Spokane with Dr. Ralph Berg, and the Berg Surgical Group became his employer. Nebraska never left the group (R. Berg 2006).

In March 1969, Dr. Everhart opened his solo practice in adult cardiology. He took an office close to Sacred Heart. He did his own catheter manipulations to enter the coronary arteries, as well as right- and left-heart imaging as indicated. He used both cine film and cut films to preserve and share his work. He generated reports on his procedures and remained annoyed that a radiologist would read over his work. He used Drs. Berg and Kendall as his cardiac surgeons, remaining present in the operating room with his patients to observe and learn the intraoperative findings. He accepted Dr. Lang's supervision of his patients on the heart bypass pump. However, he managed his own patients postoperation conjointly with the surgeons. He had great admiration for this team and its work (F. Everhart 1975).

The advances in pacemakers, the stylets that allowed percutaneous placements without a thoracotomy or need for a chest surgeon, caused turmoil. Sales representatives for pacemakers pestered the surgery desk, asking and wanting to know who the qualified surgeons were while offering tidbits that in Seattle, the surgeons were doing up to five pacemaker implants a day. Nebraska knew to discount this kind of information.

However, kickbacks to the surgeon/cardiologist teams implanting these devices was an issue. Nebraska got called in for a Saturday case, a pacemaker implant. The same thing happened the next weekend. A pacemaker case with a general practitioner—not a surgeon, not a chest surgeon. Pacemakers were typically not urgent/emergent cases, but that did not mean they were simple. On Monday morning, it was revealed by the director of radiology that one of the devices was upside down, incorrectly placed, not recognized and not corrected.

With the door shut, the administration, working to prevent subpar work being performed by noncredentialed providers who assumed pacemaker inserts were quick and easy, produced a list of surgeons who held privileges to perform pacemaker implants. Nebraska was given instructions for what to do if a doctor not on this list wanted to get into the operating rooms, especially after hours or weekends. Nebraska kept a meticulous ledger for pacemaker implants where all the pacemaker devices were logged in addition to the surgeons, several of them open-heart surgeons, who implanted the pacemaker devices.

Pleased with the pacemaker advances and the cardiologists placing them percutaneously, Dr. Berg had quit putting in pacemakers a few years prior, though Kendall continued with surgical pacemaker placements. Berg continued to do the difficult blue-baby cases, his passion. He appreciated the brilliant young cardiologists who chose to be in Spokane working with Spokane's open-heart teams.

When Dr. René Favaloro's much anticipated report on direct coronary artery bypass for treatment of chronic angina associated with a coronary artery blockage was published in March 1969, the survival and mortality numbers were stunningly good. The Vineberg was now officially obsolete. A whole new area of open-heart surgery began (Bakaeen 2018). Dr. Ralph Berg took this advance to his patients; he felt no need for a dog lab to detail this work. He invited Dr. Favaloro to Spokane for several days of direct coronary bypasses with Dr. Berg and his partners.

By early May 1969, Dr. Berg was performing direct coronary artery bypass with saphenous vein graft. Demand was up. More and more adults were getting heart catheters with coronary angiograms when they developed angina. Many of the angiograms showed partial occlusions in the coronary arteries. Some of the angiograms showed a single coronary artery with a blockage, while others had combinations of two or three coronary arteries involved. Dr. Berg, his team, and his group were busy with elective coronary artery bypass grafting.

CHAPTER 12

Is It Fixable? 1969

The trip to Hawaii in January 1969 was a treat, a reward for so many things. Ralph and Mary had five children, the youngest about to turn fifteen. They were a team with two careers. He was successful in private practice with the dog lab, open-heart surgery, two partners, published research papers, and this new direct coronary artery bypass operation for chest pain patients with imaging showing occlusions. Supportive of her husband and committed to him, Mary had a thriving real estate business. She bought, remodeled, sold, and managed real estate properties, a skill she had developed during those lean years of medical school and surgical training.

They planned this trip to celebrate their twenty-seventh year of marriage, just the two of them. Ski season—a little hectic that year with several of their children on ski teams—could go on without them. The Hawaiian Islands provided paradise and relaxation. The Bergs did some sightseeing, walked the beaches, held hands, and stood out in the breakers. Mary really enjoyed the waves and the sun. The cool water soothing her sun-tinged legs felt so good. They smiled at each other. Mary caught the flu and was sick for a day or so at the end of the vacation, but they flew home connected and tranquil.

Soon Mary noted she was tired. Odd after a relaxing vacation; yet the tiredness persisted. Mary wondered if she was going through menopause. Ralph wondered about the flu, German measles, or Hong

Kong flu. She made an appointment with her gynecologist about this issue of menopause. Instead, she got a surprise: she was pregnant. Yet when she thought about it, it was most welcome, a pregnancy late in life. She was forty-seven, and Ralph would be turning forty-eight in May. Mary was fine—a little tired but happy. She went back to work. Not much was said. Life went on. A medical doctor and wife, friends, were in a similar situation, with both expectant mothers in their late forties. All four friends noted that a generation earlier, such a pregnancy was unheard of.

Mary and Ralph went on an extended trip to the Far East that spring, visiting one of their sons and traveling. They could not get over the situation on the international flight home, where they were forced to breathe air filled with cigarette smoke in the plane cabin. No way to escape. Passengers weren't even asked to curtail their smoking. With Mary being pregnant, Ralph was upset by this.

Ralph's letter about the situation, published on April 7, 1969, in the editorial page of the *AMA/American Medical Association News,* was entitled "The Clouded Sky":

> Would you please let me know where I may obtain information on what—if anything—has been done to secure an acceptable respiratory environment for non-smokers on the nation's airlines. My wife and I just returned from an extensive trip by air to the Far East, the air travel portion of which was much less pleasant than it could have been if we had not been forced to sit surrounded by chain smokers, pipe smokers, and cigar smokers. In view of what is already known about the harmful effects of smoking, it seems inconceivable that this forced exposure to tobacco smoke in a confined area continues . . .
>
> Ralph Berg Jr., Spokane, Washington.
>
> Editor's Note: *The AMA News* would be interested in learning how other physicians have coped with this situation.

Many doctors in Spokane were still smokers. In the weekly case conference, smoking cessation was discussed, and several of the doctors who regularly attended this conference had quit. Ralph Berg was steadfast in his recommendations about the dangers of smoking, but this battle would take decades to bear fruit.

A group of friends held a baby shower for Mary in late June.

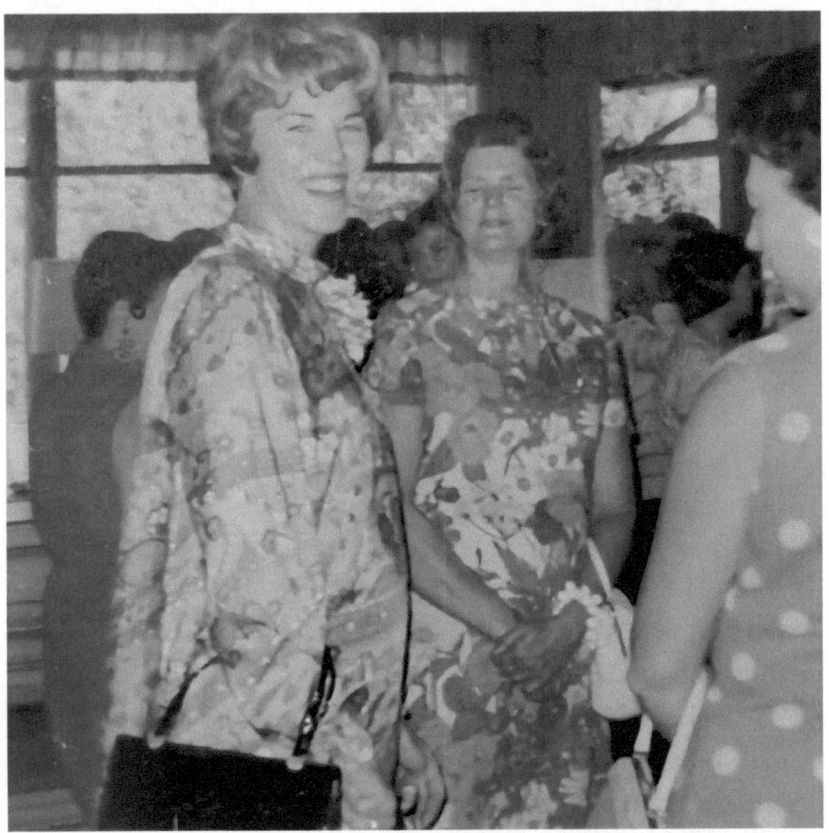

Mary's friends held a baby shower in late June 1969.

Mary took over the management of a large apartment complex that was losing money. After looking at the books, Mary felt confident it could become an asset again. She arranged a work trip for later in August with her sons as the crew. The Berg boys were ages fifteen to twenty-four, and they stayed a week in the southern part of the state, working as a team, doing repairs and maintenance. Mary worked alongside her sons and enjoyed their time together. When the Berg family returned to Spokane, job done, she was confident the apartment complex would turn a profit.

One Sunday morning in August, she awoke to labor pains; Ralph drove her to Deaconess as planned. The maternity ward inside the brick building had an elegant lobby. She delivered her baby in the usual way with little fanfare on August 31, 1969. The baby was just beautiful. They named him Jason. He was taken to the nursery, a healthy baby boy, big and round. Ralph was pleased. Mary was fine. After spending the day at the hospital with Mary and the baby, Ralph went home to get ready for the early-morning departure for duck hunting, an annual tradition, on September 1. Mary and Jason were to go home in a few days.

Alice Berg, working in the microbiology lab just a few floors away from the maternity ward, was relieved to hear all went well. Having a child this late in life was a worry (A. Berg 2010). Dr. Henry Lang, the pediatrician for all of Mary's children, was there for Mary and Jason. Then a night nurse in the Deaconess postpartum nursery noted Jason's coloring was off that first night. He turned a slight cast of blue when he cried. The color returned to pink when he was calm. This nurse alerted Dr. Lang, who arrived to evaluate Jason very early that Monday morning, Labor Day.

He looked at Jason in the nursery. He listened to his heart. Then he took a chest X-ray. The film showed Jason's heart was big, shaped like an egg. The top of Jason's heart, where the great vessels are located, was narrowed, and the vascular markings in his lungs were increased. The aortic arch was to the right instead of to the left. Henry put Jason on oxygen and gently told Mary that something was wrong with the baby's heart.

Mary listened. Then she asked, "Is it fixable?" She knew better than most that the blue babies did not always make it. Thankfully, she had the best of the best right at her side. Henry told her, "Yes, it is fixable." She was reassured. This team would fix it. Feeling well, Mary took photos of Jason's chest X-ray. She knew Ralph would want to see the films (M. Berg 2011).

Dr. Lang was concerned and needed to know more than what the chest X-ray showed. Jason was taken to Sacred Heart, where Dr. Lang had Rashkind balloon catheters and surgical backup if needed. In the cath lab that Labor Day morning, Dr. Kendall and CRNA Julie Spores were in attendance. Lang suspected complex transposition of the great vessels.

Dr. Lang sedated baby Jason with an oral liquid medication and carefully placed access lines in both groin vessels. He gave Jason an intravenous medication and then entered the large vessel that would allow the catheter to travel backward through the arterial tree to his heart. On the opposite leg he entered the large vein that would allow the catheter to travel with the venous return into Jason's right heart. Dr. Kendall watched the first images as Lang injected the dye. It was not a simple defect. There were several holes between the ventricles. They identified five ventricular septal defects and a patent ductus. The aortic arch was indeed to the right. Lang had discovered the dreaded complex transposition of the great vessels—a confusing group of defects and lethal.

The rare but standard version of transposition had not yet been modeled in a dog lab. The atrial switch procedures that were in use had high mortality. Truly this defect was not yet fixable, but Mary needed hope and reassurance that her new baby would live (Spores 2011).

Dr. Lang knew what to do in this moment: create a hole between the atria to provide mixing of the two circulations. Jason was tolerating the heart cath procedure, so Lang moved ahead and performed an emergent Rashkind's atrial septostomy. He took the large Rashkind balloon with a cutter device attached and passed it over his wire, threading it into position inside Jason's right atrium. Then he punctured through the atrial septum into the left atrium. He checked on the fluoroscopy imager for his position. Then he inflated the balloon and pulled it back across Jason's atrial septum, cutting a large circular defect. This large hole between Jason's upper chambers, an atrial septal defect, now allowed more mixing of the two circulations. Certainly a life-saving gift to have Dr. Lang's experience and a Rashkind balloon available at the hospital seven blocks away.

When Jason cried after his sedation wore off following the procedure, he remained pink. He returned to Deaconess when Dr. Lang felt it was safe, and Mary took Jason home the next day, Band-Aids on both sides of his groin. When Ralph got back from duck hunting, all seemed well, as Mary reported to her husband.

The mind-numbing magnitude of this baby, Jason, was forever on Ralph's mind; Jason was so much a reward for both Ralph and Mary and yet touched in such a way that few could understand, fix, or cope with. Their will as a family was going to be tested, and survival was the only option for Ralph and Mary. The pioneering open-heart surgeon found himself the parent of a blue baby with a complex defect without a repair and without a model.

Jason did well, remarkably well. His family worked to keep him well attended. He would get winded if he cried, so he had attention and he was carried all the time. Two of Jason's older siblings were still at home. Surrounded by adults, Jason was not stressed. He grew and was a happy, round baby. He got frequent office checkups with Dr. Lang.

During my May 2011 interview with Dr. Alvin Merendino, I revealed to the doctor my uncle's experience with his blue baby. Dr. Merendino was visibly affected and had to sit down, tears in his eyes. "Ralph Berg stayed in the game, for Jason," he realized (Merendino 2011).

Transposition of the great vessels had haunted Dr. Merendino since his first attempt at correcting a blue-baby defect using the biologic oxygenator in 1956. That case resulted in an on-table death of a child and launched transposition of the great vessels as his career focus. Merendino outlined the multiple attempts and procedures from his research lab in our interview. In 1969, there was still no durable procedure for correcting transposition.

CHAPTER 13

It Happened in Spokane for a Reason

Other things started to change in late 1969. Deaconess Hospital's open-heart team performed a blue-baby VSD repair using the heart-lung machine and lost the twenty-one-year-old patient on the table. Air trapping, a problem with the tubing and the pump, caused a bleed-out. Dr. Shields, who tracked all his patients referred for heart surgery, noted a difference in outcomes based on the facility. A cardiologist working with Shields called Nebraska and set a secret meeting in the doctors' sleep room at Sacred Heart. Nebraska recalled the cardiologist was upset.

"The Deaconess team is not going to be doing any more cases for us," he said. It was painful for this cardiologist to say. The loyalty, the respect, the pattern of practice and referrals are sacred, but they do not trump successful outcomes. The cardiologist wanted better care for their heart patients.

The cardiologist relaxed some when Nebraska brought Dr. Berg down the hall, as if Berg were the Triple Crown winner. After a brief conversation, cardiologist to open-heart surgeon, Berg agreed to provide an open-heart surgery service at Deaconess. Ralph Berg thought of it as the right thing to do and was happy to operate at another facility. Sacred Heart administration did not like this. "Bring the patients here" was her response. Ralph said, "No. We are going to Deaconess."

The turmoil of the next decade was beginning. The details of starting a new and second open-heart service largely landed on the cardiovascular pump technician. Nebraska had to pack up the instruments and go to Deaconess. "Simple" was how Dr. Berg explained it to Nebraska. Nebraska spent hours ordering new instruments. They needed another complete set so the heart teams could perform pump cases at the same time, whether at the two hospitals or in separate operating rooms at the same hospital.

Nebraska called his connection in Texas and had some of the instruments made. He was pleased when he found out he could get them at half the price from the engineer who worked with Dr. Cooley. When Nebraska told Ralph it would take thirty days to get the entire set of instruments, Dr. Berg responded, "Nebraska, make it happen in two weeks." Nebraska called all the instrument makers and got enough instruments for a half set. Ralph was still unhappy. So, Nebraska kept calling. It took Nebraska twenty days to get the instruments. Some came from Seattle. It was hard to get the vascular clamps. The eventual price for this new set of open-heart instruments was $12,000. Finally, they had three complete sets (Stephens 2011).

Meanwhile, a Rockwood Clinic cardiologist arranged a direct coronary artery bypass for one of his VIP patients with the founder of the procedure, Dr. René Favaloro. Feeling that travel with angina was life-threatening, the cardiologist accompanied his private patient with adult acquired heart disease to the Cleveland Clinic. Simpson, the senior cardiology fellow, met the Spokane cardiologist, who promptly invited Simpson to visit Spokane and the Rockwood Clinic. The patient did well with her procedure. Carroll Simpson fell in love with Spokane when he visited a short time later. He agreed to join Rockwood Clinic and made plans to come to Spokane late the following spring (Simpson 2011).

At Deaconess, preparations for a second heart team stopped. Their heart-lung machine was not certified, so Dr. Berg and his surgical group would not use it. This was a big concern for the cardiologists and administrators at Deaconess. The heart-lung machines were expensive and not easy to get.

Every year, the Berg Surgical Group's heart-lung pumps were sent to Cleveland, Ohio, for recertification. The process took about a week and involved cleaning, inspecting, and resetting the standards of all the pump's working parts. The group offered to use their own pumps at Deaconess; they would employ and provide the pump technicians, then bill the patients for the use of the pump. The hospital would take 10 percent of this collected fee. This was a situation unique to Spokane and because of Dr. Berg. Around the country, most heart surgeons operated with instruments and heart-lung machines owned by their hospitals. The Deaconess administrator relented and, to get started, allowed this.

Anesthesia was another point of concern for Dr. Berg. However, the Deaconess anesthesia group was well trained in cardiac anesthesia and eager to work with the Berg Surgical Group. So, at Deaconess, they used physician anesthesiologists.

Nebraska had an Audi Fox station wagon. He would load the pump into the back—heralding back to the "Have pump, will travel" method Merendino and Harkins had used—and head to Deaconess. Dr. Berg and Nebraska did their first case there shortly after the instruments arrived. All went well. The Deaconess administrator and the cardiologists were pleased. Referrals for open-heart cases came in more rapidly, and the open-heart surgeons in Berg's practice covered both hospitals.

While operating, Dr. Berg's teams would talk, listen to music, and sometimes eat cake—different from the prepump times of silence while Dr. Berg worked. A nurse and OR technician from this era reported that Ralph, always regal and authoritative, would tease and push the team. He would ask demanding questions like "Who killed Abe Lincoln?" to get them talking. Most of the young team members were on pins and needles amid the intensity and precision of the open-heart cases, regardless of their experience or which hospital they worked for. Ralph soothed their stresses and concerns and bantered with them as he was closing (Kappen 2011).

As 1970 rolled in, the cardiology and open-heart surgery teams moved through the list of chronic angina patients. The coronary angiograms were being done by several cardiologists who now utilized the advanced imaging of the heart and its three coronary arteries. The direct coronary bypass open-heart operations were also successful. With the new heart catheter procedure, many Vineberg patients were found to have coronary artery blockages and were referred for redo surgery with a direct coronary bypass. The coronary artery blockages in Berg's longtime patient Mr. Caruso—following his asbestos, talc, then Vineberg procedures—were impressive. He wanted a direct coronary bypass. Dr. Ralph Berg presented his case at the weekly case conference both before and after his direct bypass. Mr. Caruso did well.

Dr. Lang successfully completed the transition from pediatric to adult cardiology. His expertise enveloped multiple areas of heart disease that now had formal titles—pump technician, cardiac care unit, and all manner of cardiac imaging. Lang's new pediatric cardiologist partner arrived in Spokane, and the need for better pediatric imaging equipment was noted once more. The request was made and denied again. The congenital blue-baby cases were becoming a smaller percentage of their overall workload. Prenatal care, vitamins, imaging, and birth control helped slow the volume of blue babies.

Meanwhile, acquired disease of the coronary arteries was exploding. The Berg Surgical Group obtained coronary angiograms on all their heart-valve patients and were not surprised when many of them also needed a direct bypass. The group was doing more cases at Deaconess and talking about getting a second office there.

The population of Spokane was increasing, and huge projects were in the works, including moving the railroad depot and the rails and turning the riverfront with its islands into a multiacre park for the upcoming Expo '74. Mr. Larry Knauft and the Spokane Ambulance company were in negotiations with the city council, the mayor, the fire department, and the Spokane Medical Society.

Knauft started working for Spokane Ambulance in September 1967. He was a military combat medic during his time in Vietnam and was sent for emergency medical technician (EMT) training at the community college by his company, then to the paramedic training program. Both programs were run in coordination with the medical experts in Spokane. Spokane Ambulance trained all their personnel, drivers, and attendants this way and maintained close relations with the hospitals, the community colleges, and the Northeast branch of the Washington State Heart Association. When Larry started his job, the ambulances were large Cadillacs. The upgrade to a van with more room for patient-monitoring equipment occurred soon after he started (Knauf 2008).

Spokane Services Company owned the ambulances of Spokane Ambulance. They were a progressive company, passionate about getting patients to the hospitals alive. After the negotiations, Spokane Ambulance received authorization for a direct phone line to the hospitals. They installed a radio-phone patch system that allowed the paramedics to send electrocardiogram strips and relay other information about the patient from the ambulance to the emergency room while they were en route to the hospital. With this closed-loop communication, the paramedics were able to give medication as directed by the ER doctor, start intravenous lines, take a twelve-lead EKG, and transmit results to the hospital ahead of arrival, and the ER staff was able to prepare for the incoming patient (Knauf 2008). This kind of prehospital care is now an essential component of emergency treatment.

———

In the spring of 1970, at seven months of age, Jason got sick with upper respiratory symptoms. Dr. Lang admitted Jason to the hospital. A senior nursing student in her pediatric rotation observed and assisted Jason during this hospital stay. He was in an oxygen tent, a crib enclosed in plastic sheeting to provide humidified air with the extra oxygen. His serious congenital cardiac defect was a big concern. Was there a change in his condition? Attending pediatrician Dr. Lang's concern was that this was not a simple pneumonia. Jason was fussy and tired easily if he cried. He was not crawling yet.

An intravenous line supplied the fluids and antibiotics. Mary was there with Jason every day, all day. Dr. Berg came every day for a visit, garnering respect and attention when he walked on the pediatric ward, described the student nurse. The nurses reported the labs and gave an update on Jason. Ralph would sit and talk with Mary while holding Jason. Dr. Lang came by late every evening to make sure no issues were brewing into the overnight hours. They all noted the blueness had returned.

Normally, the patent ductus closes at birth. If it fails to close, it becomes a shunt that steals flow in an anatomically correct heart. In Jason's heart, the patent ductus was a blessing and provided mixing of the two circulations in addition to the Rashkind procedure providing an atrial septal defect. But Jason's chest X-ray and heart exam suggested his patent ductus had closed. He developed congestive heart failure, then pneumonia. Dr. Lang recommended digitalis to slow down Jason's heart so it would not work so hard. Ralph thought more could and should be done. He was vulnerable. He had given Mary his word, and he anticipated a "fix" for Jason.

Ralph settled on the Mayo Clinic, the first American institution to go from the dog lab to open-heart in a successful and enduring way back in 1955, with Dr. John Kirklin. The clinic had continued their congenital heart work and academics. Ralph and Mary made arrangements and took Jason to Mayo. Upon arrival, they discovered that Dr. Kirklin was no longer there. He had moved to Birmingham, Alabama, and was rebuilding his program, having left Mayo about a year earlier. So, instead, they met with open-heart surgeon Dr. Dwight Magoon.

After Dr. Magoon examined Jason, he recommended a Blalock-Tausig-Thomas shunt procedure to reestablish mixing Jason's blood now that the patent ductus arteriosum had closed. This procedure, to create a shunt via surgically connecting the subclavian artery to the pulmonary artery, would not require a heart-lung machine. Done outside the pericardium and outside of Jason's heart, it would create a larger shunt compared to the size of Jason's patent ductus. Both Magoon and Berg understood how important it was to buy time for Jason and to avoid opening his pericardial sac. When the definitive repair for transposition of the great vessels was discovered, Jason would not have the added concern of pericardial scarring to his heart (R. Berg 2006).

Dr. Magoon arranged for and scheduled Jason's surgery within a day or so. Ralph and Mary waited patiently and were much relieved when Dr. Magoon came out and told them Jason was pink, surgery had gone well, and the ductus was confirmed to be closed. Mary held vigil at Jason's bedside during his recovery. She was more than a little annoyed when a young surgery resident came by on morning rounds and picked Jason up, out of his crib. With his new left chest scar, it hurt Jason terribly, and he cried vigorously. The resident quickly saw his error and put Jason back into the crib—onto his left side, where his incision was. Mary turned Jason off his left side, and he calmed down (M. Berg 2011).

After Jason achieved enough recovery, the family returned to Spokane. Mary and Jason picked up their routine, and Ralph picked up his practice. The wait list for the chronic angina patients wanting the new direct coronary bypass graft was long and provided steady work.

Berg, disciplined and focused, was under pressure with Jason's situation. He was a bit distracted during the open-heart coronary bypass cases, busily researching transposition of the great vessels and learning everything that was known during his off hours.

A model for the defect, always the first clinical step, had not been achieved, though the concept of a surgical repair was simple: switching the great vessels back into anatomic position so blood would flow through the lungs and the heart could pump out the oxygenated blood into the arterial tree. The great vessel switch had been done at the level of the aorta in dog labs where the experiment was time-on-pump toxicity, but the dogs had normal hearts, normal valves, and no associated complexities. In children, the switch was at the level of the atria and without a dog model. And Jason's transposition was particularly complex (Spores 2011).

For Dr. Carroll Simpson, telling Dr. Sones he was leaving for private practice was going to be difficult. An intensely loyal person and a bit hard to get along with, Dr. Sones would "pin . . . to the wall" anyone who bluffed a response. Sones wanted Simpson to stay academic and work at the Cleveland Clinic with him. Rather than undertake a prolonged goodbye, Simpson came in early, did his case in Dr. Sones's room, finished, and was gone before Sones got there.

When Dr. Simpson left the Cleveland Clinic in the late spring of 1970, there were eight cath labs in the clinic's basement, and Simpson had performed over 400 coronary angiograms. He was flat broke, tired, and in turmoil when he drove into Spokane. Lots of things were not right in his life. But he had a great education, great training, and had landed a great job. He felt lucky. He would be working with a group of doctors who were not in opposition to coronary artery angiography. He had seen how the "Don't touch the heart" mantra had affected his mentor, exiled to the basement when he switched from pediatric to adult cardiology.

What Carroll found in Spokane was even better than he could have imagined. Not only were the medical doctors supportive and the cardiologists not opposed to coronary angiography, but the surgeons in Spokane were equally progressive. The Berg Surgical Group had been around since the early 1950s. They were proficient in open-heart, knew Dr. René Favaloro personally, and were already doing direct coronary artery bypass for chronic angina patients. The competitive environment in the Spokane medical community was also friendly and collegial. They shared and educated each other at the weekly cardiac case conference. They took care of patients, and they worked hard. Dr. Simpson was busy as a new cardiologist in Spokane's Rockwood Clinic that summer (Simpson 2011).

Dr. Everhart had completed a coronary angiogram on a patient who was not a chronic angina patient. Preinfarct, not the same as chronic angina, could evolve into a heart attack. This patient came to the ER with acute chest pain, EKG changes, and was fortunate enough to get in immediately with Dr. Everhart for heart cath. At coronary angiography, Dr. Everhart found an offending plaque in the main coronary artery. He immediately called Dr. Berg, who came to the angio room, looked at the films and the patient, and recommended a direct bypass. Everhart observed Drs. Berg and Kendall perform a direct coronary bypass on this preinfarct patient within an hour of symptoms beginning.

Francis explained,

> During my training, I was intimately involved in the pathology of both chronic coronary artery issues and acute heart attacks. One of my main interests involved coronary artery disease. The prevailing cardiac wisdom, at the time, was that acute heart attacks were caused by bleeding under a plaque. A plaque is a weak spot in a coronary artery caused by atherosclerosis. At autopsy, shortly after a lethal heart attack, these individuals would typically have a blood clot at this site within a coronary artery. It was assumed that this clot developed following the heart attack because of the impaired cardiac contractility associated with the myocardial damage.
>
> However, on several occasions, when I was involved with

autopsies done on people who died sometime after their nonacute heart attacks, there was no clot, and the plaque did not completely obstruct the coronary artery.

The body will normally dissolve clots after some amount of time, so not finding a clot in these patients was no surprise. But based on that observation, Everhart speculated that it was possible that the plaque ruptured and then a clot formed immediately. It was this clot that totally obstructed the coronary artery and was the basis for the significant degree of myocardial damage. If no clot formed at time of plaque disruption, the obstruction would not be complete, and the individual might well survive the plaque rupture alone.

But the only way this could be confirmed would be to do a coronary angiogram while someone was experiencing an acute heart attack. This was not recommended by cardiologists because they assumed that the patients would almost certainly have more complications, including death and fatal cardiac arrhythmias, during the angiography than they would with conservative medical therapy.

Everhart noted the significant improvements in the heart-lung machines and the surgical procedures designed to help people who had chronic coronary artery disease. He also noted these procedures were done electively, not emergently and on the patients who arguably needed the procedure sooner. More adults were getting coronary angiograms when they developed angina, showing occlusions of various degrees in one, two, or all three of the coronary arteries. They wanted the new bypass around those occlusions, and in Spokane, the surgeons were adept at bypassing areas of narrowing and/or obstruction of the coronary artery or arteries with vein grafts. His theory: if a coronary artery obstruction was found during a heart attack, a surgical procedure existed and could be performed to treat that obstruction.

The surgeons' installation of the coronary artery bypass graft on Everhart's preinfarct patient was swift. The patient's recovery uneventful, chronic angina did not develop.

And this upset Dr. Francis Everhart because he was being stymied in providing this lifesaving procedure to his preinfarct patients. He wanted to prevent chronic angina from developing in patients. He wanted to avoid the second heart attack for these patients. He needed to discuss this with a heart surgeon who could provide the treatment, the bypass graft, and he chose Dr. Berg, who seemed more open, more available than other heart surgeons.

At the meeting in mid-June 1970, Dr. Everhart discussed his leap of insight about heart attacks with Berg. Everhart proposed doing urgent coronary angiography on patients with preinfarct symptoms, basically an evolving heart attack. He then wanted Dr. Berg to perform emergent vein coronary bypass grafts around the coronary artery blockages. He hoped to limit the extent of myocardial necrosis and the development of chronic angina patients by restoring the coronary artery flow sooner (F. Everhart 1975).

Several heart attack models existed in the dog research labs, but they were insufficient to prove Everhart's theory. One model achieved heart attack by rapid occlusion of a dog's single coronary artery. The subsequent heart attack was severe, and when revascularized several hours later, these dogs died of ventricular fibrillation with a hemorrhagic infarction. As the heart fibrillated in electrical disarray and then shut down, a clot formed in the coronary artery. For this extreme dog model, the clot was after the fact, in both Drs. Berg's and Everhart's opinion, so its formation provided no new data. However, most felt this dog experiment supported the entrenched thinking that any attempt at coronary angiography during a heart attack was sure to lead to more deaths than would occur if patients were treated medically in the CCU. The "Don't touch the heart" mantra remained.

This idea of acute coronary artery occlusion by a clot as the primary event leading to heart attack was untested. Dr. Everhart's proposal was a paradigm shift in the current thinking. To reestablish flow in a human coronary artery during a heart attack would most likely lead to the same result as in the dog models: immediate death from electrical disarray and a hemorrhagic infarction. There was collective fear of causing death or harm while placing a catheter inside the artery already filled with hemorrhage and plaque. This fear was entrenched. It would have been easy, reasonable, and safe for Dr. Ralph Berg to say no.

Yet Dr. Berg agreed to consider vein graft surgery in acute myocardial infarction (MI)—with a condition. He wanted this work to be scientific; he wanted Francis to present the results of their acute coronary angiography, while Dr. Berg would track and publish his work with acute coronary revascularization. The meeting was short. The protocol was initiated.

Ralph found parallels to both the congenital heart patients and to vascular patients with leg artery blockage in Dr. Everhart's theory to correct the coronary artery blockage more urgently. The nihilistic fear that opening the heart would cause immediate electrical disruption or uncontrollable bleeding and death had preceded the heart-lung machines for many a millennium. Crossing the open-heart barrier, which led to many lifesaving procedures, was not that far in the past.

The thinking regarding heart attacks was progressing. The Levine care was six weeks of bed rest if the heart attack was not lethal—which worked well for blue babies. "In the congenital heart patients, after the heart-lung machines were safe and available, small procedures, then wait, rest, and grow until the definitive procedure could be done, worked beautifully," Ralph explained. However, for many adult heart attack patients treated with Levine's bed rest, "well, they died, typically of the second heart attack." Dr. Berg noted that a similar arterial occlusion in a leg artery threatened amputation if not surgically corrected with a swift bypass (R. Berg 2006).

Berg and Everhart understood that a heart attack was due to coronary artery circulation insufficiency. Of course, with there being three coronary arteries, not all heart attacks were the same. And congenital blue-baby hearts did not have coronary artery circulation insufficiency. The blue babies had shunts that overworked their hearts. However, myocardial preservation was important in both groups—in other words, avoiding necrosis, aneurysmal dilations, thinning and diffuse dilation, arrhythmias, and scarring. The concept was not hard for Ralph to rally behind.

When Dr. Berg agreed to consult for a coronary artery bypass surgery on acute myocardial infarction patients, it was a big event for Dr. Francis Everhart. He was going way out of bounds on his side of the protocol in getting the diagnosis. Most cardiologists in the United States were not doing coronary angiography, much less considering this diagnostic test during a heart attack.

This agreement was all the validation Dr. Everhart needed. His solo practice was still new, and he was also teaching cardiac physiology at the local Spokane Community College. The push and support to publish the results had a profound impact at work. He was eager for a patient on which to begin testing his new theory regarding heart attacks; he felt heart attacks would become better understood and better treated. Dr. Everhart proceeded to study, by urgent coronary angiography, those acute infarction patients who 1) presented to Sacred Heart Hospital within about five hours of the onset of chest pain, 2) showed acute changes on their initial ECG, and 3) whom he was asked to consult on (F. Everhart 2011).

The chronic angina patients on the wait list reported how much better they were after the direct vein bypass. The magnitude of the coronary occlusions on angiography was predictive and related to the patients' symptoms. Acute coronary syndrome, the surgical term for coronary artery occlusions, had more severe symptoms and became unstable compared to the chronic angina patients. The urgency of proceeding to direct bypass in acute coronary syndrome patients as the degree of the coronary occlusion and symptoms increased, predicting an evolving large heart attack and death of the myocardium, seemed clear. But to push back the nihilistic surgical and medical teaching would require scientific results.

During procedures for chronic angina patients, Ralph noted ventricular aneurysms, something that had also appeared in his congenital patients and which would become important to his understanding of heart attacks and the importance of early intervention. These would not infrequently resolve with revascularization. Dr. Ralph Berg felt the muscle was weak and thinned, therefore dilating while working in an ischemic environment. Newly developed enzyme tests could show the muscle was dying through a blood draw. At these procedures, when the arteries were opened, he would invariably find significant plaque. In the more acute patients, he would find an associated fresh clot at the plaque, which caused 100 percent occlusion. The ventricle would progress from recoverable aneurysm to infarction, and the patients would die. He felt that restoring blood flow to the ventricle muscle would be a benefit. "Simple," per Ralph Berg.

With lower-extremity arterial disease, the patients could compensate by resting. With rest, the skeletal muscle could recover from being hypoxic. With the myocardium, there is no similar rest or recovery, only less cardiac output demand. To stop the myocardium—unless on pump during an open-heart procedure—is death. As Dr. Berg put it, the only rest for a heart was on pump, not in a bed.

Nurses in the CCU noted how much better the surgical patients were doing than the medically managed heart attack patients (S. Shields 2011). However, Dr. Kendall, when informed of the new protocol, was against it. The concept of acute coronary revascularization was experimental, and he noted it was an additional and unnecessary burden to their heavy workload. Meanwhile, Dr. Simpson was pleased to hear about the new protocol and supportive.

Dr. Simpson's practice and office were based at the hospital, but he spent most of his time in the cath lab, which had been using old imaging equipment as well as arterial access at the groin instead of at the wrist into the radial artery. Knowing what equipment Cleveland Clinic had, he sat down with Sacred Heart's administration and radiology department to convince them to upgrade the equipment. At first, both administration and the radiologists were resistant. However, within that first year, they did upgrade. An image intensifier replaced the cine, and a new table and state-of-the art catheters were brought in. There was a culture of first a "no" and then a definitive "yes" to new technology from administration at Sacred Heart, according to Dr. Simpson. Once administration saw the need, they modernized.

When the upgrades were complete, it was associated with a new name: Sacred Heart Hospital was now Sacred Heart Medical Center. For Dr. Simpson, the ability to favorably compare this Spokane hospital to the Cleveland Clinic, one of the finest cardiac centers, was powerful. For Dr. Berg, the new adult angiography equipment at the new hospital also represented a painful reality: Administrators were not caregivers to the children. He mourned in silence the blue babies who were sent away from Spokane, who came home dead in pine boxes, unable to wait for or benefit from these upgrades, which did not include the pediatric radiology table.

Nebraska recalled the last board meeting where Ralph sat in "the big guy" chair. Once again, the topic of pediatric radiology equipment upgrades was presented. Once again, the funds were denied. Berg calmly told the administraor to crawl up "the side of your new building and change out the holy cross for a dollar sign." Dr. Berg got up and kissed her on the top of her head. The room went silent, tense. He left and never attended an administrative or committee meeting again. Berg and Lang themselves bought an advanced radiology table for the children.

They were interested in doing better angiography studies by using less intravenous contrast and getting better images of the coronary arteries and chamber with less difficulty to the patients. The cases were presented at the weekly cardiac conference. Information was shared and discussed, as were results. The conference was well attended. There were discussions helpful to all the providers.

Over the next several months, Dr. Everhart studied five acute heart attack patients within four to six hours of symptom onset and without experiencing any significant problems. The patients tolerated the coronary angiogram. Dr. Berg chose not to perform vein graft surgery on these first five. Ralph recalled he rejected patients if the myocardium was already damaged. He would have these patients come back later when the infarct was complete.

At the Berg home, there was some tension. Mary assumed that Jason's defect was fixable and that it would be repaired soon. She found Ralph's behavior toward his youngest frustrating; he babied and seemed to favor Jason. He did not act like this with their other children.

Ralph researched, wrote, and presented "Surgical Management of Transposition of the Great Arteries" at the 57th Annual Meeting of the North Pacific Surgical Association meeting on November 14, 1970. The paper acknowledged that this defect carries a high mortality:

> Surgery itself is the third cause of death. Transposition of the great arteries has a spectrum of associated lesions profoundly affecting the clinical course and requiring meticulous dissection, and often post-mortem, to understand the palliative and corrective procedures. Proper timing of treatment is most important. No class of congenital cardiovascular lesions has required as much research and the efforts of so many cardiologists and surgeons to achieve a modicum of success in therapy. Totally satisfactory results may never be secured, but achievements to date have changed the prognosis from 90% fatality to 50% survival in the first year of life. This fact is to the great credit of all who have worked so diligently on transposition of the great vessels. (R. Berg 1971)

After he sat down, the next presentation started, and Ralph quietly began to eat dinner. Bob Kendall, sitting next to him, said it was well done; but few surgeons in the room were interested in a rare congenital heart defect with dismal outcomes. Few, if any, were aware that Ralph was a new father, let alone the father of a blue baby with a complex version of this defect. The paper was to publish the next year, 1971.

Within the first six months, Dr. Simpson realized Ralph Berg was unique. Simpson compared him to Dr. René Favaloro, who was distinctly different from the other Cleveland Clinic heart surgeons. Favaloro was a surgeon you could reason with.

As an example of the more rigid surgical type, Simpson recalled an encounter in a patient room during his residency. Simpson had consulted a surgeon regarding a cardiac problem, and while looking at the heart patient, the surgeon said, "You either have to grow a foot taller or lose a hundred pounds." Both the patient and Simpson were offended by this denial of surgical intervention. "This was said directly to the suffering patient," recalled Dr. Simpson; it was arrogant and mean. Dr. Favaloro, in contrast, was more sensitive to Dr. Simpson's patients' needs and easier to talk with.

Similarly, while Ralph was a private person and not one for opening up, he was easy to talk to regarding work. Drs. Simpson and Berg could talk over a case and decide to not intervene. Berg, an excellent technical surgeon and not afraid to go in, had superior results. Dr. Simpson was impressed with a surgeon who said no with conviction and without hurtful words to the patient (Simpson 2011).

At the annual Christmas party in 1970, the open-heart team was congratulated on hitting 1,000 open-heart pump cases. It had taken over ten years to reach this milestone. Ralph and Mary, while pleased, were also subdued. During the party, Ralph's sister, Margaret, defended her brother from a spouse of a team member who claimed Berg was demanding and difficult. "It is easy to enjoy the heart team's successes. Also, easy to be critical of Dr. Berg's demands" (Gayda 2011).

Berg's colleagues, on the cutting edge of being able to reveal what happens during a heart attack, had varying opinions about this exacting, demanding surgeon. But acute coronary revascularization happened in Spokane for a reason; all the pieces needed to carry out the protocol efficiently and successfully were there at that time.

CHAPTER 14

Acute Coronary Revascularization (ACR)

A forty-two-year-old male came in with progressive chest pain. In the emergency room, he explained the pain was now happening at rest. He was unsettled. His chest discomfort continued despite the emergency department's evaluation and treatment. So, Dr. Simpson admitted him to the hospital's new CCU and treated him with intravenous nitrates. The chest discomfort got better.

It was early March 1971. Dr. Simpson, not alarmed, reassured the patient, explaining he was preinfarct and that Dr. Simpson would perform a heart catheter with coronary artery imaging in a few days. The patient was relieved. Simpson scheduled the catheterization as a preinfarction case for 7:30 a.m. on the third hospital day.

Over the first night, the patient had an episode of chest pain around 5 a.m. with the nitrates running. The CCU nurse did not call Dr. Simpson. On morning rounds, Dr. Simpson found his patient also had elevated cardiac enzymes consistent with myocardial damage, and he had new EKG changes with Q waves and ST-segment elevations. In an "Oh shit" moment, he realized with dread that his patient was having a massive heart attack. Dr. Simpson called the cath lab and took the patient to radiology in a rush. An elective heart catheter case was delayed by this urgent coronary angiogram, and Everhart was content to be delayed. He stayed and watched Dr. Simpson perform the Sones technique of brachial artery access and left ventricular and coronary angiography.

Dr. Everhart noted, "The left anterior descending artery was totally occluded, and the ventricular angiography was consistent with a significant acute anterior-septal myocardial infarction!" Dr. Simpson reported, "At heart cath, the LAD artery, the main artery to the left ventricle, was blocked. Maybe a trickle of flow was getting through it, with a patent end artery . . . a ninety-nine percent blockage." The front of the heart, the entire left ventricle, was paralyzed on the cine run with the left heart injection. This was a well-known pattern to both cardiologists; it was a widow-maker heart attack about to happen—like the extreme coronary artery dog model of a heart attack, lethal. "Not moving" describes both Dr. Carroll Simpson and his patient's hearts at that moment. Simpson hoped there was a chance; otherwise, this healthy young man would die or, worse, become a cardiac cripple (F. Everhart 2011).

Dr. Simpson grabbed the phone and called the heart surgeon's office. Panic setting in, he found out Dr. Berg was already in the operating room, doing a case. Simultaneously, Dr. Everhart called Dr. Kendall, who was soon on his way. Kendall consulted on an emergency basis with Dr. Simpson and agreed to perform an emergency direct vein graft to the coronary artery for an acute myocardial infarction.

In recalling this first acute, Dr. Bob Kendall noted that Dr. Francis Everhart "set it up." Dr. Everhart cared and was quite invested in his protocol. Simpson went to the operating room with his patient. On pump, Dr. Kendall opened the left anterior descending coronary artery, and a fresh clot, under pressure, came squirting out. Kendall removed the entire remaining clot and performed a single bypass, as the other vessels were fine. The patient came off pump well. He did not die (Kendall 2011). Dr. Simpson had seen many patients die with this type of a coronary angiogram and the front of the heart paralyzed. Yet the day after the emergency vein graft surgery, the Q waves were gone on this patient's EKG, and the ST-T changes had normalized.

"This was a rare event, the patient survival, and everyone took note," reported Dr. Simpson. With this case, acute coronary revascularization for an evolving anterior myocardial infarction became the preferred care. In Spokane, if indicated by the patient's coronary angiography and with the agreement of the operating surgeon, the revascularization was done emergently. Dr. Simpson's patient was sent home in a week, and everyone was relieved and amazed (Simpson 2011). The weekly case conference at both hospitals presented this case, and there was lots of excitement and conversation about the clot Dr. Bob Kendall found in the main artery feeding the left ventricle and how well the patient did. The entirety of the Spokane teams now knew this treatment was not only possible but also successful.

The tragedy of losing an otherwise healthy male to a massive heart attack was well known. A relieved Dr. Simpson repeated the coronary catheter on this patient several weeks later. He found the vein graft open, the LAD open, the EKG normal, and the ventricle also normal. This case became legend—the first successful treatment of a heart attack with correction of the occluded coronary artery. And in Spokane, all the pieces had been in place: prehospital care, advanced cardiologists who were aggressive and technically excellent with coronary angiograms, heart surgeons with excellent results on the direct coronary artery bypass, and an operating room with teams that were available.

Drs. Everhart, Simpson, and Lang made themselves available for urgent heart catheters with coronary angiogram, knowing the patients tolerated the diagnostic procedure. Drs. Berg and Kendall likewise made themselves available for surgical consult and emergent bypasses of the preinfarct patients with coronary blockages. The protocol was unique.

Referring primary doctors, internists, and ER physicians heard about the team urgently offering the two-sided protocol and procedures. The teamwork between cardiologist and surgeon and their success was impressive. Several referring physicians and other cardiologists started to send their acute patients in. Trained with Mason Sones, Dr. Simpson had no qualms about early catheterization of his patients with the preinfarct syndrome. It was a frustration to him as well as Everhart that this hesitancy still existed. It was to be an uphill battle.

Valley General Hospital had opened in 1969, and several family practice colleagues started a group called Valley Hospital Emergency Services in September of that year. In March 1971, a twenty-nine-year-old male came into the ER with crushing chest pain and an acute myocardial infarction. The young man arrested, and Dr. Charles Wolfe successfully resuscitated him. Dr. Everhart was notified, accepted the patient, and had to again resuscitate him in the cath lab after transfer (Wolfe 2011). Dr. Berg was called and performed a successful emergency direct coronary artery bypass using open-heart with pump technique. This patient, recalling his ambulance ride, reported, "I knew I was going to die." He did not die that day.

When Dr. Robert Hustrulid, a doctor who was indispensable in the creation of this book, arrived in Spokane in the late spring of 1971, what he found was a big deal. Heart attack patients having a heart catheter procedure during the event and then open-heart surgery was a dramatic change. More stunning, these surgery patients lived. "It was huge," he reported. Hustrulid joined his uncle in practice with a large group of internal medicine physicians who were already in support of the protocol (Hustrulid 2011).

Dr. Berg's transposition paper was published in August 1971, just as Jason was turning two. It reminded Ralph that *any surgical procedure was the third cause of death, after heart failure and malnutrition. For Ralph, surgical death could be avoided. He wanted to advance science for this defect. A repair was slow in coming, and the number of transposition babies was few. It was a daunting task* (R. Berg 1971).

The new hospital tower at Sacred Heart opened in November 1971. It was a huge building with long hallways, multiple floors, and multiple times more rooms for patients than the old hospital. It was to be a panacea. The base of the building, with its imaging and operating rooms, had been up and running for a few years.

Soon after the grand opening, Ralph and Nebraska met at the office one morning and walked over to make rounds. They found a new nurse on the chest ward. Instead of two nurses to one open-heart patient, as administration had promised, this nurse had a heart patient by herself and a second patient as well. She gave the precise details to Dr. Berg, who listened. Then he walked into his patient's room and found him dead, with rigor mortis set in.

Berg, calm but incredibly disappointed, shared his finding with this nurse, who was devastated. Dr. Berg went to administration. "It was not the nurse's fault," he began. Administration blamed the lack of financial resources to get the nurse training. To Dr. Berg, patient care and safety always took priority over the finances, and he angrily applied emphasis to this basic principle and the intolerable outcomes without the training. He again taunted the administrator, "Climb the side of your building, pull down the cross, and replace it with your almighty dollar sign." Calm, furious, there was no kiss on her head this time. After this Dr. Berg encounter, administration provided all the cardiac floor nurses the two-day in-service training they needed to care for post-op open-heart patients.

Teaching cardiopulmonary physiology and cardiac dissection, both human and animal, to students at the local community college fit Everhart's academic demeanor. One notable physician assistant student, Mr. Ken Galloway, joined Dr. Everhart's cardiology practice at completion of his degree.

Drs. Everhart, Simpson, Lang, and his group were aggressive and accurate cardiologists who were right almost all the time. They were reliable and excellent coronary angiographers. If they called, the team moved. Dr. Everhart, like Dr. Lang, used the femoral artery approach for his coronary angiograms. Dr. Simpson used the brachial artery exposure. Nebraska could set up the pump in about ten minutes. The operating room took a little longer. They would bring the patient from radiology to the operating room. The CRNA was right there. All in all, it took about thirty minutes to get the surgical procedure started. They had a beeper for notification.

Dr. Everhart restudied his patients with another angiogram before they left the hospital. He noted that in some patients without the second portion of the protocol, surgical treatment, the coronary blockage was opening on the repeat study. He was curious as to why. However, he also noted the heart muscle was not doing well on these repeat studies. Everhart began thinking of other ways to dissolve or remove the offending clot for patients turned down for bypass. Dr. Berg, also curious about these patients, felt the heart muscle not recovering was due to ongoing ischemia, which would explain the ventricular aneurysms he saw over the years in the blue babies and in the chronic angina patients (R. Berg 1976).

Because of his intense interest in cardiac pathology, Everhart attended all postmortems on the patients who passed while under his care. He also advocated for cardiac echo at the hospital during planning for the new cardiac catheterization suite at Sacred Heart Medical Center. He regularly attended the weekly cardiac case conference. He too was pleased when the new hospital tower opened. He liked the "Medical Center" moniker.

Another Valley Hospital ER services doctor gladly activated the new protocol and sent a patient with chest pain and EKG changes to Everhart by ambulance. This patient, who had previously survived a heart attack, was female. A fast cath was initiated, during which she had a dreaded arrhythmia with cardiac arrest. Dr. Everhart resuscitated her. As the patient was reviving, she asked, "Why are you French-kissing me?" Pleased she was conscious and talking, Everhart called for surgical consult, and she was whisked to the OR for emergent direct coronary bypass.

She eventually returned to her family practice doctor—alive, recovered, and able to report about her experience with a smile. Her doctor was incredulous and thankful. Now aware of the protocol, her doctor and family practice group sent more patients (Thiel 2012).

In one case, Dr. Everhart believes he proved, at least to himself, that clot was the causative primary event of the transition from preinfarct to acute heart attack. While imaging a male patient having an acute MI, the right coronary artery was occluded on the first dye injection. This was consistent with the EKG, which showed an inferior infarct. The right coronary artery supplies blood to the inferior wall of the ventricles. Dr. Everhart did four more dye injections, and on each run, he noted first a trickle of dye getting through, then more dye, then retraction of the clot. The patient started with the dreaded arrhythmia, ventricular fibrillation. Dr. Everhart successfully defibrillated him. Dr. Everhart called the surgeons. Dr. Kendall was able to urgently bypass the offending coronary artery with success and patient recovery.

Everhart was once again prompted to think of a clot buster. If the clot could be removed or dissolved in such a way as to immediately restore the coronary artery flow, would that stop the subsequent events of a heart attack? He aggressively treated the preinfarct patients with intravenous fluids—heparin, digoxin, aspirin, pain meds, and the fast cath—with a restudy of the coronary arteries when the patient was stable. All these patients reopened the occluded artery to some degree, but with a notable difference from surgical results. There was no improvement in the ventriculogram, thereby indicating that the performance of the heart muscle was damaged (F. Everhart 2011).

Ralph listened to his team. The nurses who worked with the open-heart surgeons and the cardiologists in the cardiac care units continually noted a difference between the surgical patients and the medically managed patients. This was the case with direct coronary artery bypass as well. Acutes, the next logical step, also had improved results. The Spokane team felt that myocardial preservation was important and that myocardial damage and death could be prevented by coronary artery revascularization in the acute situation.

Ralph was at home one evening when he got a call from one of his trusted referring cardiologists. It was dinnertime, and Mary answered the phone. She gave the phone to Ralph. A fast cath had just been done. The patient presented with an acute emerging heart attack. The results on coronary angiography showed an occlusion of the LAD, the main artery feeding the left ventricle. Ralph agreed, called the operating room, and gave the go to get a room ready. The patient would go to the OR for an open-heart procedure and a direct coronary bypass and ACR. All was set.

Administration, involved in scheduling "add on" cases, called Dr. Berg and said they could only do one open-heart case at a time. "Dr. Berg, you will have to wait," she said. Berg upped the ante and asked, "So you are saying we have to let this patient die?" The reply: "Yes, they will have to die." By the time Dr. Berg was at the hospital and in the operating room, the situation had been corrected, as the staff had prepared a second OR for an acute coronary artery bypass on pump. Berg, and the team, were for the patient.

In 1972, both the open-heart surgeons and the cardiologists involved in the protocol expanded with new doctors. Ralph Berg added the fourth open-heart surgeon to his team. He teased, "I picked him off the streets of Los Angeles and brought him to Spokane, God's country, to show him the light." Dr. John Gangi was technically an excellent heart surgeon. While they worked together, assisting each other in the operating room, Berg would tease Dr. Gangi, who embarrassed easily.

Dr. Henry Lang's new pediatric cardiologist was doing well in Spokane. That year, Henry went to Cleveland Clinic to recruit an adult cardiologist who could do coronary artery angiography. Henry met Dr. Gerry Hensley, they went to dinner and discussed the Spokane practice, and Henry, quite satisfied, asked the young cardiologist to join his practice. Gerry said yes.

Gerry Hensley had started medical school in 1957 at Johns Hopkins. After his first year, he stepped out for five years to do research. Upon his return in 1962, mouth-to-mouth resuscitation breathing was new and being taught to the medical students, who practiced on each other. They placed an IV to medically paralyze and sedate a student, thus inducing a real need for resuscitation breathing. The new cardiopulmonary resuscitation (CPR) techniques were used to sustain the vital signs of the paralyzed medical student, who was then awakened. The students were both eager and serious in their intent to learn CPR. They would switch roles of provider and paralyzed medical student. The dean of the Johns Hopkins School of Medicine thankfully stopped this part of this curriculum. Dr. Hensley graduated from medical school in 1965.

After medical school, he interned at Case Western Reserve University, then was drafted and sent as a flight surgeon to Fairchild Air Force Base in Spokane in 1967. Hensley was impressed with the medical community and the town. He returned to Case Western after military service and did a cardiology fellowship from 1970 to 1972. He learned coronary artery catheterization—entering via the brachial artery, at the elbow, with a small cutdown to expose the artery before it was punctured. After the procedure, the brachial artery needed a repair, usually a stitch.

At Case Western, Dr. Hensley worked in an older building, on older equipment. For example, the angiogram table had to be raised on blocks to gain the lateral view. The crew would raise the patient from flat onto his side, block the patient, and shoot a lateral view with a second dye injection.

Gerry Hensley arrived in Spokane for the second time in June 1972. The Sacred Heart Medical Center building was new, with new equipment, including a radiology table that was moveable. "We did good work," he reported—both on old equipment where he trained and on this new equipment. Under Dr. Henry Lang's influence and with time being an issue, Hensley cross-trained to a groin access into the femoral artery. This arterial access site did save time, as the cutdown and the artery repair were not needed. He found the groin to be quicker access for a fast cath.

Henry Lang occasionally tried to talk to his new partner about the early years of the practice, to explain the big gamble Henry had taken in coming over to Spokane from his academic position as well as needing to take outside jobs in Spokane to make extra money. Hensley listened, but the old days were not so important to him. This transition was a challenge, and there was not a moment of downtime. He was busy at work from the day he started. There were other new cardiology doctors that year also doing the advanced coronary angiograms.

Dr. Hensley recalled being startled about the protocol, both the diagnostics and then the treatment. Where he was trained, doctors still considered it dangerous to perform angiography on heart attack patients. He had never performed a heart catheterization with coronary angiogram on a preinfarct patient, let alone an acute heart attack patient. Nor had he even considered such a step, before coming to Spokane. Dr. Lang reassured his new partner, and Dr. Hensley quickly saw the logic and success of the fast cath protocol. He recalled Dr. Carroll Simpson was a master and a joy to watch while performing the Sones radial artery coronary angiogram technique. He also noted Ralph Berg and Bob Kendall were excellent surgeons.

Dr. Gerry Hensley went to the weekly chest conferences. Fridays at Deaconess and Wednesdays at Sacred Heart, he presented often and at both locations. The conferences were well attended. Dr. Everhart was pleased when Dr. Hensley arrived and tried to get Hensley to join him. When Dr. Henry Lang obtained adult cardiology privileges at Valley General Hospital, he was annoyed to learn Dr. Everhart had attempted an unsuccessful block. While collegial, these three eminent cardiologists were also competitive.

The referring doctors at the new Valley General Hospital had quickly learned to send their acute heart attack patients to Sacred Heart, and they sent Hensley many of their patients (Hensley 2012). At Deaconess, the cardiologists still did not believe in performing coronary angiography on patients with acute heart attacks. The acutes were not getting the fast cath, surgery consult, and direct revascularization at Deaconess as of June 1972.

When the main ward clerk at the brand-new CCU at Deaconess went on vacation, the young wife of Ken Galloway, PA for Dr. Everhart, filled in. Karla, not trained, was overwhelmed, and the work was intense. She said it was this work—which she quickly mastered, with the new coronary angiograms, the drama of the open-heart patients, and the heart teams coming through the doors postoperative for intensive care—that inspired her to go to nursing school for her RN degree. Lots of young people in Spokane were inspired by these teams and these heart advances (Galloway 2011).

Dr. Carroll Simpson became president of the Washington chapter of the American Heart Association in 1972. He was aware the new coronary angiograms were not widely used or accepted. When one referring doctor talked with him about a patient with any heart issue, he asked Simpson, "Right heart or left heart?"—referring to the standard of blue-baby imaging prior to 1959.

As president, Dr. Simpson made trips to Seattle to meet with cardiac providers on the west side of the state. This was when he became aware that the other side of the state "thought Spokane was nuts." The cardiologists and heart surgeons there used the Levine approach, and a few were advancing to coronary angiogram, with treatment mainly Vineberg; a few performed direct coronary artery bypass on the chronic angina patients (Simpson 2011).

Waiting was still the standard for the entire country, if not the world. Doctors delayed an open-heart surgical referral until the patient was stable and the infarct was complete. Dr. Berg commented, "The poor open-heart surgeon was at the mercy of the referring cardiologist, who would wait until the patient was almost dead." He went on, "Complications like electrical dysrhythmia, infarct extension, or organ failure before calling in a surgeon was the more likely scenario than a hope for a stable completed infarct. This new protocol was a big difference, to go straight away to fast cath, surgical consult, and then the operating room for a successful early coronary artery bypass before the myocardial damage was irreversible. The only rest for a heart is on pump, not in a bed."

During this time, Dr. Carroll Simpson and his wife were driving to visit the Seattle area in his role as AMA president when he rolled his car at 60 mph. Thankfully he and his wife were all right. Carroll was busy at the Rockwood Clinic, but he had not realized how tired he was until this dramatic wake-up call. He set up satellite clinics and took a large portion of the overnight calls. There were a lot of cardiologists in town, a lot of competition. Carroll and his wife began thinking of ways to decrease his workload.

The Spokane doctors and nurses continued to witness acute coronary syndrome patients not only surviving but also recovering and doing well. The CCU was full of both medical and surgical heart attack patients, often in beds next to each other. The surgery patients were usually up and walking around, with fewer arrhythmias and shorter times to discharge than the medically treated patients. The nurses who cared for this group frequently suggested that the cardiologists with patients in the CCU consider a surgical consult (S. Shields 2011). Many cardiologists, internists, and family practice doctors began calling Dr. Everhart to arrange surgical care for their heart patients. Everhart was known to have access to the heart surgeons. On June 21, 1972, Dr. Everhart became certified by the American Board of Internal Medicine.

At chest conference and with his research, from 1970 to 1973, Everhart and the cardiologists following the protocol studied a total of sixty-five patients with a fast cath, surgical consultation, and surgical coronary revascularization. Of these sixty-five, two-thirds were Dr. Everhart's patients and one-third were from other cardiologists. During these three years, Dr. Shields sent his acute myocardial infarct patients to Dr. Everhart. Physician assistant Mr. Ken Galloway worked on the background for this paper—the data organization and analysis. Ken also helped Dr. Everhart in the office and with patient care. This cohort generated the first research paper, entitled "Early Acute Myocardial Infarction – A Surgical Emergency." True to his word to Ralph Berg, Dr. Everhart did the research, submitted the paper, and would present this work in Buenos Aires in September of the next year, 1974.

CHAPTER 15

Father and Son, the Anchoring Shot, 1973

Before the end of 1972, Nebraska and Julie both knew Ralph Berg was focused on creating a dog model for transposition of the great vessels—Jason's defect. Ralph was happy as a lark with his plan. A switch of the great vessels was the basic concept, both to create the model as well as the planned repair. Additional shunts for mixing of the circulations to maintain the dog until the corrective switch could be done was the challenge. Berg was convinced they would eventually get the dog model to work. Dr. Adib Jatene (1929–2014) in Brazil and Dr. Augie Senning in Switzerland were also working on transposition defects.

Julie Spores, one of the few people who understood both lines of work—the blue babies, especially Jason, and the acute heart attack research—was aware of the special burden this created on Ralph. He was private at work about the dog-lab plans. When he asked Julie, a trusted team member, she eagerly agreed to help revamp the dog lab. She soon discovered that when the main operating rooms had moved into the basement of the new building, the ORs on the fourth floor of the old hospital building were left unused and available. Berg noted they were superior to the old dog lab in the basement (Spores 2011).

Frustrated over his son's dilemma, Dr. Berg held a steady course. In his own words, Ralph felt that the crown of chest surgery is open-heart. The jewels in this crown are the blue babies. Open-heart procedures with the heart-lung machine brought hope and successful repairs to the blue babies. This pioneering heart surgeon and parent of a blue baby without a surgical repair was in a dynamic that had to lead to success, to that last jewel—Jason, so much more than a child late in life.

An avid hunter and precision shooter, Ralph had talked about his ideal safari hunting trip for years. The planning was getting serious. He wanted to go for a month. Mary also wanted to go. She had no interest in hunting, but she loved to travel and was an avid photographer. Jason was doing remarkably well as a three-year-old, and the two older children still living at home were willing and able to take care of him. Bob Kendall also wanted to go. That meant the two senior surgeons would be out for a month.

The surgical work from the cardiologists doing coronary angiography for their angina patients was still growing. The fast caths for the acute heart attack patients were also growing. These cases were more complex and disruptive. Not being scheduled, they needed emergency surgical care. Dr. Berg had the acute cases covered by the surgical group in such a way that the elective cases were not impacted by the acutes, or at least minimally so. Could the workload and the call coverage be handled by the two junior open-heart surgeons? It would mean every other night on call and covering two hospitals.

Ralph looked at the numbers. The most recent addition, the fourth surgeon in the Berg Surgical Group, could operate. The coronary bypass operation was technically challenging and demanded precision, and the fourth surgeon had solid outcomes with both the elective chronic angina and the emergent acute heart attack cases. It had taken over ten years to reach the 1,000 open-heart cases they celebrated at Christmas 1970. It took just two more years to reach 2,000, marked with another big celebration at Christmas 1972. Now it was early 1973, and the Berg Surgical Group was on pace to perform 1,000 cases that year.

Ralph's records predicted eight cases a week at Deaconess, twelve at Sacred Heart. Drs. Everhart and Simpson were both looking for partners, younger cardiologists who could do the coronary angiograms. Dr. Henry Lang's pediatric cardiologist and Dr. Gerry Hensley were both working, yet Dr. Lang was still too busy. Berg realized the surgical work, particularly the coronary revascularization cases, were growing so rapidly that regardless of the monthlong safari, the Berg Surgical Group needed a fifth pair of hands.

Berg committed to the safari. Ads looking for a locum tenens open-heart surgeon for that month of May, with the hope to hire on permanently, went out. Three surgeons who could operate would be safe while Berg and Kendall were gone. Before too long, Dr. Lloyd Rudy, chairman of surgery at the University of Georgia, answered the advertisement. Salaried at $46,000 annually, working twenty-hour days with all the responsibilities of teaching residents and operating, he wanted to leave Georgia and get back to his home territory, the Northwest.

Lloyd had researched Dr. Ralph Berg and was pleased when Berg called. He reported, "Berg got through the pleasantries quickly." Berg listened as Lloyd told of his connection to the Northwest. Then Dr. Berg asked him, "Can you operate?" which took Dr. Rudy aback. It was more than a challenge. Dr. Rudy let Dr. Berg know he could operate, including the coronary bypass procedure. Berg hired him for the monthlong locum position. Lloyd was going to show Berg that not only could he operate, he could operate better than Dr. Ralph Berg.

Influenced by Dr. Merendino, Dr. Rudy had watched open-heart cases from the observation deck of the new university hospital while in medical school back in 1959. He went on to train in general and chest surgery at the University of California, San Francisco. He "got boarded" in 1966, in both thoracic and general surgery. Then drafted, he went to Thailand and ran a MASH unit. He came home in August 1969. The University of California decided he needed additional training, a reflection of the advances in open-heart and the impingement of acquired coronary artery disease. Lloyd did an additional year of training with Dr. Shumway at Stanford University Medical Center.

Dr. Rudy arrived in Spokane for the month of May 1973. His first impression of Ralph Berg: "Here is a guy with five other kids. Jason was his sixth. Ralph appears to have the world by the tail, all the positives, including beautiful wife, lots of money. He was hard to figure out" (Rudy 2011).

May went well enough from Dr. Lloyd Rudy's perspective. The African safari also went well, for the first two weeks. Then, Kendall reported, he woke up at camp one day, expecting to hunt, and found Ralph and Mary gone. The guide came back from the airport and reported that a sandstorm had prompted the Bergs to leave. Kendall noted the hunting was good in the days after the sandstorm.

On the weekend that Secretariat won the second leg of the Triple Crown at the Preakness, Ralph and Mary showed up unannounced in Belgium to visit with his brother, Mike, Virginia, and their kids. First, they had hopped a plane from Africa and headed to Switzerland to visit with Dr. Augie Senning, who was having some success with the next level of great vessel switch, above the atria for transposition defects. Unfortunately, Senning was away. Disappointed, the Bergs flew on to Brussels. Ralph's brother was happy to pick them up at the airport.

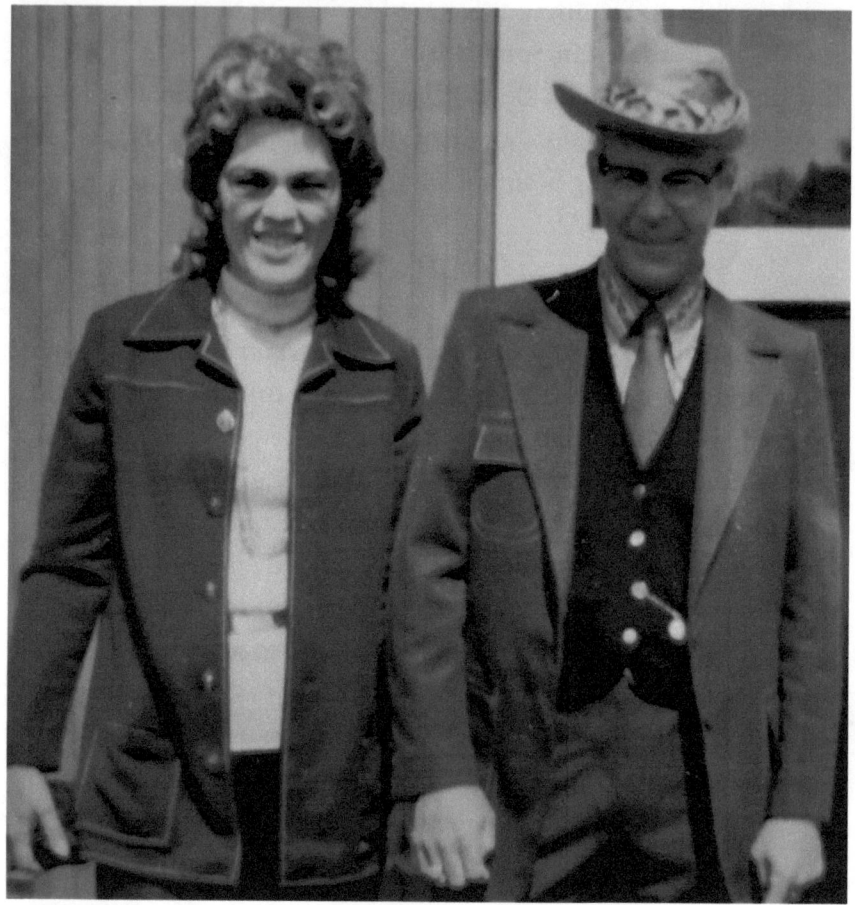

Disappointed during their safari, May 1973, Ralph and Mary flew on to Brussels. Ralph's brother, Mike, was happy to pick them up at the airport.

Virginia was stunned at the magnitude and spontaneity of the visit. It was a whirlwind weekend visit with a trip to Chateau d' Havre, champagne, fresh whipped cream and strawberries, sightseeing, and the next day the men were shooting at the range. Mike was finishing his three-year military service at Supreme Headquarters, Allied Powers Europe (SHAPE), and planned to move his family home to Spokane that summer. At the time, I was on a school field trip to Weimar,

Germany, to see Buchenwald. I learned of Ralph and Mary's surprise visit later from my family.

Upon returning to Spokane a few days earlier than planned from their safari, Ralph and Mary found their Melinda Lane house had sold. With the three older boys moved out, they no longer needed the multibedroom home, and Mary was in the process of having a house built on Sunset Hill. In the meantime, she and Ralph moved to a condominium on Twenty-Ninth Avenue with their three youngest children. The condo next door was also available, and Mary asked for a hold, thinking about Mike and Virginia. Rory soon opened a record store, Looney Tunes, about four blocks away.

Dr. Berg reviewed the work of the locum surgeon. He talked with the cardiologists and his established Berg Group surgeons. The report was good. He hired Dr. Lloyd Rudy on a one-year contract, with an option to make partner.

A brief respite occurred amid the whirlwind of Spokane life. The Bergs arranged a "Welcome to Spokane" pool party for Dr. Rudy and several other doctors who were coming to Spokane. Cardiologist Dr. Tom Mouser, who had left Spokane for an academic position at West Virginia University School of Medicine, was returning to work with Dr. Simpson. And Spokane itself was getting ready for a historic event, Expo '74. It was a beautiful, sunny day in July 1973. All the families and children at the pool party were swimming, relaxing, getting to know each other and Spokane. The success at work with the heart attack patients was openly discussed. No one talked about Jason's condition; Ralph and Mary were private, especially about Jason.

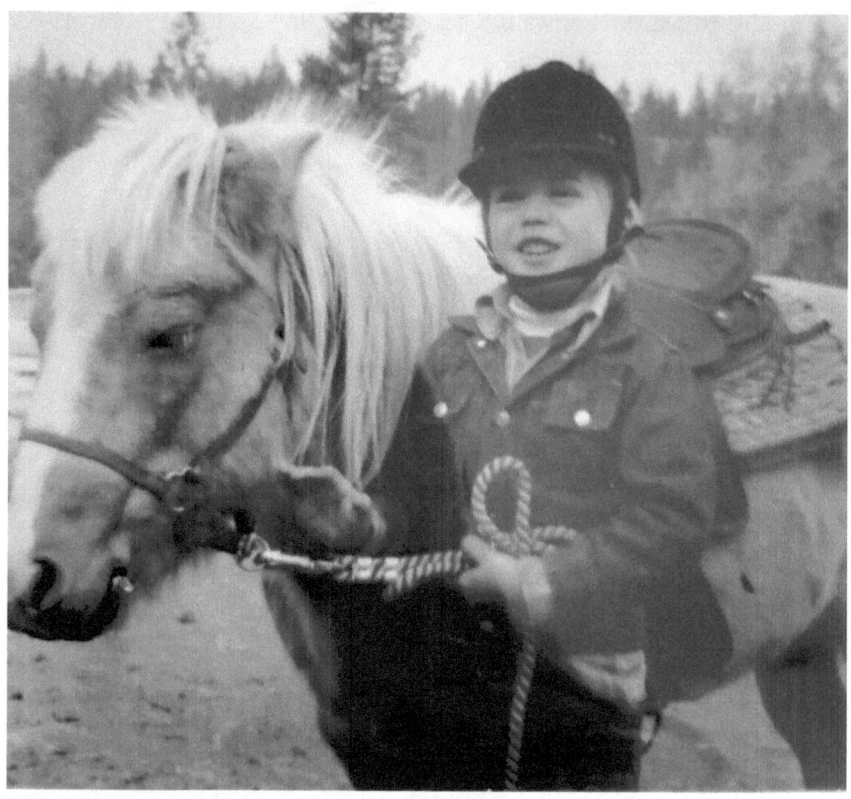

Jason on the pony, late summer 1973.

Cardiologist Dr. Mouser quickly settled into his work with Dr. Simpson. They shared the on-call burden, taking every other night call at the hospital. Fortunately, their group, Rockwood, only covered one hospital, Sacred Heart. One or more fast caths for acute heart attacks could be performed on any given night. The acutes happened anytime. Their large cardiology group had many patients with chronic angina, and the occasional conversion into an acute heart attack was not unexpected.

Dr. Mouser, calm and scientific, was an excellent angiographer. "As a new field, coronary arteriography brought questions over the science of heart attacks," he explained. At the weekly case conference, he saw the value of myocardial preservation by correcting with a saphenous vein bypass. Their team understood the newer care delivery of coronary imaging and direct coronary bypass for the adult acquired heart disease patients (Mouser 2011).

Myocardial preservation was the key. Infarct completion was associated with permanent heart muscle damage, so they went into the hospital for middle-of-the-night fast caths with patients who came in through the emergency department with all varieties of chest pain and EKG changes. It was busy. It was exhausting. It was successful, and it changed medicine forever.

Shock Trauma, a unit of the University of Maryland Medical Center solely dedicated to the care of trauma victims, opened in 1973. The Maryland Institute for Emergency Medical Services System, MIEMSS, was also started. This statewide entity to coordinate, improve, and develop the delivery of emergency services to the residents of Maryland is based on the "Spokane Experience"—the emergency medical service plan in place that allowed the Spokane Ambulance company drivers and attendants to provide lifesaving medical care and give the hospital all the information it needed to ready itself.

A young anesthetist in training, Maggie Myers, was interested in hearts. She liked the challenge. Her training was to finish in the late fall of 1973. Julie Spores, Carmen, Donna, and Ester were the nurse anesthetist team at Sacred Heart, and Julie was looking for a nurse anesthetist they could train for the heart team, as one team member was leaving.

The invitation from Julie was casual. "Come to the dog lab this Saturday," Julie said after a Monday case. "The researchers pay twenty-five dollars. Ralph is doing a procedure. You may as well get paid."

Maggie knew the team did research and that Julie did data collection for their research of heart attacks. However, it was a surprise to Maggie that there was a dog lab. But Maggie agreed. She knew the dog was already on "death row" at the pound and that the potential value of the information gained from this work was real.

She went that Saturday with Julie Spores. They arrived at 7 a.m. The lab was in a caesarean section OR in the old hospital building, not yet remodeled. The lab was a single isolated operating room with a substerile room and a supply area attached. It was a full operating room, with all the plumbing, lighting, and an anesthesia setup. There was the same type of bypass pump machine as was used in the main operating room.

They started an IV on the dog, induced, intubated, and put all the same lines in the dog as they did in the main OR. All the equipment was sized for the dogs. They used Seratol instead of Pentothal as the paralytic agent. There was a standard ventilator. It took about a half hour to prepare the dog. Julie placed a femoral line. They had two peripheral intravenous lines and a central line. Julie had an anesthesia cart with all the necessary supplies needed. While they were getting ready, Ralph would walk in and see how they were doing, make his comment—"Fits and starts, fits and starts"—and walk out, not bothering them. The surgical scrub technician and sterile technique were no different from what Maggie had trained to do in her schooling and in the main OR.

Finally ready, Ralph made a chest incision. He used a hand sternotomy knife instead of the mechanical saw; the dogs almost never had a thoracotomy. They went on pump. Ralph was transplanting the coronaries. This was stage one of an attempt to create a dog model for transposition of the great vessels and then reverse or correct it. He was doing a technical procedure to create this model on a healthy dog who was not born with the defect. Dr. Berg anticipated cutting the great vessels below the takeoff of the coronaries for the repair (Myers 2012).

Anticipating stability and grateful to Mary, Virginia Berg moved her family into the condominium next door to Ralph and Mary. It was late summer in 1973, and school was starting in a few days. Virginia hoped to move into a nice house before too long.

Mike arrived a week later. The two Berg couples arranged the first meeting with Jason and his closest cousin in age, Cathy, just eight months younger and second daughter to Mike and Virginia. The four parents were anxious. Jason, with his complex heart defect, was fragile. Yet at times, he was indomitable. The adults hovered as the three-year-old cousins met on the living room floor in Mike and Virginia's condo.

Mike's youngest daughter was curious about Jason because he was blue. She found it confusing. "It was like having an alien plopped down with me, then being told, 'This is your cousin Jason.'" *What is a cousin, and why is he blue? thought this young Berg.*

Jason picked up a little plastic elephant figurine and held it in his hand. His younger cousin had a whole set of these animal figurines and had never noticed the bluish cast of the elephant until it was in Jason's fingers. Suddenly she was sure Jason was getting his blue on her toys. She did not want him to touch anything else. However, she was also fascinated by him, and from the view of their parents, all seemed to be going well (C. Berg 2010). Soon Jason was walking next door by himself. He liked the chaos at his cousin's house.

Dr. Rudy found work with the Berg Surgical Group intense. There was a huge backlog of chronic angina/chest pain cases where an elective surgical coronary bypass was needed. The cardiologists, referring physicians, and nurses all noted that some of the acute patients were previously on the chronic angina list. Drs. Lloyd Rudy and John Gangi, the two youngest Berg surgeons, took weekend call at the main hospital, Sacred Heart. They split this call obligation into one week on with a weekend day followed by one week off with the other weekend day. It kept them in town working for a week, and then they each took a week off. Lloyd and John got to know the cardiologists, as the work was intense, fast paced, and demanding at all hours of the day and night and for all the doctors. The history of the work—the foundation with the blue babies and the heart-lung machine development and implementation—did not seem relevant to Lloyd nor to the other heart surgeons. The crush of heart attack patients was the pressing work at hand. To them, unaware of the dilemma Dr. Ralph Berg faced with complex transposition, Ralph certainly looked like he had it all; his extreme intensity was therefore a mystery (Rudy 2011).

Nebraska brought a dog for each lab. He made the rounds to the local animal shelters, picked a dog, paid for it. The concept: to switch the great vessels congenitally attached to the opposite sides of the heart, resulting in two separate circulations instead of an in-line circulation with pump functionality. Creating the model was done in two stages. First, they created both an ASD and VSD. They changed or altered the intrachamber pressures by banding the pulmonary artery with a piece of Teflon. They would take the intrachamber pressures and adjust the band. When the pressures were close to even across both septal defects, they would sew the band down at that position, then wait to see how the dog responded. If the dog was okay, they would come off pump and awaken the modeled dog.

They had created and used both an ASD and a VSD model before, with a couple of weeks in between for the dog to recover. But the model with both an ASD and a VSD was difficult. Still, Dr. Berg loved to figure things out. As the dog labs pushed on, the work was slow. Not all the dogs made it through the recovery. At the second staged procedure, the dogs died, most with lethal arrhythmias. Berg expected failures, but when there were no successes, it was humbling. Ralph, successful with esophageal atresia, blue-baby repairs, acquired coronary artery disease, and heart attacks, was struggling.

The schedule for the lab stated 7 a.m. to 12 noon. Maggie was never involved in the dog recovery. She did about eight of these labs over the summer of 1973, on Saturday mornings when Dr. Berg was not on call. "Ralph never talked about Jason in the dog lab; however, there was no question what he was doing," said Maggie. Henry Lang was there with Dr. Berg but not at every dog lab. No other doctors or surgeons were in the dog lab. Maggie was aware that she was not to talk of these dog labs; she was also aware the dogs were not surviving (Myers 2012).

Berg kept adding more modifications to the two shunts. Jason's future repair was always on his mind.

Frustrated, Dr. Berg called his colleagues in Switzerland and Brazil. He learned both were unencumbered by litigation and animal cruelty advocates. He also learned neither Drs. Senning nor Jatene were using a model. Dr. Jatene in Brazil, as part of his definitive repair, wanted to move the coronary artery takeoffs from the aorta. Ralph understood this aspect of the problem. The new direct coronary bypass had started on the proximal coronary artery, landing past the offending plaque onto the distal coronary artery. The proximal was moved up onto the aorta as the takeoff point during the dog-model phase, for its better blood pressure and supply. Dr. Senning figured out how to reimplant the coronary arteries onto the corrected or switched great vessel.

Toward the end of the weekly dog labs, obtaining a dog became an issue. Nebraska had a harder and harder time answering the shelter workers about why he needed a dog every week. Worried, he resorted to grabbing stray dogs if he could. He was under suspicion at the dog pound facilities. Maggie noted with humor that Nebraska, a big Black man, was the most notorious team member for this job.

When Maggie graduated from anesthesia school with over 100 open-heart cases on her case list, she was hired by Sacred Heart to work with the open-heart team.

Panic was not an option. Ralph did not talk much about it. He was deeply in this race; as far as he was concerned, a repair *would* be available. But these research sessions were painful. The team kept quiet.

Every day that Jason was okay was a positive. But by late summer, Ralph Berg painfully realized that he could not make science move for his blue baby. He only ever expressed his deep grief about this situation indirectly.

At Jason's fourth birthday party in late August, the extended family got together. Jason was to start preschool at the local grade school. Virginia had found a house—later affectionately called "the Big House" by the teenagers who likened it to a prison because they knew it rankled Virginia—and they were moving. Ralph marveled at his son, a happy child who carried on. Jason was a mystery to Ralph.

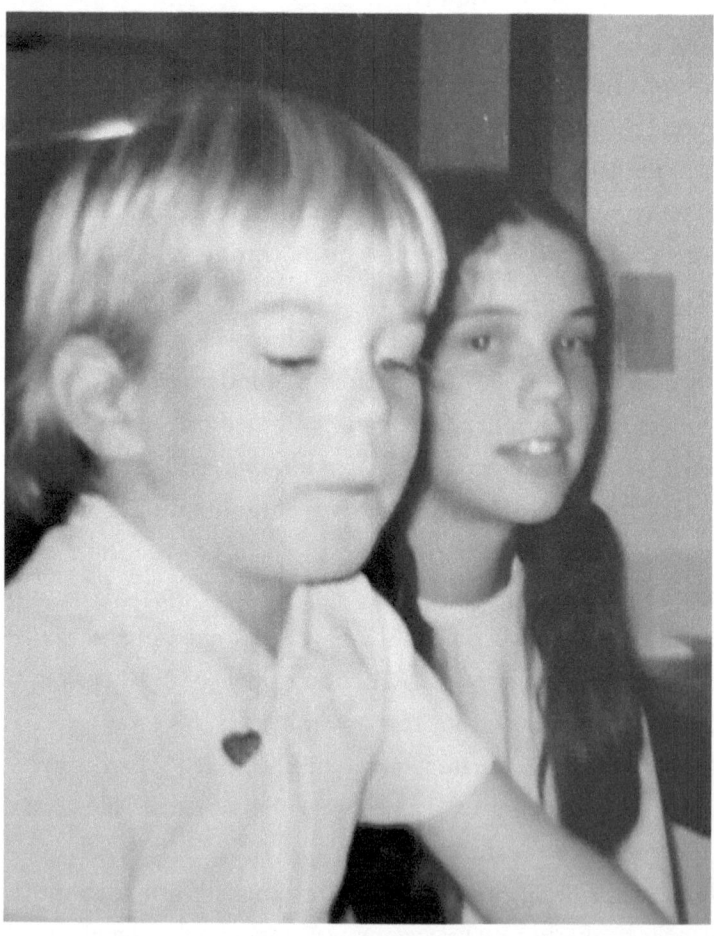

Tracy and Jason at his birthday party, August 1973.

CHAPTER 16

Rejection

Expo '74 opened in May. The population of Spokane had more than quadrupled in preparation, and it exploded with visitors. Mike and Virginia, now the parents of four children, got passes for their three oldest. The first several times, they went as a family, noting the similarities to their years in Belgium. Soon the kids went with their friends. At Jason's fifth birthday party in late August, Expo '74 was in full swing. Mary warned Virginia, my mother, to keep a close eye on me, as I was tall and rail thin. Mary knew from her years of watching Jason that something was wrong. My dentist had found seven small cavities and told Virginia as much.

Acute coronary revascularization in Spokane was in its fourth year, being done well and successfully. However, far from being accepted or taught in the medical schools or chest surgical residencies, many centers were just starting open-heart surgical care. Focused on valve replacements, the simpler intracardiac septal defects, and maybe coronary artery bypass for chronic angina patients, most centers felt acute heart attack patients carried too much risk. The approach to hearts and heart attacks for the broad medical community was still a no-touch, "do no harm" philosophy.

Dr. Everhart, preparing his first scientific research paper, noted that the first sixty-five acute coronary artery bypass patients on the protocol had a 5 percent mortality. This was before intra-aortic balloon pumps and included ten patients who were turned down for surgery and were therefore treated only medically. Dr. Everhart said the group of surgically acutely revascularized patients' mortality dropped over the four years and came to an average of 5 percent. The patients treated only medically had a stable 20 percent mortality for the same lesions shown on coronary angiography. Everhart was excited and wanted to share these results.

On September 3, 1974, Dr. Francis Everhart presented this work at the World Congress of Cardiology in Buenos Aires, Argentina. Dr. Everhart was medically aggressive, giving intravenous fluids, heparin, digoxin for arrhythmias, rest, and pain meds and restudying the blocked vessels via angiography. All ten patients turned down for ACR as being too high risk for surgery showed reopening of the artery to some degree, but a notable difference was there was no improvement in the ventriculogram. With the clot shrinking, Dr. Everhart felt the clot was a consequence of the ruptured plaque in the coronary artery. The performance of the heart muscle was still impaired. He explained that Dr. Berg felt this was due to ongoing lack of blood flow.

At the end of his presentation, Dr. Francis Everhart's scientific results were not accepted by the audience of cardiology experts. At the conference he was called "a fool." These cardiologists were not able to get beyond their impression of the fast cath as foolishly dangerous. However, despite the audience's reaction, the presentation titled "Early Acute Myocardial Infarction – A Surgical Emergency?" would be published. Drs. Everhart and Berg continued the protocol. Each voluntary addition of a referring doctor or a cardiologist brought patients and their families into the two-tiered program. As the success grew, so did the number of patients, and the scientific data grew. The rejection was real, and yet the diagnostics and treatment saved lives and was known to be successful (F. Everhart 2011).

Dr. Kleaveland, chief of staff at Sacred Heart Hospital that year, got pulled into a committee set up by administration to deal with Dr. Francis Everhart. Everhart defended himself. He questioned how a limited and nonmedically-trained understanding of their ACR work could be a platform for the administration to attempt to force patterns of behavior between any doctor and patient. The gap between them was tense. Kleaveland, of course, wanted Dr. Everhart to continue the ACR work. "We need someone like Dr. Francis Everhart to take on this work," he reminded the administrator. He recommended that Dr. Everhart's work continue and felt that he had mellowed administration's ire. Unfortunately, she loaded her committee with young, impressionable doctors, including Dr. Hustrulid, which would come into play later.

A newspaper article came out November 1, 1974, in the morning *Spokane Review*: "Heart Attacks Cut" by Bill Salquist, who had interviewed Dr. Everhart about his first research paper with the protocol.

> A fifty-year-old man in apparent good health experiences sudden chest pains and slumps to the ground while running to catch the bus home. Heart attack? Perhaps. A health care professional would know. The prognosis? Nationally, a person who suffers a true heart attack, one which involves death of part of the heart muscle, has about a 70 % chance of survival, providing he reaches the hospital.
>
> If the patient is hospitalized and receives the usual medical treatment in a coronary care unit, his chances of survival increase dramatically. Only 15 % of those so treated die as a result of the damage to the heart if they are under age 65. But a new technique being pioneered here suggests that the mortality rate may be cut still further—perhaps by as much as two-thirds. The evidence from a study which began here in 1971 was presented by Spokane cardiologist Dr. Francis Everhart last month at the Seventh World Congress of Cardiology in Buenos Aires, Argentina. The paper was entitled "Early Acute Myocardial Infarction—Surgical Emergency?"

Bypass Used: The procedure, which has demonstrated so much potential here, explained Dr. Everhart in a recent interview, involves early coronary bypass surgery to restore blood circulation to the heart and minimize subsequent damage to heart muscle. Time is apparently the critical factor in achieving the lower mortality rate, 4.6 % in the study of 65 patients. If the emergency bypass is performed within six to eight hours of the heart attack, the lower mortality rate appears likely. Beyond that critical time, the advantages of quick surgical revascularization are less certain and traditional medical treatment may offer equal or better chances for survival, he said.

Experience Cited: Had the operated patients received traditional medical treatment, which usually includes two to three weeks of hospitalization, nearly three times as many would have been expected to die, according to statistical evaluation, if the surgical experience in Spokane continues with the present results. With a six-to-eight-hour time limit between the onset of symptoms and the surgical procedure, quick response is necessary on the part of everyone from the victim to his physician. "The only way this procedure can be successful is with a completely organized city. Spokane is about five to ten years ahead of its time in this respect," said Dr. Everhart. The prompt actions necessary for the success of the early surgery likely could not be achieved in a larger city where distances are greater and reaction time, necessarily, slower.

Group Credited: Dr. Everhart credited the local chapter of the Washington Heart Association with helping to speed the reaction time. The association has been active in promoting emergency medical training for ambulance attendants so they can spot suspected heart attack victims and react quickly. The association also has been active in public education programs to help individuals recognize the tell-tale symptoms of a heart attack and seek immediate medical care. Dr. Everhart noted that quick surgical treatment of heart attack victims is not indicated in all cases: "The suggestion is that if the heart attack only involves one vessel, the risk is the same whether the person is treated medically or surgically. But if two or three vessels are involved, the chances appear better with surgery."

Procedure Risky: The extent of involvement can only be accurately assessed by catheterization, a procedure which some cardiologists reject as too risky on persons who have just suffered heart attacks. While bypass surgery is generally accepted procedure for various coronary heart diseases, the treatment of heart attacks as surgical emergencies remains highly controversial, Dr. Everhart said. Preliminary evidence, however, indicates that Spokane residents who undergo prompt surgical treatment for heart attacks have a better chance of survival than others for whom such treatment is not available. (Sallquist 1974)

It was an accurate article, and Dr. Everhart was pleased. Scientific findings and changes to older established therapies are never easy. Francis hoped this positive press might help with his problem at the hospital. Regardless of the administration's follies, it was an exciting time. The public took note and sought out this care for family and friends with chest pain.

Meanwhile, my mother was worried about me and acted on Mary Berg's advice. At the pediatrician's office, I explained how much I was eating—more food than anyone in the family—but I was getting thinner and thinner. The doctor examined me and said to both of us, "Tracy is starving herself because she wants to be noticed."

At the dinner table that evening, my brothers shared how impressed they were by how much water I could chug. My dad consulted with Ralph. About a week later, I was taken to see Dr. Henry Lang, who knew my diagnosis before we met. He was kind, knowledgeable, and accurate. Lang explained the hunger, the thirst, and the weight loss, then admitted me into the new Sacred Heart tower with type I diabetes.

This diagnosis felt like a failure on my part. Dr. Lang skipped over my negativity and projected my success. He visited me every day, often in the evening, sitting on the bed and talking to me like his equal: "Tracy, you will do well. You are smart, and you will be able to manage this." He taught me the history of insulin's discovery, the improvements since 1921. He offered details about how to succeed with my new condition and advised me to never be afraid of it. Lang further boosted me: "Expect new technology and embrace it." I missed Thanksgiving, had few visitors, but loved my nurses, and on the last day, Dr. Lang arranged an office appointment in a few weeks, explaining he wanted to know how I was doing.

Dr. Rudy noted that the majority of the acutes came in at night; he and John Gangi did the night calls. "As surgeons, our mortality for elective direct coronary bypass operations was only 1.5% to 2%. We had a mortality rate of only 2.5% in our first 100 acute coronary revascularization patients," he explained. Dr. Rudy shook his head as he accentuated how difficult it was to convince his colleagues outside of Spokane to take acute heart attacks to the operating room.

He recalls that the Berg surgeons would meet regularly, separate from the hospital case conferences. At one of these meetings, concerned with a disparity in surgeon results, Berg and the other open-heart surgeons discussed the golden time to reperfuse the myocardium via a direct coronary artery bypass after myocardial infarction: six hours. Dr. Lloyd Rudy stated, "Spokane, Washington, with a surrounding population of 300,000, is actually a small town of 10,000. Anybody who worked for us had to live within ten minutes of the hospital. We say the golden period is six hours. If they have chest pain and get to the ambulance, the EKG shows ST changes, and fast cath shows coronary artery occlusion, well, let's operate" (Rudy 2011).

The second research paper from Dr. Everhart showed more of the fast cath angiographic data and had seventy-one patients. Titled "Angiography of the Acute Evolving Myocardial Infarction," it was presented in San Juan, Puerto Rico, at the annual American College of Cardiology meeting on February 25, 1975. In both of Dr. Everhart's papers, the acute myocardial infarction mortality treated with urgent coronary revascularization was well below 10 percent and decreased if other vessels were revascularized. The reaction to this paper was again flat-out rejection—difficult to accept in the face of superior results.

For his paper on the surgical treatment of the preinfarct or evolving myocardial infarct patient, Dr. Berg wanted to have one hundred patients; he had ninety-six since data collection started in 1970 with the first acute emerging heart attack and coronary revascularization (R. Berg 1975). But the success with ACR was clearly high. Dr. Ralph Berg presented the work in May 1975 at the annual thoracic meeting in New York, and the presentation went well. Mary and Jason were in the audience. There was silence when he finished speaking. Ralph had expected some criticism and certainly discussion. Instead, he got shock, awe, and silence from his audience of thoracic surgeons. He walked off the stage, and the program moved on.

This moment changed Ralph Berg's life. When this paper was published, the world's reaction was much more effusive than that audience of surgeons. It needed to know more. The phone calls and letters from heart surgeons all over the country started. Years later, when Ralph talked about this, he reported that the scientific standards had changed. A paper with close to a hundred cases was a profound piece of work; however, the new scientific standards demanded case controls. The mechanics of a heart attack were still not understood. The ongoing debate about the clot and what it meant needed to be answered before treatment, mortality, and survival could become the focus.

After the presentation, Ralph, Mary, and Jason went to dinner. It was Jason's first trip to New York, and he liked the big buildings. While riding the elevator back to their room at the end of the day, all three were quiet. Ralph and Mary were winding down, tired. The person riding in the elevator with them broke the silence by commenting on Jason. "He is short, lips dusky; he has a major problem with his . . . ?" It was a bold query from a stranger. Before the person could finish or his parents could protect, Jason retorted, "At least I'm not a fat cow!" Apparently, the person was chubby. Both his parents cracked slight smiles, quietly staring. Even then, Jason had a keen awareness of his dad's influence on his longevity and sought to protect his parents with a blunt, humorous diversion.

Upon returning from New York, Ralph and Mary found their new house on Sunset Hill was ahead of schedule on construction but not ready for move-in. The Berg family would stay at the condominium until the house was finished.

Severe criticism locally and regionally of ACR was followed by international recognition. The era of acute coronary revascularization had arrived. Dr. Ralph Berg received invitations to speak at academic and community hospitals with open-heart programs. Many of the hospitals and medical groups implemented Ralph Berg's ideas, protocols, and procedures. Many letters asked about how his heart team was constructed.

In 1975, Dr. Gerry Hensley, now chairman of the cardiology department at Sacred Heart, was aware that administration thought Dr. Everhart was mean, possibly mentally disturbed, and had come before committees previously. Dr. Hensley shared in this opinion and advised the committee to vote to suspend Dr. Everhart of his privileges. Despite strong objections from many in the committee, Hensley held the committee's "feet to the fire." The committee was forced to vote; a split decision resulted, and the chair called for a suspension of

Dr. Everhart from the staff of Sacred Heart Medical Center for four months, from July to November 1975.

Dr. Everhart knew the ACR work was saving lives and the demand for it would endure. His side of the two-tiered protocol showed the occluded artery was the cause of the heart attack, and the entire group of doctors that liked the results were eagerly engaging the protocol. Francis had privileges at Deaconess Hospital, and so he worked there exclusively for those months. After he was reinstated in the fall at Sacred Heart, he continued to practice unlimited invasive cardiology (Judge 2012; D. F. Everhart 2011).

About the same time as Everhart's suspension, Ralph Berg was surprised when the Berg Surgical Group embraced the local rejection of the ACR work. The local rejection did not last long. However, the four junior Berg surgeons felt empowered by the rejection. They informed Berg that they found him difficult and demanding. They did not want to perform to this level of emergency surgical care for the acute heart attack patients. Using a clause in Dr. Berg's original contract with Kendall, they excused Ralph Berg from the Berg Surgical Group.

When Drs. Berg and Kendall had started their practice as partners, they had drawn up a partnership agreement. They both had attorneys. Ralph's attorney died during this process, and the final contract was not reviewed by an advocate for Ralph. There was a clause that allowed a partner to be terminated without cause. This clause was used at this time to retire Ralph Berg early. There were other issues. Kendall particularly did not like the name Berg Surgical Group. The four surgeons did not like the retirement financials. To avoid lawsuits, the issue was taken to arbitration. Arbitration ruled in favor of the breakup.

Of course, Ralph had no intention of retiring. He said, "It was the best thing that ever happened." He was not concerned. He understood how the competition and the success of ACR would advantage his surgical skill and keep pressure on the former surgical partners, who despite their complaints needed to perform surgery to stay in business. Ralph went off with one pump and one pump tech after the split.

The ACR work continued, and soon the demands for acute revascularization were such that Dr. Berg needed to devise a call arrangement, as all the cardiologists called Dr. Berg for their patients. The Berg surgical call for acutes evenly involved all the heart surgeons at both hospitals. In this way, the former Berg Surgical Group heart surgeons were not able to avoid performing emergent coronary artery bypasses.

Berg knew Dr. Everhart's theory about heart attacks and their treatment was correct. He described Dr. Everhart as someone who pushed the envelope and took risks. Ralph said Francis was logical, smart, and treated patients as well as the lab animals. He had survived polio, with one leg shorter. His bedside communications, however, were not the best. Ken Galloway, PA, provided the bedside manner for Everhart, as well as assisting with his data collection and writing of the scientific papers. Galloway had a gift for talking to the patients and explaining to them the details of the cardiac exam, tests, and care.

The cardiologists had good reason to stand behind ACR. They recorded the results of their work and surgical referral results and continually learned and updated their knowledge and skills with weekly heart conferences. They assembled records of patient lists, which coronary arteries were blocked on coronary angiography, the clinical scenario, what had been done, the surgeon, the type of bypass, and the outcomes. It was a huge database and a part of the Spokane Experience.

One of those doctors in the trenches with patient care, Simpson, did not have the academic interest that Drs. Berg and Everhart held. He simply knew the results after emergency surgery were better for heart attack patients compared to medical-only care. Operative mortality was low in Spokane because of the high caliber of the heart surgeons. Patients benefited. Simpson reported he was too busy to remain president of the American Heart Association. Too busy to write up his results as a research paper or to even lecture about this huge change in care for heart attacks. He remained pleased with the level of care in Spokane and felt all the medical fields were excellent there, perhaps partly due to its isolation and surrounding beauty, which attracted excellent doctors.

The rejections were tough: first the cardiology care and now the surgical care. But group think, group dynamics, disloyalty, and naysayers did not trump the lives saved and restored. Rejection became a motivator to move forward. Dr. Berg easily assembled his second team for ACR . Members of the new team had been youngsters on the first team—the surgical and physician assistants. The work to save heart attack victims continued. The work was demanding. With their broad base of success as the foundation, the lead heart surgeon, a parent of a blue baby, now working solo, continued.

On December 5, 1975, Dr. Everhart became certified by the American Board of Internal Medicine's subspecialty board on cardiovascular diseases, certificate no. 29725. Everhart worked in both the practice of cardiology and internal medicine.

Julie Spores noted the other heart surgeons from the Berg Surgical Group did not appreciate how Ralph gave each of them a start. He brought the cases, the teaching, the surgical mentoring, the introductions to referring doctors, the validation of competence, and the guidance that led to their successes. Julie stated, "We all loved him very dearly. Ralph was a class act," adding, "He has always been generous about nurse anesthesia as a part of his success." After the breakup, Ralph gave the team members a hard time for working with his competitors. It was tough for all of them. Yet Ralph, always pushing, knew he could not hire the team as a solo surgeon (Spores 2011).

It was no longer considered science to show survival of patients like they did with the esophageal atresia and the doomed blue babies. The science had changed. They now needed to show comparison between the two types of treatment. The nurses noted that the heart attack patients with a Vineberg or a direct coronary bypass did better than the bed rest group, but these observations did not meet this new scientific standard.

Additionally, Ralph noted, the close-knit group of pioneering open-heart surgeons was no longer so close knit. Dr. Kirklin had moved to Alabama in 1969 and was building a new program from the ground up, on his terms. This master of congenital heart defect repairs did not attend the annual thoracic meeting. Dr. Starr was not at the thoracic meeting either. Dr. Lillehei had been demoted at the University of Minnesota and sent to New York, where he was trying to start over. The younger heart surgeons—Dr. Barnard particularly—were being made into media celebrities for basically "jumping the gun," said Dr. Berg; installing a heart transplant on a human without doing any of the immune suppression groundwork nor acknowledging the surgeons and teams who did the groundwork was a significant change. Meanwhile, Dr. Merendino had left the country after deciding he was not going to perform the new coronary bypass operation. He thought the procedure was too demanding, too technical. He moved to Saudi Arabia in 1973 to develop a heart program there.

Dr. Berg's former surgical group was not connected to the congenital blue-baby defects. Neither did they want to come in at all hours to perform emergently the direct coronary bypass on acute heart attack patients. The era of the research lab and the pioneering open-heart surgeons was at an end.

Dr. Ralph Berg saw the rejection and breakup of his group as an opportunity. After going solo, he was flooded with consults, all day and night, as well as invitations to give speeches about ACR. At Deaconess, the heart surgeons had split prior to the Berg Surgical Group's split. Ralph reported that "seeing the writing on the wall," the younger faction had already brought in a new partner. The large hospitals with open-heart programs were eager to learn how to set up an ACR program. Better outcomes demanded well-trained heart surgeons; excellent with the coronary bypass procedures. The two young open-heart surgeons agreed to cover call with master heart surgeon Dr. Berg and were appreciated.

The naysayers, the uninitiated, were not able to stop ACR. The protocol of fast cath followed by surgical consultation for emergent coronary artery bypass continued. For patients suffering a heart attack, acute coronary revascularization was the right thing to do. These patients survived. They returned to their families and to work.

CHAPTER 17

Another Meeting of Minds, 1976

Julie Spores, CRNA, a scientific mind, could and did work with all the teams, regardless of personality or status. There was a gap in the ACR work. The scientific data needed case controls for the work to be validated. Julie Spores found ways to bridge that gap with matched case controls, and she needed help.

Dr. Marcus Dewood was early for his morning meeting on his first day at work since coming home to Spokane. It was a crisp early-September day, and he had walked to the hospital from his mom's house. He had made this walk many times when he was in high school at Gonzaga Prep and worked in the Sacred Heart Hospital cafeteria. Working in the intensive care unit with surgical heart patients for $800 per month sounded interesting and challenging. He was content to be back in his hometown.

When his brother first called and told him their mother was sick with chronic lymphocytic leukemia, it still sent chills of fear through him. He had finished medical school at Creighton and was starting his second-year internal medicine residency but told his brother he was driving home. When Marcus arrived from Omaha, Nebraska, all the light bulbs were burned out; the house was dark and almost ninety degrees inside. His mom was alone. Worried she was dying from this combination of heat, loneliness, and CLL, he wanted to give her better care. He planned to stay home for a year and take care of her. A year's leave of absence from his internal medicine residency was arranged. He delayed his marriage. Thankfully he had some savings from his moonlighting work so he could do right by his mother, and she was getting better now.

When Marcus got to the meeting room, he realized he was the first one there. He looked around—a typical doctor conference room and lounge on the first floor. He waited. The next person to enter the room was a lady with a metal cart on wheels, delivering coffee, donuts, and ashtrays to the doctor lounges. When Marcus said, "Hello," she fell over, gray. Panicked, he realized she was in trouble. He grabbed her by the ankles and dragged her out of the room. Looking for help, he got her to the nearby emergency department. The ER team immediately assessed a severe heart attack with cardiovascular collapse. Oxygen, bag ventilation, and chest compressions, then intravenous line, fluids, medications, EKG, paddles, and a shock. She responded. She was about forty years old.

Dr. Henry Lang was called and came immediately. He had been on his way to meet Dr. Dewood. Dr. Lang took the patient to the cath lab and performed the fast cath. Dr. Lang called the chest surgery office, and Dr. Kendall came over. He looked at the cine films, talked to Dr. Henry Lang, and made the decision to operate. It happened so fast, so smoothly. Amazed, Dr. Dewood went, or perhaps was sent, to the operating room. He followed Dr. Lang.

The surgeon found and pulled out a fresh clot from the patient's main coronary vessel. A direct bypass with vein was done around the remaining plaque. The OR team gave young Dr. Dewood the clot, and he took it down to pathology. There he found Dr. Ditman, the pathologist, a friend from high school. An exciting reunion. Dr. Ditman sent Dr. Dewood back to the operating room.

The surgeon could not get the patient off the heart-lung pump. Therefore, an intra-aortic balloon pump was brought in and successfully installed, and the woman was taken to the ICU on the second floor.

Dewood stayed with her until she was stable. There Marcus met Julie Spores and attached himself to her. She was so smart and answered all his questions. He was surprised and amazed; they had successfully revascularized an acute heart attack on a Friday morning. He finally left the hospital on Monday. His new job was intense from day one, as was his interest in the clot (M. Dewood 2011).

During his first-year medicine internship, Marcus had been taught about counter-pump timing and how these intra-aortic pumps assisted the heart. This was a new technology, and Marcus was curious about the science of heart attacks.

The cardiologists welcomed Dr. Dewood into his role providing postoperative care for the ICU patients, most being post-open-heart cases, with a few acute coronary revascularization patients. Busy, he saw the labs, nursing concerns, and small changes in real time and wrote orders. The team consisted of both a cardiologist and a surgeon and all the supporting members. Marcus became close with CRNA Spores. She worked well with all the doctors, and she was also interested in the science. Marcus noted the political firestorm due to the divorce of the Berg Surgical Group. At first he felt pressured to pick sides, but he quickly understood he was there for the patients and not the controversy.

The post-open-heart care was largely directed by the referring cardiologist. However, dysrhythmias and chest tube outputs were a concern for the dreaded postsurgical bleeds with tamponade, whose management was directed by the surgeons. Dr. Berg, for instance, replaced blood lost in the chest tubes in a two-to-one ratio—one unit out the chest tube and two units transfused back to the patient. Both groups of surgeons and all the referring doctors were happy to have help and easily turned over care to Dr. Dewood. They had office patients and diagnostic procedures to do. Dr. Dewood filled a need as a dedicated physician in the ICU, an intensivist for these patients.

Julie suggested he meet with Dr. Berg. Marcus and Ralph met at the Park Inn, a pizza joint and bar across the street from Sacred Heart. When they sat down, Marcus told Ralph about his childhood heart cath. He was held out of sports due to a heart murmur and sent for a heart cath, which was normal. Ralph chuckled and asked if he was okay. Then Marcus found out Dr. Ralph Berg would not drink alcohol due to his hepatitis B infection back in 1947. He also learned that Berg did not like the aortic balloon counter pump. He felt swift surgical technique could avoid a failing heart that would need support by the balloon pump. Particularly with the acute heart attack patients, Berg felt the struggling heart could rest while it was being repaired on pump, and swiftly getting on pump was essential. If the time to get on pump was too long, the heart damage became too extensive, and the heart would struggle to come off pump.

The two doctors talked about the next step in the research effort to scientifically show the benefit of ACR. They got the first enzyme value from the ER blood draw, considered to be a metabolic marker. The value of the marker often coordinated with the ER EKG changes that showed an ischemic heart. However, doctors could not use this value as part of the surgical consult and decision to move ahead with ACR for the simple fact that it was not available from the lab when the decisions were being made.

Berg and Dewood wanted another diagnostic tool to improve diagnostic indicators for ACR that would also help with the follow-up and results and was scientific. If they could obtain sequential values of this metabolic marker as the protocol unfolded, Berg felt the additional data might reveal what was happening during a heart attack and after revascularization. Would the metabolic value from the ischemic myocardium stay the same, get better, or get worse with emergency direct coronary bypass?

Ralph and Marcus discussed how to collect this data from the heart patients in the post-open-heart ICU. They discussed sampling blood at the coronary sinus located at the back of the heart. With these extra data points, the value of urgent revascularization could be shown independently of a case-control patient treated medically. Berg agreed to add to the ACR protocol. The catheter in the coronary sinus would have to be placed in the operating room by the heart surgeon in such a way that it did not fall out but could be pulled safely prior to patient discharge. It would then be used for postoperative collection of blood samples coming back from the heart muscle as venous return through the patient's recovery from heart attack. After their meeting, the metabolic measurement was added (M. Dewood 2011).

At the next weekly case conference, Dewood discussed the need for medically diagnosed and treated control patients and the broader picture of what was happening during a heart attack and after acute revascularization. Dr. Henry Lang argued each detail, which helped everyone to understand. They all agreed the additional cardiac enzyme labs from the coronary sinus or the venous return of the postrevascularization myocardium could be helpful.

Marcus Dewood went to the operating room to watch Dr. Berg place the coronary sinus line, learning how to maintain the line and how to collect blood samples from these lines after surgery. He collected data while managing the post-open-heart patients. The cardiologists continued to perform fast cath and request surgical consultation. The surgeons did the ACR cases on pump with direct coronary bypass graft for the acute patients. Dewood tracked the patients for similar types of infarcts in regard to the three coronary arteries being similarly affected by blockages that were managed with medical therapy only. The protocol was not randomized, but there were matched case controls. There were still many patients and referring docs who refused a surgical evaluation and some who refused a fast cath (M. Dewood 2011).

Julie and Marcus pulled the cine films and charts to add objective patient information to the study. The heart attack cases were labeled emergent, nonemergent, and nonoperative. All the cases were followed. Marcus noted that Ralph Berg put his name on the line and followed the data closely.

The medical records department was a frequent location for Dr. Dewood. First, he needed the chart, then headed back for the cine films of the coronary angiogram, then repeat. With Sacred Heart not being a research institute nor an academic center, Medical Records was crazed by his enthusiasm and needs. Dewood got case controls, patients in the facility at the same time, EKGs, and coronary angiograms with the same coronary occlusions. He and Berg compared anterior and inferior infarcts managed two different ways, with and without revascularization.

Dr. Dewood soon became aware of the difference in recovery between the medical-care-only and the ACR-treated groups. The ACR group did better. In the operative group, for the first year after the protocol, it was clear that anterior infarcts did better with surgery. At the close of the second year, the difference was bigger, as it took longer for the inferior infarct patients to show superior results with surgery.

Dr. Berg wanted to see the data from the metabolic study. A bump in the metabolic lab indicated myocardial damage with a significant arrhythmia. Julie would pull in the lab work as it became available. The delay in getting these data points back from the lab had made this information moot in the decision to proceed with ACR treatment. However, after the treatment, these data points were revealing, showing the metabolic status improving with ACR. Ralph put the coronary sinus catheter in with finesse and ease. Some of the other heart surgeons had trouble putting this catheter in and would occasionally put the heart into fibrillation. Julie worried this would mess up the results (R. Berg 1976).

It was an exciting time. ACR cases were exploding in 1976. The protocol gave the cardiologists and referring primary doctors the information needed to make better referrals. Any delay or hesitancy to refer their acute MI patients was winding down. The data made it difficult to not believe in the benefit of treatment versus aggressive medical care alone. The patients poured in.

Dr. Ralph Berg was the whole package. He never just operated. He saw the patient, the process of how they became sick, the interventions, the recovery, and the reasons why. Ralph was a thinking man, and success for him was each patient recovered. Dr. Berg continued to educate, fundraise, and support the protocol.

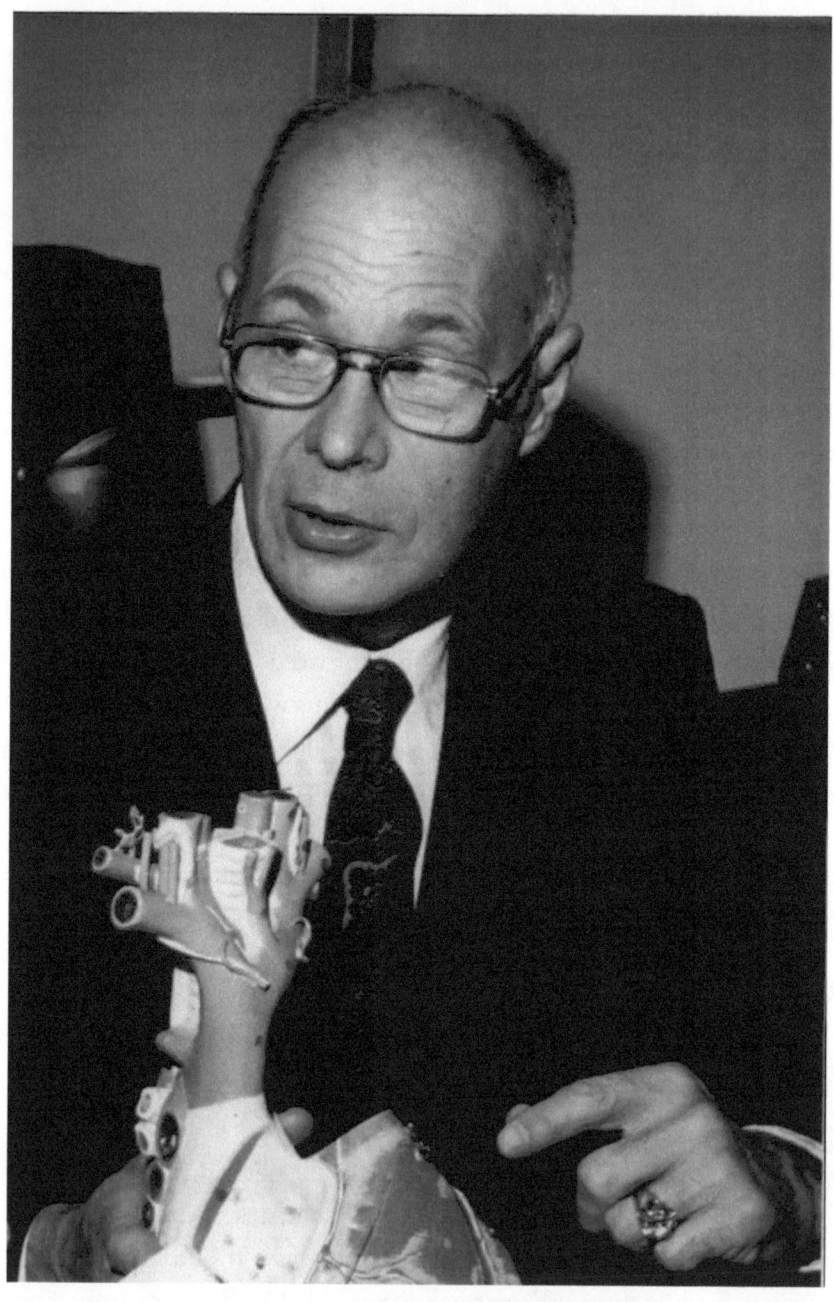

Ralph educating and fundraising, 1976.

Jason's heart was awaiting a repair, but somehow he carried on. He had humor and patience.

Because of his heart, Jason's level of oxygen was always low. To compensate, his body made lots of extra oxygen carriers. He made so many red blood cells that it became a separate problem. Jason's doctors handled this problem by removing the excess oxygen carriers. Every three months or so, Jason would drive with his dad to work early in the morning. At the hospital, they walked together into admitting, and Jason got dropped off, then admitted. The blood removal session, phlebotomy, would start. After his first case in the operating room, Jason's dad would stop by and check on him. If all was well, and usually it was, Jason's mom would come pick him up in her car.

Over the fall of 1976, Jason, now seven, was big enough to get the blood draw without being admitted. Although it was still traumatic, the ER was better for Jason. The hustle was distracting. A young doctor, Dewood, who worked with his dad, would come down to the ER and find Jason, draw his blood, get a chest X-ray and EKG, talk to him, and listen to his heart. When the evaluation was complete, the young doctor called Dr. Berg and reported. Jason's mom arrived shortly to pick him up. As a relief and a reward, Jason's mom would take him to Geno's Italian restaurant over by Gonzaga University. They had spaghetti for lunch. Even Jason's friends knew about Geno's spaghetti (M. Berg 2011; M. Dewood 2011).

The ongoing work to develop a surgical repair for transposition was slow. In 1976, Dr. Augie Senning published a paper on his repair. He was using a patch of great vessel wall, which included the coronary ostia. As the aorta was transected, Dr. Senning included this posterior patch to move the coronary ostia onto the other great vessel, the pulmonary artery. Dr. Berg explained that in this way, the two great vessels were transected differently from each other and from all the previous transposition repairs, which were done at the level of the atria.

The pulmonary artery, a great vessel, was also cut above its valve, but without including any artery takeoff. Dr. Senning thereby definitively moved the ostia, which supplied pulsatile blood flow to the myocardium, onto the proper great vessel to match the higher-pressure ventricle and its valve. Then, through the right ventricle, the VSD was repaired with a patch. The blood flow reversed to the correct circulatory anatomy, and then the patient was brought off pump.

Berg noted the mortality reported by Dr. Senning was less with this repair, compared to the atrial switch procedure, but still well above the mortality of standard open-heart congenital defect cases. Coming off pump was often difficult, requiring prolonged on-pump times. Dr. Abid Jatene had done a similar and successful great vessel switch about eight months earlier in Brazil, using deep hypothermia in addition to open-heart machine. However, none of these reports were on patients with a complex version of transposition.

Dr. Dewood left Spokane to return to his medical residency at Creighton in 1977, lugging along suitcases full of data. For Dr. Berg, choosing to become a chest surgeon simply meant saying yes to the father of chest surgery. Dewood had said yes to ACR, which naturally led to a cardiology fellowship and ongoing investigation about what a heart attack is, the clot, and which of the three coronary arteries led to severe myocardial damage. Marcus Dewood continued to analyze their data. In many ways, he took over the role of Dr. Francis Everhart.

CHAPTER 18

Marvalene's Paid Assassins, 1977–1980

One evening, Dr. Berg—on call for his turn on the rotation for providing surgical treatment if the fast cath was positive for an evolving MI—needed to schedule an acute at Deaconess. Berg had not done many acutes at this hospital, and the operating room team was stressed at having him as the surgeon. Not everyone understood the flow of care with these acute emerging heart attack patients. The OR manager, Marvalene, did a great job. Her young operating crew took direction well from the master open-heart surgeon. However, Ralph, frustrated with some minor blocks that came up while getting the patient to the OR, then into the room, then on pump, called them "Marvalene's paid assassins," a tease to push them. His older tease, "Fits and starts," just did not work anymore (Kappen 2011). This team came back with "Big Daddy," a nickname that stuck.

Working solo, Dr. Berg was under stress but pleased. Not one to buckle, not likely to turn to alcohol or self-pity, Ralph would tease and push the teams to perform (Simonsen 2011). Despite the divided and now competing Berg Surgical Group, work was steady. In his responses to surgeons and cardiologists sending him letters to congratulate him on ACR, invite him to talk, and ask him questions, Berg would always say, "There are now ten open-heart surgeons in Spokane who perform this procedure, ACR." The ACR work was not going to be stopped.

Ralph Berg felt ACR was the correct therapy for acute infarction or heart attacks, especially the heart attack involving the left anterior descending artery—the widow-maker.

Ralph, Mary, and Jason finally moved into their new house on Sunset Hill. Mike came to visit, bringing along several cousins to play with Jason. It was a great house in a unique location, close to downtown Spokane yet tucked up on the hill. Jason could continue at his same elementary school, and his brother Rory, having graduated from the local high school, was always there for him. Rory took care of Jason in a way that only brothers can, pushing him, protecting him, connecting with him. Rory's record shop up on South Hill, Looney Tunes, had become a success and a local hangout for teenagers and young people.

Thoralf Berg, retired for over ten years from the bakery, had remained active, hunting, swimming, and gardening. His eightieth birthday was approaching. In June 1977, the family gathered at Ralph and Mary's new house with a huge celebration focused on the eldest Berg's birthday. Thoralf's good health and active life was amazing. The two sickly cousins, Jason and I, were holding our own, with the doctors in the family guiding. Any worry about health issues were understated. After the birthday party, Thoralf water-skied at his lake place. All the grandchildren clapped as they watched.

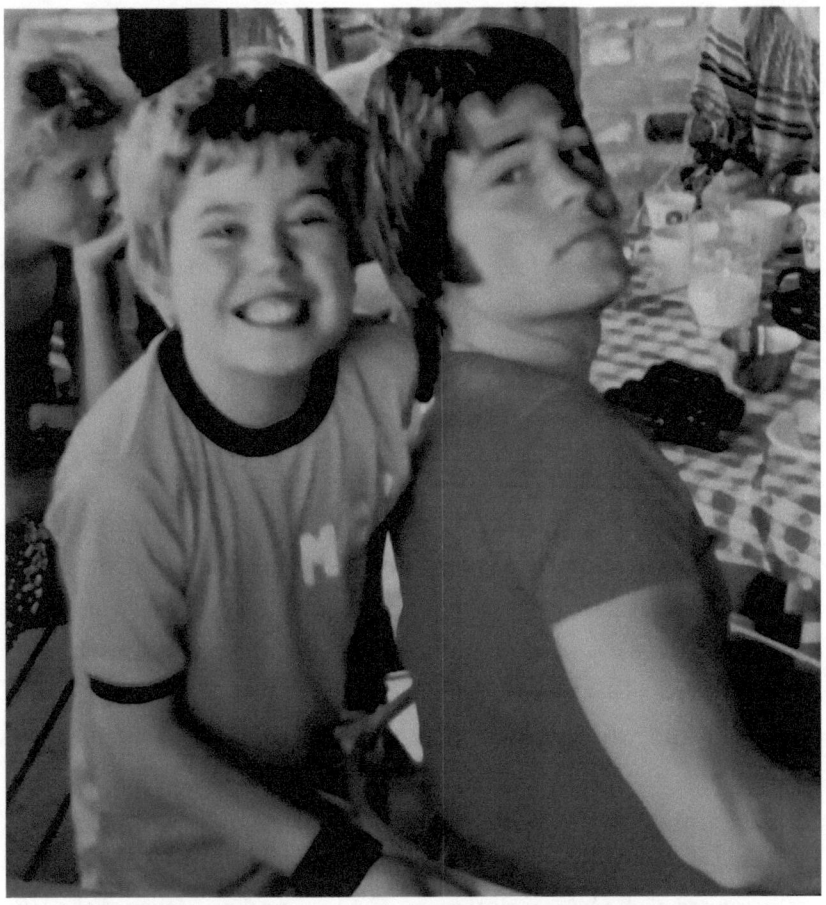

Jason and Rory at Thoralf's eightieth birthday party, 1977.

Exhausted but present at the party, Ralph was intent on building a new group of heart surgeons.

Shortly after Thoralf's eightieth, Mary held an eighth birthday party for Jason. He was set to start third grade that year and would take the bus to Hutton Elementary School. Jason was eager. He was gifted with keen eyesight and loved to get out. If his dad was going anywhere, even to work, then Jason would want to go.

The two parts of Dr. Henry Lang's original practice, adult and pediatric, had successfully split by 1977. Dr. Hensley continued working with Dr. Henry Lang on adult coronary catheterizations and adult cardiology and had little interest in the pediatric side of their practice. The new pediatric cardiologist likewise had little interest and no privileges for adult cardiology. Both sides of the practice left the medical building located between the two hospitals and moved close to Sacred Heart. At the same time, for personal reasons, Dr. Everhart left Spokane and relocated to another state. The magnitude of Dr. Everhart being away from this work, the Spokane Experience, was somehow not discussed by the heart teams who remained.

That September, a large review study of over 600 patients from fifteen Veterans Administration hospitals, assigned randomly to surgical or medical treatments for their chronic angina pain, came out. The report looked at one outcome: death at three years after elective coronary bypass for chronic angina compared to medical management only. This study showed that direct coronary bypass versus the newer aggressive medical treatment of chronic angina patients was the same— 13 percent mortality in both groups at three years.

Immediately, Ralph believed this was due to inferior surgical performance of the VA surgical teams. The surgical mortality of the VA study was higher than the mortality being reported by other surgical groups around the country. However, this large report had an impact in Spokane. The referrals of chronic angina patients for a surgical consult for the coronary artery bypass declined, for a time.

―•••―

In the cath lab, while performing an adult coronary angiogram, Dr. Lang was coughing. His voice had been hoarse for a while and was not resolving. It was 1978. Since he was at work, he got a chest X-ray, and it showed a lung mass. Henry, a nicotine addict, was still smoking cigarettes. He was so busy that the symptoms and diagnosis of lung cancer came fast and as a shock. He consulted with his sacred friend and colleague, Dr. Berg. The surgery was set with no delay.

When Ralph operated on Henry Lang, Julie was the anesthetist. Both Ralph and Henry requested her. It started as a lung resection and turned into a sixteen-hour surgery. Ralph did not cry, but Julie did as they discovered how advanced the cancer was. While crying, Julie worked. First, Ralph took the lung out. Then, finding cancer below the diaphragm, into the tail of the pancreas, Dr. Berg felt the affected part of the pancreas should be removed. Dr. Berg went out of the operating room and talked to Henry's wife, Pauline, and the Lang family for thirty-five minutes before proceeding.

Other surgeons came in during the case to observe and weigh in on the decision to do more. Ralph found cancer spread into the back half of the pancreas, and the lymph nodes were affected. Despite some of his surgical colleagues suggesting a less aggressive approach, Ralph resected the lung and the distal half of the pancreas with the nodes. After the case, Henry was stable and did well. It was 2 a.m. when he got to his hospital room. Julie went up to talk to him in his hospital room. She chatted on about the case until Henry fell asleep.

Henry Lang's living room was set up for him postsurgery. He was happy to be able to go home. Henry did not return to work after his cancer surgery. Drs. Hensley and Lang had just brought in a new cardiologist before this devastating diagnosis. The three adult cardiologists had worked well together. Henry's illness and not being able to return to work became the motivation for his Spokane Heart Clinic group to merge with a second, larger group of Spokane cardiologists. Together this group formed Heart Clinics Northwest.

Mary stood by Ralph and cared for him. She knew how painful it was to lose Henry from their day-to-day work relationship. Ralph had also been criticized for the extent of his operation. However, he sent Henry home alive, with his family. Ralph continued to work alone, sharing call with two other heart surgeons.

The former Berg Group surgeons continued accepting rotating referrals for the acute patients. Most of the elective cases were still going to Dr. Berg: The cardiologists all kept results of their referrals by surgeon, and Berg, at the top of the lists for outcomes, was easy to work with and available.

In March 1978, the *Spokane Magazine* article *"Bypass Surgery, Spokane's Dr. Ralph Berg in Action"* by William Stimson was published (Stimson 1978). The entire magazine was devoted to Dr. Berg's work. It was beautiful and colorful, with lots of pictures. Mary and Ralph's sister, Margaret, were so proud of it that they got multiple copies.

Ralph read it several times. It got him thinking. And not about the naysayers focused on the expense of a coronary artery revascularization—a.k.a. CABG—on a chronic angina patient while complaining there was no study on acute anterior heart attack. Not about chronic angina surgical treatment. Not about heart surgeons elsewhere still struggling to perform the coronary artery bypass operation with acceptable risk. Berg Surgical Group had been performing the coronary bypass since three months after Dr. René Favaloro initiated it on humans at the Cleveland Clinic in March 1969 with a low mortality. The transition to the ACR work being used in selected cases did not enter the chronic angina debate because, according to Ralph Berg, "we're so far ahead of everybody else, they haven't caught up with this one yet." This realization sent Berg back to the VA study.

Everhart's theory that a heart attack urgently required a bypass operation to prevent development of chronic angina was being validated. Spokane was now in year seven of the two-tiered protocol, which remained radically different from the protocols of other locales; and most cardiologists still did not perform the coronary angiogram when a heart attack was occurring, let alone an emergency open-heart, on-pump procedure to treat. However, the soundness of the treatment was obvious, and Ralph Berg felt that "eventually it will be standard."

To restore the circulations prior to myocardium necrosis, Ralph needed to scientifically prove the treatment—restoring the blood flow through the coronary artery—and prove that the treatment was safe, durable, and low risk. His plan: to look at the Spokane Experience database by surgeon and by years after the treatment. The obvious treatment, absent any other alternative, was replacement of the clogged artery with a new one.

Many in Spokane and the state of Washington read this *Spokane article* (Stimson 1978). Referrals and business picked up again when it became obvious to most referring physicians that surgical revascularization was better than nonsurgical approaches for the chronic angina patients. Dr. Berg knew ACR would be validated. The naysayers were dramatic.

When interviewing candidates to build his new group of surgeons, Dr. Berg looked for the highest quality and performance in regard to education, training, surgical skill, ethics, and devotion to profession. Patient care delivery was his guiding light.

The first heart surgeon Ralph interviewed and hired did not work out. A Harvard-trained cardiothoracic surgeon was the second to interview. For Dr. Sam Selinger, this interview consisted of following Dr. Berg for a few days in 1978, in the office, in the operating room, and on call. Dr. Selinger realized how advanced Ralph's techniques and how successful his outcomes were and wanted the job. He spoke to Ralph about needing additional training to get his skills up to a par with Berg's and went back for an additional six months of open-heart surgical training at the Cleveland Clinic. Selinger was anticipated to arrive in 1980.

Dr. Selinger represented the gap between what was happening in the surgical training of young surgeons in academic institutions and how fast the technology was being developed in some centers around the country. Ralph was on the cutting edge and motivated to be there.

Dr. Ralph Berg had been planning his next presentation and research paper in support of the two-tiered ACR protocol, particularly the surgical revascularization piece. There was no doubt the movement on the medical side of treating heart attacks had progressed and improved. From the Levine approach to this point, with prehospital diagnosis and treatments with EKG, IV fluids, pain medication, oxygen, coronary angiography, and aspirin, the mortality had come down significantly. Berg had well over a hundred patients this time. He planned to report on all of his cases—as they had presented to him when he was on call—with the most serious acute evolving myocardial infarcts and ACR.

Berg also knew Dr. Marcus Dewood was coming back to Spokane when his training as a cardiologist completed in the spring of 1980. He had ongoing presentations and research papers on the Spokane Experience work. Dr. Dewood's focus was on the cardiology side of the protocol. Always fascinated by the clot found in the most critically occluded artery, his research explained why not all heart attacks are the same. The Spokane Experience heart teams arranged a research position for Dewood.

Dr. Dewood presented the Spokane Experience work at the American Federation for Clinical Research in Washington, DC, in May 1979. He lectured on the topic of heart attacks, the differences in heart attacks, and their treatment. On invitation from Dr. Eugene Braunwald, husband of pioneering open-heart surgeon Dr. Nina Braunwald, Dr. Dewood lectured at the Cleveland Clinic. Eugene assisted Dewood in submitting the research paper to the *New England Journal of Medicine*.

Spokane's development as a major medical destination was due in part to innovators like Ralph Berg. Dr. Berg had been invited and traveled to seven centers before 1980, lecturing, advising, and helping set up for ACR. He continued to answer the call. All who did the work, especially the work on an acute evolving heart attack patient knew it was not a matter of if but when the rejection would be resolved and the benefit accepted. The patients who received ACR knew it worked (R. Berg, Curriculum Vitae 1995).

Ralph's deep feelings for Mary and Jason guided his work. What he came to do and what he actually did are profound.

CHAPTER 19

The Jewel in the Crown of Hearts, 1980

Rory's newborn was at Jason's tenth birthday party in August 1979. Estee was chunky and round, the perfect baby. Jason, adoring his niece, noticed things about her that others could not see. She calmed in Jason's arms. He became her devoted uncle. When pictures of the birthday party came back, the color contrast with the new baby was startling. Jason was blue again.

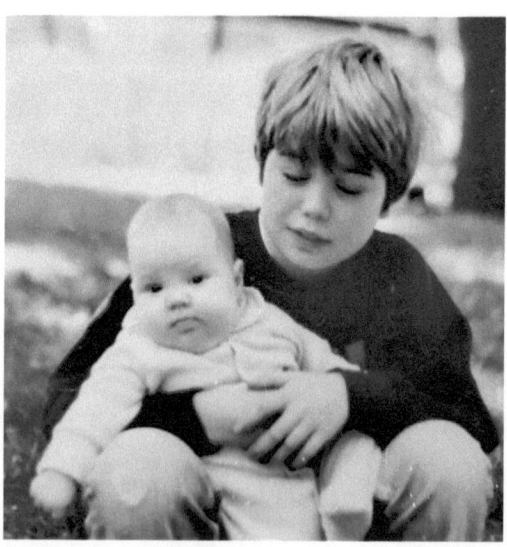

Jason with Rory's new baby, August 1979. The contrast with the new baby was startling. Mary noticed Jason was blue again.

He missed some school that fifth-grade year, and his best friend, Tola, worried.

Jason's parents took him to the annual thoracic meeting in late April 1980 in San Francisco, afraid to leave him in Spokane. At the meeting, Dr. Berg read his latest research paper. This time 227 consecutive patients with acute evolving myocardial infarctions had experienced his surgical technique. Dr. Berg shared that the mortality of conventional medical management of these types of heart attacks was between 22 and 27.5 percent at one year. Dr. Berg reported, "The largest published series of acute evolving myocardial infarction patients treated with emergency coronary artery bypass grafting had mortality at one year of 3.2 %." This was a tenfold decrease in mortality compared to medical management. The results were stunning for these patients. The surgeons in the audience were astonished. They questioned Ralph about his team, and he explained that he used two surgical assistants for each case, both trained in open-heart procedures (R. Berg et al. 1981). At the same meeting, Dr. John Kirklin's work was honored: twenty-five years working on blue babies.

As grand as Berg's ACR work success was, it was offset by his ever-deepening realization that a repair for Jason's heart was a race. The competitor was time. Buying time with small, lower-risk procedures might always be the best option. Berg could not talk about the risk of submitting his son to a definitive repair. The lethal complications were real.

Ralph's friend Dr. Augie Senning sought him out after his presentation and advised him about the new surgical options for transposition—for treating Jason. Augie had done grueling work in this field. The latest switch procedure, in use since 1976, was done above the valves instead of at the level of the atria, with the coronaries moved as a single patch onto the correct great vessel. But Jason had not been imaged, and Ralph was hesitant. Augie advised Ralph to get something done. Under Augie's encouragement, Ralph acquiesced to the first step, a heart catheter. That information could only be helpful.

Jason got his heart catheter procedure the next day. As they were already in San Francisco, the procedure was arranged with one phone call. Afterward, Jason recovered at the hospital. Mary waited for the cardiologist or anyone to come talk to them. Finally, when it was getting late in the day, they were released from the hospital. Mary and Jason returned to the hotel room. Jason was doing okay, but Mary was irritated that the cardiologist who performed the procedure had not talked to her, so she did not know the results. She had expected news and a plan.

The Berg family left the hotel the next morning for the airport and flew home. Neither Ralph nor Mary was impressed. The fancy heart catheter procedure did not change anything except that Mary knew Jason was not the same, not well. And Ralph knew that, if needed, Dr. John Kirklin would be his choice of open-heart surgeon.

So, Jason went back to school.

Jason's heart catheter procedure from San Francisco was not officially read for about eight days. The report on the procedure noted Jason's history: the Rashkind atrial septostomy at birth, the Blalock–Taussig–Thomas shunt at seven months, the digoxin, normal growth and development, and the recently increased cyanosis and decreased exercise tolerance. The report recommended an atrial septal switch procedure. However, the detail needed to understand the recommendation for an atrial rather than a great vessel switch was not in the report (Rudolph 1980).

The repair, regardless of the level, would need to be open-heart with hypothermia, and Ralph Berg was not convinced. For the most part, Jason was doing well. The surgical option was filled with unknowns and associated with a high chance of morbidity or worse mortality for his son. Ralph and Mary planned to hold. Ralph was not ready to commit to surgical repair, as it remained the third highest cause of death for this defect, and Mary agreed.

Toward the end of that school year, Tola learned Jason was dealing with an issue larger than the condition of his heart. Their grade school, nestled in a quiet, secluded area, offered security and privacy, and the two friends reflected together. Jason confided to Tola that as he was the baby of his family by many years, his birth may not have been planned. His parents, having to deal with a child late in life, might find him a burden. Driven by this uncertainty, Jason sought connections with his friends, his cousins, and his niece. Together, Jason and Tola made a life plan: to never be too serious and to say yes to everything with friends.

The family made plans to travel over the Fourth of July holiday. Mary continued to note that Jason was not himself after the "fancy" heart cath.

It was some relief for Ralph to have in his corner Dr. Augie Senning, who pushed for imaging. Senning's atrial switch repair for transposition defect was done by sewing a new atrial septum made of pericardium. He and several other heart surgeons in America had success with the atrial switch procedure and had rolled out great-vessel-switch procedures for humans in 1976, with little to no fanfare. The "heavy hitters," the pioneering open-heart surgeons, with their slow, methodical work, often slide under the radar and are not celebrated.

Before the May 1980 trip to San Francisco, managing Jason's heart had been a lot of work and worry but steady and almost smooth. It hit Mary hard when Jason's condition showed signs of slipping. Leading up to Independence Day, Jason did not feel well, and he had a fever. Ralph arranged for him to be admitted into the local hospital in mid-June, after school ended for the summer. The hospital did blood draws, blood cultures, X-rays, and EKGs, then released him, having found nothing. Before leaving for the July 4 trip, the family checked his blood cultures at the hospital. The hospital reported the cultures were negative. So, they went to the holiday celebration at Friday Harbor, a relatively isolated locale.

Jason had chills, shakes, and a fever of 105 degrees that Saturday night. Stuck with his parents on an island off the west coast of Washington, they could not leave until the next morning. They were dependent on the ferry and the ferry schedule. Ralph tried to get a pilot and a plane without success.

They got the ferry the next morning and drove back to Spokane, where they raced to the hospital. Jason was admitted and started on antibiotics intravenously. The blood culture grew strep viridians. On recheck of the first set of blood cultures, they too had been positive on June 28 for alpha streptococcus. Ralph and Mary had never been notified of this result. Worse yet, the hospital said they had reported the positive results.

Ralph was upset. Everyone was upset. Jason had contracted spontaneous bacterial endocarditis, an infection of the heart. Whether truly spontaneous or caused by a procedural manipulation such as the heart cath, which Mary suspected, this condition was a major cause of death. Regardless of age or defect, blue babies did not tolerate one more insult to their hearts, and heart infections were often their killer.

Jason responded to the antibiotics, and the fever came down. His first cardiac echo on July 7 showed an overriding great vessel, his pulmonary artery, confirming his transposition was complex. Ralph did not hesitate: He contacted Dr. John Kirklin by phone. Kirklin's advice was to put Jason on penicillin for a month and then proceed to a Senning atrial switch procedure. As Jason's condition involved his heart valves, he was not a candidate for a great vessel switch.

A few days later, Jason was sent home on oral antibiotics, with plans for Dr. Kirklin to repair Jason's blue-baby defect in Alabama. Jason, about to turn eleven in August, was ready. Jason seemed much better with the penicillin. Mary made plans to arrive in Birmingham the last weekend of July.

When the Berg family arrived at the Spokane airport, it was an unwelcome surprise to find the airline pilots on strike. They returned home. Eventually, they were able to get a flight and arrived in Birmingham on Monday, July 28, 1980.

Both Ralph and Mary were impressed with the hospital in

Birmingham. They were well treated, and the program was set up to comfort and help the family. They met with Dr. Kirklin, and Jason's case was set for Wednesday.

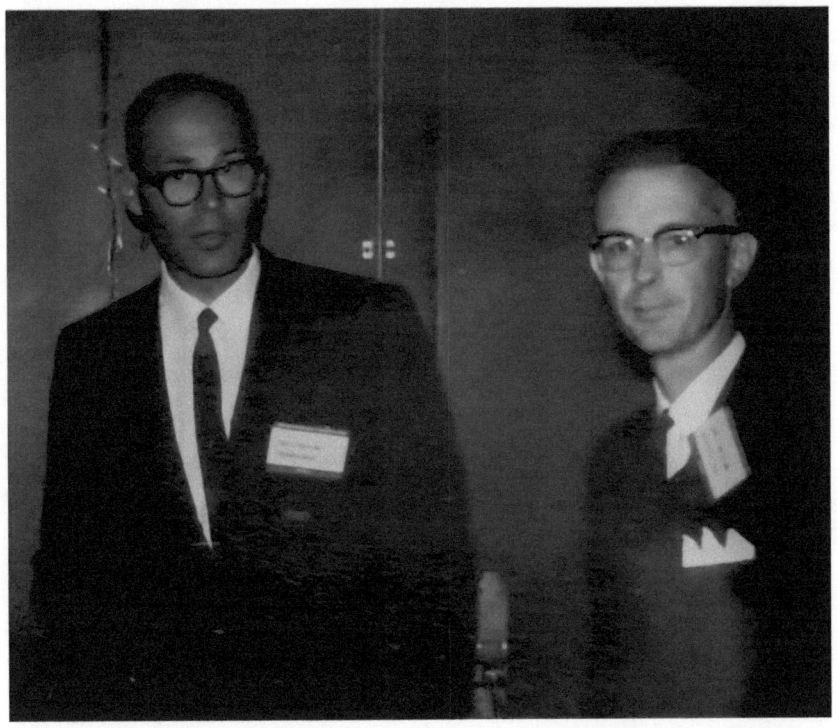

Berg and Dr. John Kirklin in hospital Birmingham, Alabama, July 1980. Dr. Kirlin performed the harrowing operation affectionately called "the big one." This operation gave Jason eleven additional years of life.

They met with other parents of blue babies. Mary recalled one young mother from Paris, France, with twins who were five years old. The twin with transposition was also set for surgery on Wednesday. As an older mother, Mary was moved by the child's young mother and her seemingly desperate situation. Mary insisted that the five-year-old child should be the first case on Wednesday. Jason was doing so much better in comparison. He had been in school, and he was growing and active. Mary knew Jason's heart was "fixable."

Waiting in the preoperative area the next morning, they were called in much earlier than expected. Jason was taken back to the operating room, and Ralph and Mary were sent to the waiting room. There they were horrified to learn that the twin had died on the operating table. The young mother was inconsolable. Mary held her and cried with her. Eventually, the young mother left with her family. Ralph and Mary waited on pins and needles for hours. Ralph paced. Mary wrung her hands. She was quiet with her worry. Finally, someone came out and told them Jason was slow to come off the heart-lung machine and that Dr. Kirklin would be out shortly. They waited again.

It was a rocky case. Kirklin did not like to lose blue babies. With the loss of his first patient that day, he would have typically walked away to clear his mind. He would sometimes leave for a day, sometimes longer. The cases would have to wait, be rescheduled. That day, Dr. Kirklin moved ahead with Jason's case. He worked tirelessly in the operating room. The anomalies in the heart's anatomy were more than the imaging suggested. Then Jason would not come off the heart-lung machine. His heart was not starting. Kirklin did everything he knew. Then he just waited. Not wanting to lose a second child that day, and not having another option, he waited and watched Jason. Dr. Kirklin could not let go. For fifty-seven minutes, almost an hour, Jason was clinically dead, his circulation not switching and his heart not picking up a rhythm.

Then Jason turned pink. The team checked and rechecked. The circulation, the flow to the lungs and to the systemic circulation, became anatomic. It corrected. Jason was able to come off the pump after those fifty-seven minutes. He was on his way to the ICU post-open-heart, and he would stay on the ventilator overnight. Kirklin was visibly tired when he told Ralph and Mary that he had used all the therapies he knew to get Jason off the pump. Ralph stayed in the ICU that night with Jason. His son's heart was working. It was a new beginning. Kirklin was thankful. Ralph and Mary were thankful.

Kirklin talked to Ralph privately the next day. At median

sternotomy, Kirklin found Jason's pericardium was native. There was little to no scarring around Jason's heart. The overriding pulmonary artery was accompanied by a subpulmonic stenotic aortic valve that was underdeveloped and several large VSDs. He explained his procedure: After ligation of the previous Blalock–Taussig–Thomas shunt, Kirklin placed Jason on the heart-lung machine, still not sure what he would find. On cardiopulmonary bypass with profound hypothermia—total circulatory arrest with cold cardioplegia myocardial preservation— he proceeded inside Jason's heart. He repaired the two largest VSDs and inserted a 25mm-valved heterograft in the position of the poorly developed left valve and ventricle so the left ventricle would pump to the pulmonary artery. Kirklin called it an "extracardiac conduit." The interatrial transposition of the venous return was done with a large pericardial patch by Senning's procedure. The work had taken hours.

Ralph walked the University of Alabama Hospital floors every day. While pacing, he learned there were twenty-five post-transposition-repair children in the hospital with Dr. John Kirklin. Ralph was impressed: that was a huge number of cases for such a rare blue-baby defect (R. Berg 2006; J. M. Kirklin 1980).

Jason's ICU stay was rocky, fraught with hallucinations, pulling out lines, and jumping up and down on his bed. Ralph was called in and spent many hours and overnights at his bedside, talking and reading to him, advising the nurses on sedation and pain management (Garabedian 2013). Jason got better slowly. He moved out of the ICU and to the post-open-heart-surgery floor. He walked with his parents. He was hungry and ate. The temporary pacer wires and chest tubes came out. He was released to go to the hotel and then later home to Spokane.

The corrective heart surgery in Alabama with John Kirklin was a success. However, some time was needed for Jason's parents. Still not sure if it was safe or smart to let Jason return to school, Ralph and Mary arranged a trip to Europe, a retreat. Ralph's sister, Margaret, met them overseas. There Ralph and Mary reported to Margaret how wonderfully they had been treated at the University of Alabama Hospital. They shared about how desperate they had been, waiting to hear how Jason came out of the repair surgery (Gayda 2011).

While at a restaurant in London where the tables were small and there was not enough room for all of them to sit together, Jason did not hesitate to separate himself and head for the table next to his parents. The adults were deep in conversation. Jason sat down next to an older lady, who was sitting alone. Before too long, he lifted his shirt and showed his tablemate his new chest scar. She was clearly impressed. Jason learned she too had such a scar, and they discreetly examined her scar for comparison. Together the two open-heart survivors enjoyed their dinner. They chatted away about their experiences under the knife. The adults at the next table, now aware of Jason's activities, were mesmerized watching him make such a personal and profound connection with a total stranger. They came to believe he would be just fine at school.

Jason turned eleven in August. He understood his second chance at life, as well as the toll it took on his parents. He named his surgery the "big one." He wanted to return to school and be with his friends. Having made it past the life expectancy predicted by his doctors, to age ten, eleven became his number.

CHAPTER 20

Myocardial Preservation, Decades Ahead

Myocardial preservation is the unifying concept for all heart patients. The myocardium, an older term from Ralph Berg's chest-training days, is the heart muscle. Ralph Berg explained that whether it is acquired heart disease with coronary artery blockage or the congenital blue-baby hearts that are stretched and dilated, both groups end up with poorly contracting heart muscle. The lack of blood flow into the myocardium via the coronary arteries and the high chamber pressure from shunts with hypoxia and extra demand for the heart muscle to work against both lead to dilated, thinned heart muscle that cannot pump blood into the next chamber.

Acute occlusion of the main coronary artery (LAD) with massive heart attack remains terrifying and lethal. In Spokane, the two-tiered protocol not only prevented heart attacks, but it also provided emergency treatment with coronary reperfusion to achieve myocardial preservation. Yes, it was a bold, even radical concept in 1970. The Spokane Experience was innovative, successful, and well established. The subsequent body of work happened in one decade—1970 to 1980. The direct coronary artery revascularization with emergent open-heart surgery is a technically difficult procedure, and Dr. Ralph Berg's results, 3.2 percent mortality at one year, remain remarkable. Dr. Ralph Berg did for the acute heart attack patients what he was desperate to do for his son Jason: preserve their myocardium.

The responses to Dr. Berg after his presentation at the thoracic meeting in spring 1980 surpassed the responses he had received after his 1975 presentation. Letters bearing accolades and invitations to speak and present his work came from all over the United States and Europe. The improved outcome and preserved myocardium compared with controls of the same type of infarct treated medically remains enduring. Berg's paper was the basis for Dr. Dwight Magoon's chapter on acute coronary revascularization and the admiration of many generations of heart surgeons.

Both hospitals in Spokane, their associated open-heart surgeons, and Dr. Shields on behalf of all the cardiologists welcomed Dr. Dewood back to his hometown in the spring of 1980. Although Marcus Dewood had stumbled into the ACR work as an intensivist in 1976, he then chose to study in the science of heart attacks and the field of cardiology. Dr. Dewood's October 18, 1980, publication in the *New England Journal of Medicine*, "Total Occlusion During Infarction," was well received by Dr. Ralph Berg and the medical community at large (Dewood MA 1980). It evolved into a landmark study, explaining what happens during a heart attack. Absent an academic medical institution, the Spokane Experience became its associated name.

Both Ralph and Mary were thankful to the cardiologists, the heart surgeons, Dr. Dewood, Julie Spores, and the rest of the somewhat dysfunctional Spokane Experience teams that had done this enduring work. Uninterested in accolades, Berg remained focused on Jason and work. The jewel in the crown of hearts—blue baby Jason—was "fixed," alive, and doing well. In so many ways, Ralph and Mary felt lucky.

With his knowledge of what he could and could not do, Dr. Ralph Berg managed his son's defect. Complex transposition remained without a durable repair, but for Mary, like all mothers of blue babies, Ralph stated, "It was important for her to believe Jason's defect was 'fixable' so she wouldn't fear." Ralph's desire to "fix" Jason's blueness was reflected in the bold work for acute coronary revascularization.

The Spokane Surgical Society met in April 1981 in Spokane. Dr. René Favaloro attended and at the meeting endorsed ACR and the work done in Spokane.

———•••———

Dr. Ralph Berg had chosen his first surgical partners for their ability to operate. In building his second group, Berg sought more. There was Dr. Selinger, Harvard trained with additional open-heart coronary bypass training at Cleveland Clinic. Then Dr. Jack Leonard, a Spokane native, who had trained with Dr. Lillehei. Next, Dr. William Coleman was signed up two years before he finished his thoracic surgical residency at Harvard. Then Dr. Leland Siwek came, also from Harvard. This surgical group brought comfort to Ralph, with their steady yet aggressive work and ethics.

Still active in his surgical practice, Ralph was always available for his family. Mike and Virginia called him needing his advice. Ralph went and sat with one of his nephews after emergency bowel surgery. It was February 1982, and his nephew had pain and hallucinations and was jumping on his postsurgery bed. Ralph assisted the nurses, and soon his nephew was calm, then sound asleep and getting better (R. Berg 2011). By late 1982, Ralph cut back at work and started making dinner for Jason every night. Ralph stepped aside from the managing-partner position of the new group. He took his earnings from his cases and from his assisting fees but stopped taking profits. He stopped taking overnight calls. He took Jason with him on hunting trips.

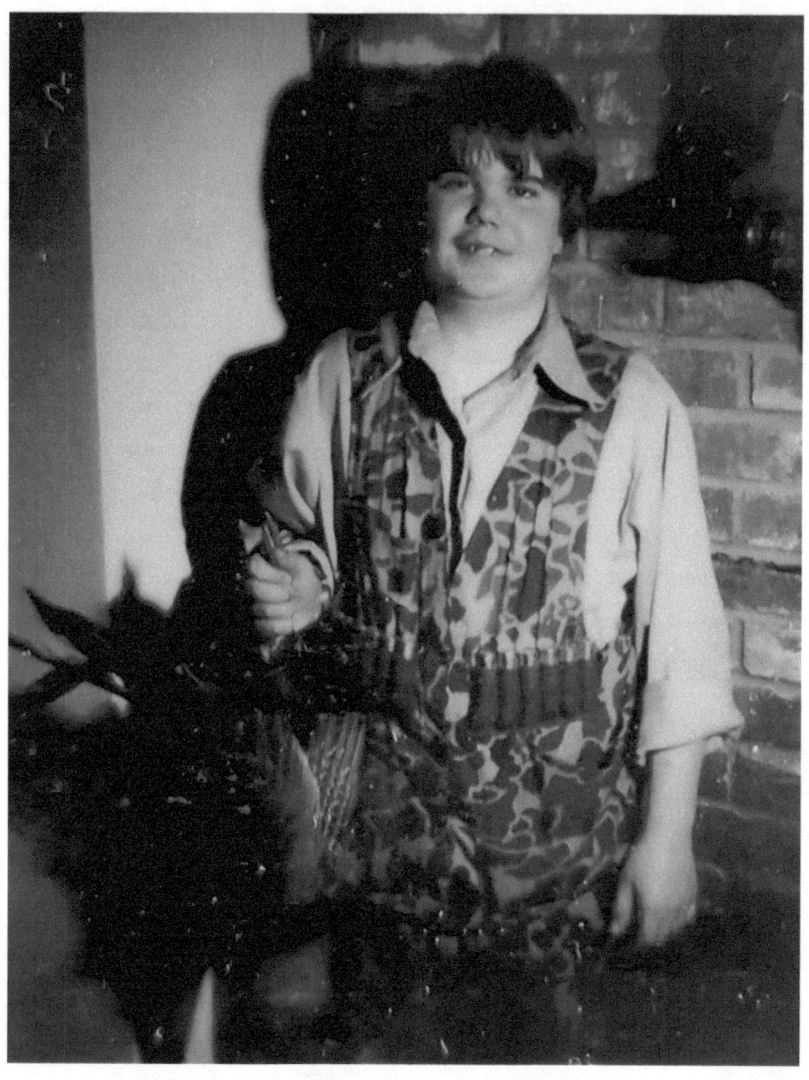

Jason with his front teeth missing, birds in hand, after hunting with Ralph, fall 1982.

Basically, Ralph pulled up. Still working, not fully retired, but no longer pushing for the lead.

Invited to Washington University at St. Louis in 1983 to be recognized as a distinguished alumni of the university and its medical school for his ACR work, Dr. Ralph Berg gave a talk and recognized his mentor, Dr. Evarts Graham, as well as Dr. Burford who followed Dr. Graham as chairman of the surgery department. Ralph was given a green jacket by the current chairman. By the end of 1983, Dr. Ralph Berg had traveled the globe on invitation to speak about ACR at twenty-six separate locations (R. Berg, Curriculum Vitae 1995). A ten-year follow-up study from the database was published in the same year (M. Dewood 1983).

An Overview of ACR

Trained in chest surgery by the father of chest surgery, Dr. Evarts Graham, Berg opened a private practice with a dog lab when he returned to Spokane in 1952. Then, with the insightful support of Sister Mary Bede, this lab was upgraded, and a heart-lung machine arrived for lab use in June 1956. With hypothermia and swift surgical skill, Berg had results comparable to open-heart surgeons. He became concerned the heart-lung machine itself was problematic. With upgrades to the oxygenators and pump leading to favorable results with the dogs, which were "no longer goofy, post-pump," the heart-lung method was applied to congenital heart patients in Spokane in early 1959, with mortality below 2 percent.

It was June 1970 when Dr. Everhart first sought Berg's opinion regarding emergent intervention on patients and his theory of a myocardial infarct. Everhart—a risk taker and willing to cross a line and boldly perform the coronary artery angiogram on patients in a new category, preinfarct or acute coronary syndrome—felt Dr. Berg's opinion was critically important. Both doctors wanted to increase blood supply to the choking myocardium. Dr. Ralph Berg agreed to perform the new bypass operation urgently on a case-by-case basis. In the spring of 1970, this theory and protocol was viewed as close to crazy when compared to traditional heart attack treatment: six weeks of rest. Ralph understood and found the protocol simple and logical. At the time, Jason was recovering from his second intervention to buy time to grow and preserve his myocardium regardless of the cause, ischemia or blue-baby defects. In a vise to buy time for his son, Dr. Berg said yes, and the protocol was launched to quickly do for others what he wanted and needed to do for his son.

It took the first cardiologist and heart surgeon team, Drs. Everhart and Berg, to realize that acute coronary revascularization was the necessary treatment for the pathologic process of heart attacks—a sudden coronary artery occlusion. Their unique two-tiered protocol, initiated in March 1971 and leading to the first success with a widow-maker heart attack, remains legend. Everhart and Berg stayed true to their scientific purpose. Their first research papers from 1974 and 1975 were rejected by academics but embraced by the public in need. At the end of the pivotal decade, in 1980, ACR became an enduring concept and the standard therapy for acute evolving heart attacks, with the patient care in Spokane standing decades ahead.

Dr. Ralph Berg led the teams to cutting-edge excellence. Cardiologists Lang, Shields, Mouser, Everhart, and Simpson came to Spokane for this trailblazing medical care and worked well with this surgeon. Dr. Berg, exacting and demanding of himself and the heart teams, dealt with and solved the vast problems that arose, using nurse anesthetists for his cases.

Despite the work, the two publications, the acceptance of the work with the knowledge of what comprises a heart attack, the different types of heart attacks, and the emergency treatment, there was still Jason. There was no weakness, no lack of faith. However, there was ongoing vigilance.

CHAPTER 21

Jason

Once upon a time, there was a special and unique young man named Jason Berg. At his heart checkup in late May 1983, the ultrasound (echo) was unchanged from the year before—fixed after what Jason referred to as "the big one" back in 1980. He knew it was not a "normal" heart, but it did not matter, and he felt lucky. At appointments with his heart doc, both he and his mom were quiet. Jason confided in Tola that again he was told he would not live long, maybe to age seventeen, because of his heart. It did not really matter. He and Tola had a lot of fun together, and his mom was guiding him to become a fine young man.

That summer, Jason was fourteen, and his niece Estee, four years old, came to visit with her dad, Rory. Jason had a huge set of Star Wars toys, a great attraction for Jason's niece. Pulling her father by his hand, she led him into Jason's room, hoping to play with them. Instead, the room was dark, and a video was playing. Jason was watching porn.

Holding his daughter by the hand, Rory glared uncomfortably at Jason. It was awkward. Jason immediately turned off the television and focused on his niece. Estee was worried about spiders and wanted to see the Star Wars toys. Jason questioned her about spiders and then responded: "Never be scared of spiders because *you* are bigger than they are." Uncle Jason's advice was comforting. While she did not know why he was treated special by others, her uncle made her feel special, which was all that mattered. She adored him (E. Berg 2010).

Play is children's work, and Jason excelled at play. He played like he lived, which was to the fullest. He figured out how to make relationships work. If he was tired, he rested. If he had trouble moving quickly enough to keep up as a toddler, he rode in his older siblings' arms. His friends slowed down for him; then he took up skateboarding and later drove his own car. He was funny, wickedly funny. He could verbally level any playing field. From the outside looking in, it appeared that Jason lived big on borrowed time. His friends and family adored him, and his father knew everything about his heart. Ralph attended to every medical detail, which was comforting.

Tola and Jason, best friends from kindergarten, were now incoming freshmen at Lewis and Clark High School. Jason had kept a lower profile in middle school because of his tutoring schedule; his parents had been slow to relax after the big one. His dad cut back at his work and made dinner for Jason on an almost nightly basis. Jason's mom was growing her real estate career.

Jason fit right in with Tola's crowd when high school started. They had a couple of classes together. Jason loved to poke fun at himself, and his new friend group could do and say anything with him. They hung out together, and everyone became protective of Jason.

Toward the end of freshman year, in late May 1984, it was again time for Jason's annual heart checkup. His heart checked out "okay" with the cardiac echo.

Dr. Henry Lang passed peacefully in May 1984. It was comforting to Ralph that Henry had enjoyed several years with his family and got to see Jason repaired, me in medical school, and ACR validated. Dr. Marcus Dewood wrote the obituary for the pediatric cardiologist who had converted to an adult cardiologist. For the Berg family, Henry Lang remains an icon as their pediatrician and sacred friend.

Throughout the summer, Jason and his friends skateboarded on flat concrete pads under the freeway. His friends helped celebrate his birthday each August—a celebration of life was the way Jason saw it. He claimed eleven as his lucky number, marking his second life. Neither Jason nor Tola had girlfriends, but their interest in girls intensified as they started sophomore year. Jason was not athletic, but he had a presence.

Meanwhile, Jason's younger cousin Cathy and her group of friends began their freshman year at Lewis and Clark High. Acutely aware of Jason in middle school, Cathy had a vague and unpleasant memory of him turning blue like her toy elephant during a family visit. Jason would notice her between classes during middle school and boldly call out her name. In the self-conscious "everybody wears the same clothes and sports the same hairstyle" world of middle school, this was a nightmare for Cathy. He nicknamed her "Beautiful."

One night, while she was expressing intense embarrassment at being related to that oddball Jason, Mike had some stern words. He informed his daughter that Jason had almost died during surgery for a serious heart issue that he had been born with, a blue-baby syndrome—a condition she was not aware of at the time. Mike demanded that she consider how "normal" she might look, feel, and act if she went through something like that.

From that moment, Cathy's perspective on the situation changed. After questioning her dad further and then thinking it over, she stopped being the "prissy snot" and befriended her cousin. She soon discovered how incredibly sweet Jason was. Behind his offensive, obnoxious exterior, he was hilarious. When she and her friends became freshmen, Jason was instantly an attraction. All at once, Jason and Tola had many "girlfriends" (C. Berg 2010).

After school, Jason hung out with Rory at Looney Tunes. Rory liked the company at his record shop and was always happy to see Jason.

Then Rory started to detect some issues with Jason's relationships with these skateboard guys. When a few of the guys in Jason and Tola's circle got out of line, the situation changed for Jason. In discussing it with Rory, Jason realized the guys were tearing down the honor of his group of girls.

Jason planned to scare some sense into them. On his way out of

Looney Tunes one afternoon, he quietly opened the desk drawer and removed the pistol Rory kept there, tucking it into his pants. He did not tell his brother. When Rory opened the store the next morning and realized his gun was missing, he decided to wait for Jason before doing anything.

Meanwhile, Jason called his guys together after school. He told them where they were wrong and insisted that he would defend his girlfriends. One of the guys challenged Jason, demanding what he was going to do about it. Jason pulled the gun and told him. The message delivered, the out-of-line guys backed off.

As Rory listened to Jason's story, he worried about Jason's choice of friends and his vulnerability and mental health. He recovered his gun from Jason.

Their parents were not understanding. Jason had planned to say nothing to them about the gun, but the school had notified them. "Waving a gun at school? No!" After a brief parental discussion, Jason was promptly sent off to a boarding school in Arizona. Tola, who was not told what had happened to his friend, missed Jason terribly.

The first letter Jason sent to Tola described boarding school and the goings-on. He had met a girl. With each letter, Tola became more alarmed. The boarding school sounded like a drug rehab center. He imagined that Jason's new girlfriend had a real drug problem and was not simply dabbling in drugs because they were available, like Jason and he had experienced. Tola was sure that Jason was not an addict, but it bothered him that his friend might go down that path with this girl.

When Jason came home for Christmas break at the close of 1984, he informed his parents that he was not returning to Arizona. They already knew this information. The boarding school had notified them that they would not take Jason back and he was not welcome to return. Life moved forward with he and his parents at odds over next steps.

That year, the whole Berg family got together at the Big House for a Christmas celebration.

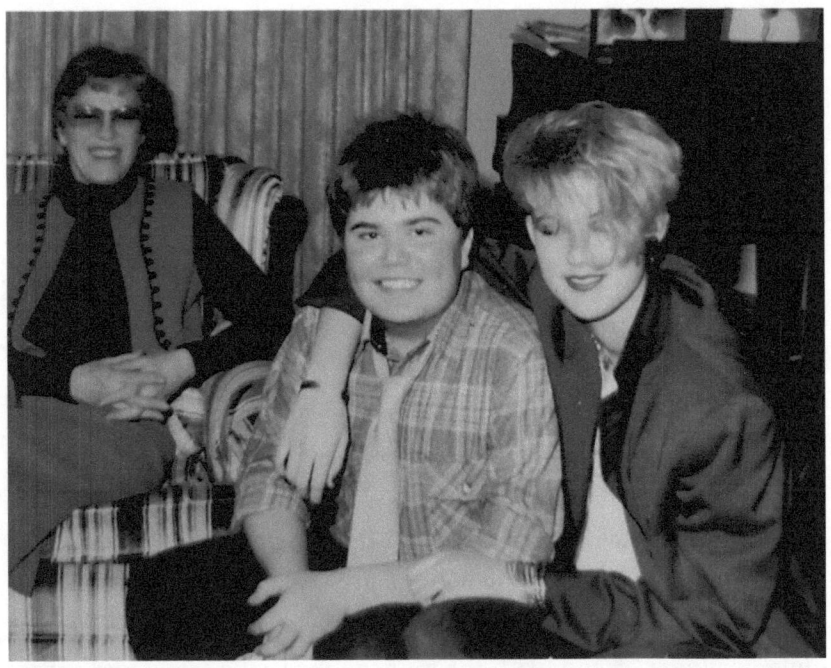

The Berg families at the Big House for a Christmas celebration, 1984.

Jason and Tola easily reconnected and picked up where they left off—enjoying life, chasing beautiful girls, skateboarding, and punk rocking. Life was good again.

As 1985 rolled in, Mike visited Ralph and Jason on a weekly basis, and Ralph made dinner for the Berg men. The manly dinner nights occurred around a formal, properly set dining table with freshly cooked meat, vegetables, and dessert. Mike brought along his youngest son, Steven, now ten years old. The Berg men talked hunting, work, guy things. Steve was fascinated by fifteen-year-old Jason.

One beautiful spring weekend day, Jason and Ralph visited the Big House. Surrounded by formal gardens designed by the Olmsted brothers, the large house had been built in 1933 by a wealthy Spokane lumber and mining magnate. Young Steve stopped in his tracks when he heard Jason say, "We hate her, don't we, Dad?" Ralph, who was dressed formally, hat in hand, casually answered, "Yeah, we do."

No one said a word, not understanding. Turns out, Jason was still in trouble with his mom over the gun-at-school incident. Mary had expectations for Jason, established by her belief that his heart condition was fixable and had, in fact, been "fixed." Therefore, Mary treated Jason like her other children and believed in the highest prospects for his future. Left unsaid were mixed messages about Jason's schooling and his future. With Mary, Ralph would hold standard parental expectations for Jason but then let them slide when he was alone with his son. The gun incident and today's trash talk provided examples, and Mary's irritation was real.

A moment later, the conversation shifted to a different topic, and soon Ralph and Jason left to go visit with Thoralf and Leila up on North Hill. Ralph wanted to visit his parents and ask his dad to come hunting. The youngest Berg men, Steve and Jason, were being introduced to the hunting world. Thoralf decided not to go. That trip the following weekend, with the raunchy jokes, the camaraderie, the focus, and the precision, was strangely fun for Steve.

Jason, developing into a young man, had a big chest and a long body but was not as tall as his four older brothers. An old scar on his left chest was contracted onto his ribs and made it hard for him to move his left arm and balance on the skateboard. He complained to his dad, who arranged to get it fixed. When school ended mid-June, Jason went in for surgery to revise the left chest scar, then was out of hospital and back on the skateboard within days.

Rory's sales at Looney Tunes continued to grow. He needed to move into a bigger store. In July, with the Scorpions' song "Gorky Park" playing, Jason helped Rory relocate two blocks away. The new store had broad street exposure and additional parking. Rory named it Video Unlimited. The two brothers enjoyed themselves, and the grand opening went smoothly. Rory's daughter, now six, helped her father and her uncle. Tall and stunningly handsome, Rory knew he would not have Jason forever and agonized over the reality whenever they were together (E. Berg 2010).

Jason resisted returning to any boarding school, no matter how fancy his mother claimed the next one would be. Ralph remained on the fence about the matter. Knowing he was not meeting his mother's expectations, Jason went to the Big House and found his aunt Virginia in her sewing room, all alone, working away on my wedding gown. Jason asked, "May I please move in with you and Uncle Mike?" He explained that he was not doing well at home and figured living with his aunt and uncle was a better alternative than another boarding school. Aunt Virginia told Jason to ask her again when the wedding was over in a few weeks. She explained to Jason how overwhelmed she felt, and he was relieved that she did not give a flat-out no.

My wedding was held in mid-August in the formal back garden, with about a hundred guests in attendance. My grandparents Leila and Thoralf were sitting on the porch for safety, arguing with each other during the vows portion of the ceremony. Following the ceremony, and with the reception barely underway, Jason found my mother and asked again if he could live with them. This time Virginia's response was "Yes, but there will be rules." Jason made a cursory acknowledgment to the familiar comment about rules; mothers were all the same. Quiet but happy, Jason returned to the reception and enjoyed the party. When Jason walked up to me, the bride, he said, "You look" —then paused dramatically—"normal." I knew immediately what Jason meant. Appearing normal and being sickly is a different condition from looking as sick as you really are. After hugging, he left.

Mary phoned Virginia after Jason's sixteenth birthday party. She needed to confirm Jason's news. The two sisters-in-law spoke about the conflict Mary had with Jason and the options they were considering. Neither woman knew that Cathy was listening in on another line. She heard her aunt ask, "Is it true? It is alright with you and Mike that Jason moves in?" Mary was still in favor of sending Jason to another boarding school. However, she was grateful to have this option. Both Ralph and

Mary were hopeful that the new environment would lead to success, though Mary clearly had higher expectations—graduation and a job. Ralph simply liked that Jason would be close to him and with family.

Cathy was simultaneously excited and somewhat apprehensive about her cousin moving in, as Jason was a handful and most people did not understand him. They couldn't get past his abrasive exterior. Jason would go through phases of poor health followed by astonishingly improved health in between the surgeries, a fact that seemed like a roll of the dice to Cathy. She worried her force field—her Star Wars term for her private space—would be upset by Jason's arrival. But a few days later, when her mother announced that Jason would be moving in, Cathy was calm and said nothing (C. Berg 2010).

Jason moved in when school started up again in the fall.

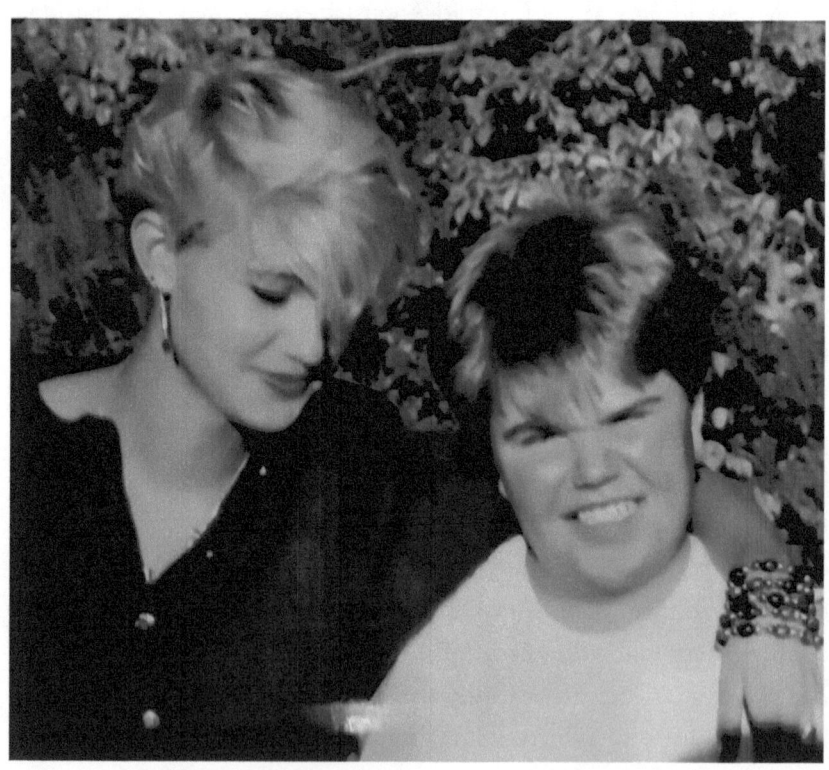

Cathy and Jason, first day of school, fall 1985.

A recent surgery had repaired a minor problem, and the "big one" was quite a few years in the past, allegedly fixing the blue-baby problem permanently. His apparent health fueled his rambunctious teenage attitude and behavior. While he appeared to be living the life of a normal and active teenager, Jason was painfully aware that his time was limited and that he was not destined to live a long life. So he really didn't care about what people thought about anything, and especially about him. He considered social conventions such as manners to be pointless and fake, and he simply disregarded them. This irreverence made him simultaneously refreshing, wonderful, endearing, shocking, and maddening, depending on the circumstances.

No one at the Big House was sure how living with Jason would pan out, yet they weren't overly concerned (C. Berg 2010). Somehow, everyone seemed to believe that the environment would be better, healthier, for Jason. Perhaps Jason would blossom under the care at the Big House. Possibly he would live forever under the stellar influence of the extended Berg family.

Jason's new room was a bedroom above the garage. It did not take long for Jason to settle in, and he made a point of hanging a special poster on the wall: a simple, small, repeating pattern. Virginia assumed he had a tender attachment to it. Jason and Cathy lived in cocoons of their own construction. They kept out everything that annoyed them, which was relatively simple since Cathy's older siblings had moved out long before. Only Steve was left in their orbit, whom they referred to as "Stop-it-Steve." He was tolerated within Jason's force field.

The house had two staircases, which helped the two cousins avoid the "cocoon busters," Virginia and Mike. They could go for days without seeing the adults, even though they all lived under the same roof.

Ralph came over one Saturday and picked up Jason to go out driving now that he was old enough to get his driver's license. Steve, tagging along, sat quietly in the back seat of the blue Mercedes with powder-blue leather interior. Ralph was in the passenger seat, and Jason drove with his learner's permit. They drove the freeway heading west toward the ranch, where Ralph and Mary had purchased land and cattle. Soon Jason was driving the Mercedes on a dirt road. Then he pulled up to a gate in a barbed-wire fence. Jason stopped the car, and Ralph got out to unhook the gate and move it aside. The ruts in the dirt road were deep. Ralph walked over to his son, who rolled down the window, and gestured with his arm: "Go this way. I do not want you to knock the oil pan off." Despite Jason's careful driving, the undercarriage scraped the road. Ralph began swearing and blaming his son, who fired back in a taunting fashion, "Is that right, Ralphie?" mimicking his father's authoritative voice and out-of-control demeanor. Jason was the only person from whom Ralph would tolerate such disrespect.

"God damn it, you shut up!" yelled Ralph. They turned around and headed to the dealership in downtown Spokane. Silent in the back seat, Steve was in awe at how Jason had stood up to his father.

Despite the mishap, Jason passed his driving test and received his driver's license. Ralph bought him a 1954 Land Rover 109 with a short chassis, a rare and unique car. It came with conditions, however: If Jason's grades dropped, he would lose the Land Rover. The car, essentially a metal box on wheels, was both a joy and a disappointment for Jason. He loved having a car, but Ralph had previously promised him the blue Mercedes, which was now in the shop and in need of major repairs.

With his license and the Land Rover, Jason drove to school the next day and took Tola four-wheeling; this basic vehicle with metal bench seats and less-than-ideal suspension was purportedly indestructible.

Evenings after dinner at the Big House, Jason entertained with stories about his parents, teachers, friends, and family. He was darkly, melodramatically humorous and made his parents out to be ogres. There was the time his mother had pushed him out of a moving car and he broke his arm. Many of the stories included his dad threatening him with guns. Best of all was Jason's self-reported backtalk, which had his cousins, aunt, and uncle in stitches. After the entertainment and dinner cleanup, Jason would drive with Steve to Video Unlimited to pick up movies.

They got *Texas Chain Saw Massacre* and other movies they probably should not have been watching, as Steve was a fifth grader. Spending time in Jason's room, Steve noticed that Jason's poster was more than a simple repeating pattern. It was a poster designed by the musician Sid Vicious, and the imagery was pornographic. Steve thought it hilarious that Virginia had failed to notice the detail.

Meanwhile, Cathy was intrigued by Jason's chest scars. They talked about life, his heart, his surgeries. The teenagers noted that the scars ran from the base of his throat to his lower abdomen. They overlapped in the middle, but at each end they could see the separate individual scars, as if he had multiple entries into his chest. Cathy noted they were like a stack of strings that slid untracked at the ends. She and Jason joked about installing a zipper for easy access.

At this point, Jason's love-hate relationship with his parents tipped a bit more to hate but still was not unusual for a teenager. Virginia was pleased about how things were going. Each time she cleaned Jason's room, she looked at his special poster and smiled. She thought that Jason's attachment to the poster was sweet.

Jason was not afraid of dying, but he did fear dying without having had sex or a girlfriend. He spent lots of energy hatching plans to get girls to notice him. But almost always these plans had unintended and unhappy effects. Sometimes Cathy would tactfully explain to Jason that he was aiming out of his league. Then she would advise Jason to try for someone suitable.

Cathy suggested he work on himself, go with her to the gym. Jason eagerly accepted. Mike and Virginia had a family membership at the Spokane Club downtown. It had two restaurants, a swimming pool, a sports club with gym, and rooms available. Cathy and Jason went there most days to work out after school. Jason, who had been overweight with his fast-food overeating and beer, liked getting into shape. Virginia bought him the book *Eating to Win*, and Jason dropped more weight. His acne cleared up. He was making positive changes, and everyone was pleased.

Jason was into his car, skateboarding, punk rock, and smoking weed. Steve enjoyed tagging along when Jason drove. When Jason spent time on the phone, his young cousin would bug him to get off and drive him somewhere. Jason controlled Steve with his "stinky finger," inserting his index finger into a stinky body part, then waving it at his cousin to ward him off. Steve was forced to wait patiently for a ride (S. Berg 2011).

Franken Christ, the Ramones, the Clash, and Butthole Surfers were the bands Jason and his buddies liked. Jason played guitar. There was a huge amplifier in his room, and he and Tola were messing around with it one weekend when Cathy walked in. "Watch this," said Jason as he stuck the microphone down the back of his pants and cut a huge fart. They thought the windows would shatter at the sound. Virginia, who was outside gardening, nearly had a fit and yelled as she stomped into the house, "What was that . . . noise?" The teenagers cracked up so hard they could barely breathe (C. Berg 2010).

One morning, as Jason went off to school in the Land Rover, Virginia watched him from her kitchen window. He drove too fast, and she always worried. Jason fired up the Land Rover and started backing out of the curved, bush-lined driveway much too fast. At that same moment, Mike came flying into the end of the curved driveway in his new red Porsche, stopping home for breakfast after his surgery cases. Virginia gasped in anticipation of a collision. Both sets of tires screeched as they braked. The Berg men jumped out of their vehicles, offered greetings, inspected their vehicles, and then continued their separate ways, barely noting the incident.

One of Jason's older brothers was in town visiting Mary and Ralph and came over to the Big House to take Jason out. He had heard that Jason was down and could use some brotherly therapy, but Jason balked. "Therapy" meant beating up on Jason when he was depressed. Jason walked away from his brother and drove off with Steve. Both cousins were surprised when Jason's brother gave chase in his car. For Steve, it was an exciting cat-and-mouse game. Finally, Jason was caught, and his brother pulled him out of the Land Rover and gently beat him up. Later, they all met back at the Big House, where the brother boasted about the incident to the family. Although Jason was fine and it didn't seem like such a big deal to him, for a brother who was so much older to get away with something like that seemed unfair to Steve (R. Berg 2011).

Tola also loved to ride with Jason. One weekend in mid-November, they were heading down Twenty-Ninth Avenue. They had a movie to watch, but driving had become Jason's all-time favorite activity because of the control, the freedom, and the mobility it provided. The Land Rover started to slide on black ice. Out of control and heading toward a stone wall, Jason hit the brakes, and the car stopped abruptly. The car was fine, and Jason remained cool after the inspection. He backed up and carried on.

At lunchtime during school days, Jason and Tola occasionally went out four-wheeling in the Land Rover. With the fun they had and the stories generated, soon the noontime escapes became a ritual and the envy of their friends. Jason was approached by a kid in their school group who wanted to drive the Land Rover. During the next outing, Jason turned over his driver's seat to this kid. Tola and Jason sat in the back, bouncing around on the hard bench seats. On the way back to school, the car stopped in the McDonald's parking lot and would not start up again. They abandoned the car to rush back to the school, just across the street, on time and undetected. Jason's Land Rover was towed away for blocking a business.

For Tola, it was fun to be in Jason's circle of friends. They went to the Big House after school and on the weekends, watched movies, played pool, walked downtown, and went to neighborhood parties. Tola had crushes on the entire group of girlfriends, and Jason was honest with his aunt and uncle about where they were going and what they were doing. Tola felt weird about acting so direct and self-assured around adults but was impressed by Mike and Virginia's tolerant and loving ways toward Jason.

Winter arrived, and there was snow and ice on the ground. For Cathy, having wheels to drive to school was much better than walking. The Land Rover was a car, never mind the lack of padding on the seats, carpet on the floor, seat belts, and heat! Off they went one morning, flying down the hill to school. As Jason made a hard left into the student parking lot at Lewis and Clark, which was a sloped, muddy field full of potholes and parked cars, Jason and Cathy bounced around as if skiing a downhill mogul field out of control—except the moguls were parked cars. They jerked dramatically to a stop. Cathy, now upset, was sure they were on top of another car, and when she opened her eyes and got off the floor, she saw only an inch between her door and the next car. They neither hit nor scraped it, but she opted to walk to school from then on, regardless of the weather. Around this time, Virginia figured out that his beloved poster was obscene. She proceeded to tear it down and throw it away.

Virginia's oldest son was home from college one weekend, and it was a beautiful ski day. Jason wanted to go. While Steve was skiing with Jason and Virginia was off skiing on more difficult runs with her older son, Jason was suddenly unable to hold back tears. He told Steve that he had chest pains. Quickly, they found Virginia, and Jason informed her that he felt sick—"Like when I had the blood infection," he said. They were at Silver Mountain in Idaho, and Virginia panicked while her college-age son kept her and everyone else calm. She got to a phone at the lodge and dialed Ralph, who answered immediately. Virginia shared what Jason had said.

They left the mountain immediately with the oldest son driving and dropped Jason off at the hospital, where Ralph was waiting. Jason was admitted and stayed a few days, but no surgery was indicated at this time. He did have a blood infection that required intravenous antibiotics. By this time, Ralph had been invited and traveled to thirty-two different locations to give talks on ACR (R. Berg, Curriculum Vitae 1995). He stopped traveling but continued with the follow-up studies on the ACR patients.

Jason needed to keep his grades up to keep the Land Rover, and his aunt and uncle believed him when he brought home grades in the B range at the end of the semester in January 1986. Aunt Virginia and Uncle Mike were beaming with pride. Unfortunately, it was short lived. Jason had made a small miscalculation, discovered only when Mike and Virginia went to his parent–teacher conference a few days later. There they learned that the coveted B was really an F in multiple classes. Jason had not expected them to attend the teacher conference. He thought he had been clever, forging his report card with a copy machine at the local grocery store. It was a good forgery, but he was caught, and the Land Rover subsequently disappeared.

Virginia became suspicious of Tola; she worried about Jason doing drugs with him—at least, smoking weed. Jason started getting into trouble after the blood infection episode. After she confronted Jason with her suspicions, he left the Big House for his parents' house. He needed time to think.

His initial streak of being in a pleasant mood and trying to be healthy began to fade after the Land Rover was taken away. Soon Jason returned to snarfing junk food and drinking beer. It drove Cathy nuts to see him falling back into his old self-destructive behavior. She did not know what to do. He even picked up smoking cigarettes. As his mood deteriorated and he regained the weight that he had lost, his face broke out. It was sad and seemed unstoppable. Jason had not formally moved out of the Big House, but he stopped living there. Yet he remained close to his cousins (C. Berg 2010).

A month or two later, he wanted to return to the Big House and discussed it with his aunt Virginia. Virginia, still under the impression that Jason was getting into trouble, turned him down. It was spring 1986, and both his mother and aunt were pushing him hard to improve.

Perhaps as an incentive, Ralph bought Jason a new blue Ford Bronco. Suddenly, Jason was back. Steve was impressed as they drove around in the Bronco to buy cigarettes. They even tried to buy a case of beer. One day they were cruising around Manito Park near the Park Bench Café. Jason stopped to admire a motorcycle and wave at the riders. The biker had a young lady on the back, and Jason rolled down his window to comment, "God, I hope that's your sister," implying that the young lady's looks did not meet Jason's criteria for a girlfriend. With that, he sped off. The two cousins laughed.

Jason pushed back hard against the formalities of life that he felt were irrelevant to him. He went where the action was, where he could connect with his friends, and he tormented anyone and everyone in the process. As he grew older, he learned to approach difficulties by arriving at some understanding, but structure, manners, and boundaries were never his concern.

Jason owned a Skulls skateboard. Awkward on the small board, Jason loved to skate despite the obvious risk of injuring himself. He led his parents to believe that because the board was small, it was safer. Then, in late May, Jason and his friends were under the freeway at a skate park near their high school. Jason tumbled off his board and slammed hard onto the concrete. He was short of breath, which frightened Tola and the others.

They watched and waited to see what Jason would do as he lay immobile on the ground. They were close to two hospitals and decided to phone Jason's parents from a nearby public phone. Jason admitted to feeling poorly, and an ambulance was called to the scene. Barely holding it together, Tola knelt close to Jason when the paramedic inserted the intravenous into his arm. Jason reassured his friend by telling him that he had received intravenous injections on numerous occasions.

After the ambulance drove off with Jason inside, Tola drove the Bronco home to Jason's parents. The next day, he and their friends went to the hospital to pay Jason a visit. The group was traumatized by the incident. At the hospital, they learned that Jason had punctured a lung and had a pulmonary embolism, both potentially life threatening. Still, Jason looked good and was cracking jokes. The doctors ran his annual cardiac echo, which showed a stable repair. Unbeknownst to all was the reality that the right ventricle is not durable when burdened with the work of the left ventricle, and chest X-rays show the right ventricle size better than a standard echo.

Jason was only hospitalized for a few days before being discharged. Everyone at the hospital was keenly aware that he was on borrowed time and would not have a long life. He was treated with abundant kindness and compassion. He returned to school one week later (Rogalski 2011).

The ferry on Lake Coeur d'Alene had so influenced Ralph as a youngster that he vowed to keep its memory alive. When a float house from this now long-gone ferry system came available, Ralph purchased it. Early that summer of 1986, Jason was working with an older brother on this float house. Rory and his daughter came out to the lake. Jason's niece was awed by the dramatic unveiling of his bare chest, exposing the scars that extended from his neck to his groin. Before the conversation got too intense, Jason changed the subject. He commented on her cool long, straight hair. He demonstrated how to "head bang" like the metal band musicians did. She immediately tried it while dramatically tossing her hair from side to side. It was cool but made her dizzy. Jason cracked up, and his laughter was infectious (E. Berg 2010).

Later that summer, when the weather had turned hot, Ralph drove Jason and Tola up to the cabin at Berg Bay. As typical independent teenagers, the boys wanted to stay a week to rough it and be by themselves. Tola, Jason, and Walter the dog remained alone without a car or a phone while Ralph went home. Ever the avid hunter and outdoorsman, Ralph was pleased they wanted solitude for a week. He would pick them up the following weekend.

As soon as they were alone, Jason informed Tola that there were girls at the lake. Tola figured this was the driving force behind the lake trip, and he did not mind. They could do both. As they were exploring along the beach, with sticks in the sand and toes in the water, Jason explained that Cathy and her friends were at a cabin about a mile south, near Spokane Point, which was easily accessible by boat. Since they had a rowboat, they decided to visit. On the following day, they rowed down the shoreline, eager to spend time with the girls in their skimpy bikinis. It was a fun and exciting day. Uncle Mike gave them a lift and towed the rowboat back to their cabin.

The next night, only three days into the week, they ran out of food but had some pocket change and were able to get to a store across the lake in Harrison, Idaho—about two miles. The journey went well in the rowboat. After purchasing supplies, they walked next door for some ice cream. There they saw a storm rolling in over the lake, with gale winds and white caps forming atop huge waves. Ominous clouds filled the sky; they would be unable to get back across the lake in their small boat. Fortunately, a friendly stranger offered to get them back to the cabin in his speedboat. The rowboat remained in Harrison, Idaho. When Ralph arrived as planned a few days later, it seemed that the boys' week at the cabin had been notably quiet until Jason explained about the missing rowboat. Ralph was visibly annoyed on the drive back to Spokane (Rogalski 2011).

Jason's seventeenth birthday was a big success. Having been told that he might not live beyond age ten, eleven became Jason's magic number. After the big one, his doctors revised his life expectancy to seventeen. And here was that birthday. Another year beyond his heart doctor's best estimate of life expectancy was not just a gift but an exception to the rule. Jason loved this annual celebration of life with all his friends.

Now high school seniors and still without girlfriends, Jason and Tola remained close with Cathy and her group of friends. One of the girls in this group, Erin, had admired Jason since junior high.

Jason always treated his friends and parents in a tough but lighthearted way, the way he treated everyone, including himself. His friends tried to reform him but to no avail. Although there was no serious trouble, Tola felt bad about the incidents that disappointed the adults. Still, he and Jason enjoyed the school year together.

When Tola graduated Lewis and Clark High School in the spring of 1987, Jason was not present to walk with him at the ceremony. Although Tola was sure that Jason had graduated, he could not explain his absence. Tola went off to college. Jason stayed in Spokane and worked.

Over that summer, Jason stayed at the lake. He worked on the float house, fixing it up with his older brothers, and he played guitar. Rory, who played in a band, had hired Jason to play with them and act as road crew. They traveled by car and van to the gig, set up, played, and then dismantled the sets and packed up to go home. They played in Coeur d'Alene, Spokane, and the Spokane Valley.

On his grandpa Thoralf's ninetieth birthday that June, Jason attended the big party at the Big House. It was a grand celebration; lots of family came in, including me, though I was in medical school. Leila and Thoralf sat together on the back porch, holding hands and new babies.

It felt a bit awkward, returning to Lewis and Clark High School without his friends, with Tola off to college and Cathy spending her senior year in Japan as an exchange student. But Jason did return and walked up the front steps and into the front hall as if he owned the place. In the fall of 1987, Jason needed a few credits to meet graduation requirements. Erin, one of Cathy's friends, was pleased to see him. It never dawned on her that he had failed to graduate on time.

When Erin and Jason met back up in World Affairs, Jason was smitten. She was stunning, with big blue eyes and wavy red hair, and full of energy. He sat next to Erin every day. Her reaction—"Who is this crazy guy?"—with his devil-may-care attitude he was refreshing to her. Erin, seventeen and living independently, made the last year at Lewis and Clark High School the best for both. She was reasonable, responsible, and had an apartment with a roommate to lower her expenses. They had a thing for each other. For Erin, it went back to junior high; for Jason, it was big and new.

After a few weeks, Erin saw the difficult side of Jason and became conflicted. He showed up late for school every day, entering with a grin. She soon realized that he came to school stoned, and she did not approve. Yet they enjoyed their time together. That same fall, Steve saw the difficult side as well. They were out cruising in Jason's Bronco and spotted a kid sitting in the grass with his legs stretched out, catching some late summer sun at a bus stop. Jason turned the Bronco slightly and drove up on the curb and straight toward the kid's legs. At the last moment, the kid freaked, and Jason turned back toward the street. The kid shook his fist at the Bronco, and Jason laughed and drove on. Steve was not laughing.

After winter break, Erin did not return to high school. Both she and Jason received their GED certificates independently of each other and seemed to drift apart. Later, there was some talk of Jason going to technical school to become an open-heart pump technician. His parents thought it would be a suitable career choice. Instead, he started at Spokane Falls Community College, taking art classes (Meenach 2011).

The summer of 1988, I was able to make a brief visit home to Spokane, and Uncle Ralph was interested in my decision to train in surgery. He advised me to "stay general." He also said, "You should go to Seattle and get a transplant." Ralph was neither joking nor rude, just matter-of-fact. We had our longest conversation to date. By then, I had figured out his communication style. A few years earlier, when we talked about my decision to go to medical school, Ralph said, "It's too bad you're not a man." He had worried that medical school would be too much for me. Speaking with him now about transplants and surgery training, I just listened. He knew so much.

He held the opinion that organ donation would never be a resolved issue. Without aggressive donations, organ replacement could not become a standard. I let him know my plan—to keep my organs healthy, preserve them. Preservation leads to prevention. I understood that he was concerned about both me and Jason. My illness, with its potential for organ failure, might accelerate under the pressure of surgical training. It is possible Ralph considered heart replacement for Jason. Heart transplants started in Spokane in 1985. At the time, I had a million questions about Jason and hearts, but Ralph did not want to talk about his youngest, who was fine.

Cautiously, I entered the world of surgeons in 1989 and almost immediately learned of Dr. Ralph Berg's distinction and brilliance with acute coronary revascularization. The long-term follow-up studies were published from the Spokane Experience database that same year (M. A. Dewood 1984, M. A. Dewood 1989).

When Jason accidentally bumped into Erin at a party in late December 1988, they had not seen each other for nearly a year. They fell into an intense conversation until Jason excused himself to go to the bathroom. Erin impatiently followed him in because she had something to say. He laughed, they exchanged phone numbers, and their relationship started again. With Erin's help, Jason moved out of his parents' house on Sunset Hill. His new apartment was nice, close to the hospital and to his aunt and uncle's house. Erin would come over with groceries and make them dinner. Jason would rent a movie. They loved to talk about music and art.

A book and video store opened called Hastings that Erin was eager to check out, so they drove there to get a movie. Jason knew Rory considered this store a competitor but didn't share his worry with Erin. It was a warm, early-summer day in 1989, and Jason got antsy as Erin lingered in the store. When she left to use the restroom, Jason fled. Erin walked around in search of Jason, who was nowhere to be found. He had ditched her.

Erin called her mom, then Rory. After forty-five minutes, her stepfather arrived to collect her. He drove her to her mother's house. Erin was livid. She had her limits about self-care, self-respect, and wanting to be together. They'd had a great time, but she was done with Jason.

Jason showed up at her mother's house thirty minutes after Erin got there. Rory had let him know where Erin was and to not worry about loyalty to Video Unlimited over Hastings. Jason parked the Bronco, walked up to the door, and knocked. Erin's mother opened the door. There was a pause, then "I have nothing to say to you, Jason."

"I got sick of waiting for her," Jason told her mother. Dead silence. Finally, Jason returned to his car to retrieve Erin's stuff from the passenger seat and brought it back to her mother. Erin watched the scene play out from an upstairs window. It was hard to stay mad at Jason; she could tell he felt badly. Then, as he was leaving, he turned momentarily to utter a quick joke: "See y'all around."

"No," she screamed, "we're done" (Meenach 2011).

After art classes at the local community college, and with Erin pissed and done, Jason moved out of his apartment and out of town to Medical Lake, a small town about twenty miles away, where he would live with his friend Nathan. It was a beautiful and rustic place, a working ranch with lots of open land and cattle. Jason and Nathan were going to run the place as ranch hands. The work was nonstop and physical. Late in the fall, Jason grew tired again, and following a battery of heart tests, Ralph finally informed him that he needed another surgery. For Jason, it was no big deal. He would be readmitted to the hospital, but at least he would be in Spokane and near his friends.

Cathy came home for Christmas break in 1989 to find Jason in a hospital bed after undergoing another open-heart surgery. His fresh, scabby scar on top of the old familiar pile of scars both fascinated and horrified her. Unbeknownst to the family and friends, the younger open-heart surgeons had closed a VSD defect between Jason's ventricles with Dr. Berg's approval, increasing the load on his right ventricle. But Jason seemed remarkably the same, and Cathy let herself relax.

He begged her for junk food. He wanted greasy Taco Bell and a large chocolate malt from Dick's. He asked Cathy to make a list and was specific about what he wanted and did not want. No mistakes! The list had foods from three different fast-food drive-ins, which seemed like a bad idea to Cathy. She phoned Uncle Ralph, who told her it was fine for Jason to have outside food and everything he requested on the list was okay. So, she fetched it all and brought it back to the hospital for Jason. They chatted, got caught up, and chowed down. Soon he was sound asleep (C. Berg 2010).

Jason slowly recovered and began to feel better. His friend Nathan visited Erin regularly. When she understood that Jason was sitting out in Nathan's car, she said, "Why don't you have him come up?" It was spring 1990, and it was good to see him. Jason invited Erin to visit him and Nathan at the farmhouse. Susan, Erin's housemate, had a car. Wasting no time, Erin bought food and drinks for a barbeque, and Susan drove them to the farmhouse. The great dinner set the stage for not just one but two new couples.

For Erin and Jason, it was a wonderful reunion. He was pleased that she took him back. "I am Virgo, earth; and Erin is Pisces, water. Together we make mud," he would say. Erin stayed with Jason that night, a night that was years in the making. Jason was still a virgin. They were game on, together, happy. Erin noted, "After we made love, we did it a lot." Jason felt he had years to make up for and was ecstatic. Shortly thereafter, the ranch hired a full-time keeper, and Jason and

Nathan moved out (Meenach 2011).

Erin's friend Janet returned to Spokane in May. She had been modeling in Tokyo and had recently met Cathy, who was also modeling, at a trade show outside Tokyo. The two models hung out together at the clubs, noting how small the world was. When Janet contacted Erin, she was surprised to hear Erin's stories about Jason Berg, Cathy's cousin. Janet, who had previously heard from Erin that Jason was an obnoxious guy who had ditched her while she was in a restroom, was amazed that Erin and Jason were dating. Janet and Erin discussed Jason at length. He received money from his wealthy parents, was unemployed but talked about finding a job, and had only his GED certificate and some community college courses. Both young ladies agreed that Jason's parents would not approve of his partying with drugs and alcohol. They assumed all parents would be opposed to this type of behavior. Janet warned Erin to be cautious.

Jason could be so frustrating. He was moody. "More than Words" by Extreme became their song, and they weathered their storms by singing those words to each other. Jason turned twenty-one that summer, 1990. Rory surprised him with a guitar and amplifier (Meenach 2011).

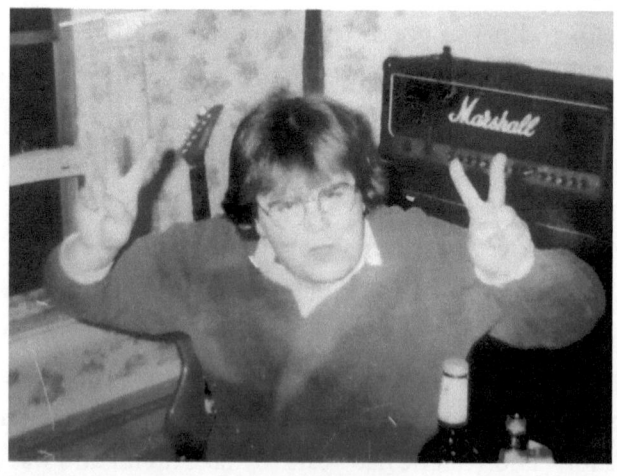

Jason at his twenty-first birthday with guitar and amplifier from Rory, August 1990.

One day, Steve ran into Jason, who was out driving his blue Bronco. Jason had a blown stereo and wanted a new one. When Steve offered to repair the stereo to save Jason money, Jason was thrilled. Steve began to recognize that his own resourcefulness and ability to achieve valuable new skills contrasted with Jason, who was on borrowed time and lived each day as if it were his last (S. Berg 2011). Jason had no use for rules, decorum, education, or anything to do with getting ahead. He lived only in the present.

Janet was delighted when she finally met Jason. She soon realized that her initial opinion had been unfairly colored. When she sat down to join the group of friends gathered to watch a movie, she appreciated Jason performing crowd control so all could enjoy. "Shut the fuck up," he commanded, and the room instantly quieted down. It was effective, a relief, and kind of funny (Robel 2011).

By spring 1991, they were all twenty-one and of legal drinking age. Having cocktails together was fresh and fun. Life was good, and Janet enjoyed hanging around with Erin and Jason. They laughed at Jason's black humor and enjoyed a break from the grind of work and low finances. They appreciated Jason's willingness to share his parental stipend (Robel 2011).

When Jason went in for his May heart checkup in 1991, his doctor said the echo was the same, perhaps a little better since the last surgery. Jason never too worried about these checkups, as they seemed to not matter much. His number, eleven, had passed a decade ago.

Two weeks later, Jason phoned his father to report that his heart was racing and he felt kind of weird. They met at the doctor's office, and the EKG indicated a racing heart. Jason was diagnosed with supraventricular tachycardia, and both the pediatric cardiologist and Ralph agreed on the diagnosis. Medication was the next step. Jason was started on digoxin, a medication to slow his heart. Jason had been on digoxin previously, before his major surgery in 1980.

When Jason told Erin that they had been invited to his parents' house, she realized that she had no idea about his family. Jason frequently talked about getting married and running away to the Hitching Post in Coeur d'Alene for the ceremony. Now Erin realized that meeting his parents was the first serious step toward that future. On the evening of the invitation, as Jason drove Erin to the house, he apologized, and she did not understand why. She did not know that Jason came from a medical family and assumed his parents would be casual and have a great sense of humor like he did. She reassured him that the meeting would be fine. When they arrived, Erin got out of the car and walked with Jason to the door to greet his family. She felt relaxed, and their home was both beautiful and grand.

Mary and Ralph were much older than she expected, and formal, which left Erin almost speechless. They were exactly the opposite of Jason. She found herself unprepared. It was awkward and overwhelming. Erin and Jason left as quickly as they could, politely extracting themselves from the situation.

Something shifted after meeting his parents, or perhaps after the racing heart scare. Jason's parents talked, and they began looking at houses for the couple. Erin and Jason were excited to move out of the party house where they had been informally living together. Knowing that Jason was on borrowed time, Erin wanted him to stop his excessive behaviors. He began to put the drinking and smoking behind him. Now they were moving into a beautiful vintage home on Twenty-Ninth near Regal on South Hill; Jason's parents purchased it for them. Jason and Erin made the move with relative ease. It was fabulous. Erin took care of him. Jason asked Erin to elope, but she declined. She loved him, but marriage was a step she was not prepared to take this soon.

Erin wanted Janet to join them at the lake one weekend. For Janet, it was so lovely to see Erin happy. It was a beautiful day, a beautiful drive, but still cold when they got to the float house. They walked down the slope and across the long dock. The float house felt like a place out of history. As Janet stepped onto the decking, Rory came out to greet them (Meenach 2011). Rory was funny and welcoming, joking with the girls. He had the same dark, dry humor as his youngest brother. Yet Rory's demeanor became serious later in the day as he explained that Jason would have been the same as Rory had it not been for his heart. Jason had the same chest size as his brother, but his heart condition had affected his legs and stunted his growth. His legs were smaller and shorter than his four brothers'.

Janet finally began to relax about Jason. She herself was in a stable long-distance relationship with an older gentleman from France, whom she had met during her time modeling. She wanted Erin to have stability too.

Two weeks later, Jason and Erin again took Janet to the lake. It was a Saturday, and this time they went to the cabin on Berg Bay. Janet was well prepared to meet Jason and Rory's parents. Ralph and Mary were kind and seemed pleased to have the company. Mary commented to Rory, who hadn't been in a relationship with his daughter's mom for years, that Janet was pretty. It was obvious Rory and Janet liked each other.

The next week, Janet called Jason and Erin, sobbing and upset. Her boyfriend had broken things off. Jason and Erin were taken by surprise and took special care to protect Janet, who was now emotionally fragile. Empathetic about Janet's breakup, Jason made her smile through her tears as he pranced around the living room of their new house, wearing one of Erin's skirts while humorously describing the virtues of wearing one. He was wickedly funny. Erin noted how Jason loved her skirts, which were like his hospital gowns, flowing and large. He seemed to feel safe and secure in them (Meenach 2011).

Janet began to struggle, working nights at the Silver Grill bartending and waitressing. She hated to be alone after the breakup. Jason and Erin would come in and sit with her at the bar. Janet started calling in sick to work and would instead hang with them at their house. She was profoundly depressed about the breakup, and in her grief clung to her friends. Rory also started hanging out at the Silver Grill in support of Janet, and soon she began to calm down. In a minor episode, Jason's guitar was stolen by people whom he thought were friends. When Rory found out who had taken advantage of Jason, he retrieved the guitar for Jason. Janet was impressed by how these two brothers looked out for each other (Robel 2011).

The 1991 July 4 weekend at Lake Coeur d'Alene was busy and beautiful, and lots of people arrived to take pleasure in the lake's many features and entertainments. Many in the Berg family were at the float house. Folks were boating, visiting, and spread around the lake: the float house on Kidd Island Bay and the family cabins near Spokane Point and Harrison, Idaho, with the gas station and store.

A sudden skirmish occurred, and Ralph got knocked out. Jason instantly grabbed for his father and slammed into the deck under his weight. Terrified for his dad, he started to sob. Erin, not knowing what happened or what to do, stood close by, waiting and watching. She thought the collapse had been the result of too many people crowded into a tight space (Meenach 2011).

When Ralph came to, he was furious at his older son, who had hit him. No one knew exactly what had happened. Nor had anyone paid attention to the skirmish until Rory and his daughter returned from the store to discover Jason injured. Then everyone panicked (E. Berg 2010).

Any trauma to Jason's chest could become a fatal event, and Jason's pain was dreadful. Later that evening, Ralph took Jason for X-rays, which confirmed rib fractures at the lateral left fifth rib. The chest X-ray also showed a change. There was progressive enlargement of Jason's heart, cardiomegaly, compared with the last films made in December 1989. Ralph knew the cardiologists were working off the annual echo of Jason's heart, not chest X-rays, but had it been that long since Jason's last chest X-ray?

In mid-July, Ralph informed Jason that Cathy was back in Spokane for a visit and wanted to hang out at the lake. Rory drove his boat packed full with Jason and friends. Tola was with them, all waving at Cathy as they pulled up to the dock. She was elated. Then Cathy spotted her friend Janet from Tokyo. Janet was with Erin, a friend from seventh grade. She looked fabulous, and it was a fun reunion. Cathy could tell Rory was moving in on Janet, who seemed to be into him. But Cathy was most interested in seeing Jason.

Her cousin looked great. Even better, Erin was a great partner. "I am so happy for you, Jason!" said Cathy. It appeared he had grown up quite a bit. Cathy had never seen him so happy or calm (C. Berg 2010). They spent the day in Harrison, Idaho, pigging out on ice cream and hanging out together. That was when Erin decided to throw Jason a surprise birthday party for his twenty-second.

Rory helped her stealthily arrange the party. She phoned Tola to explain the details. The night before the party, Erin and Rory remained mum while out on a double date with Jason and Janet and said nothing to either of them. It was a great evening, with live music playing at the local bar. Afterward, all four went back to Rory's house, from which Jason and Erin left shortly to return home. Rory had converted his garage into a large family room with a huge open window, where he and Janet, perched on the couch, sat watching Jason with his arm around Erin as they walked away. Jason turned to smile back at Rory and Janet. Janet was taken by his smile. Jason was content and happy for Rory and Janet.

Early the next morning, Rory picked up Janet and took her to the lake. They were still getting to know each other, and it would be their first time spending a weekend alone together. Rory was serious about Janet, and Erin knew that no one would be able to reach them until the next day. Rory had helped Erin plan the party, right down to the detail of *not inviting him or Janet so they could have this weekend.*

As the morning progressed that Saturday, Jason had just stopped to gas up his truck when he spotted a car driving by and honking. It was a cousin and his wife (R. Berg 2011). *That is small-town Spokane!* he marveled. When he finished his errands, he drove the truck home and returned to work at Little Caeser's. He liked making pizza. It always smelled good, and his customers were happy. He had been awarded with a golden coin for his steady work. Once his shift was over, he walked home.

"Honey, I'm home," he yelled, which was met with a chorus of "SURPRISE!!!" It was his birthday, and Jason was twenty-two years old (Meenach 2011).

Erin had arranged a spectacular party. "This is the best day of my life," Jason said, beaming for all to see. He greeted each of his friends, saying it again and again—"the best day of my life." All his friends, some of whom he had not seen for a few years, showed up. The party was vibrant, and everyone enjoyed themselves. Jason told Tola about his last heart procedure, and Tola was again struck by how giving Jason was. He affected so many people in a positive way.

The life plans Jason and Tola had made back in grade school were all about having fun. Nothing serious had ever occurred to them. Not then. Now they were hanging out again, and it felt as if they hadn't missed a day together. Jason looked good all summer, and it was the best time of their lives. Everyone was joyous and in a celebratory mood. As the party wound down and people were leaving, Erin was pleased. There had been no drama, no fights, and it felt like she and Jason were a married couple. Rory's advice about the mechanics of the party had been spot on. She would call to thank him later.

That night, when Jason broached the subject about plans for the upcoming holiday weekend with Erin, he teased her about being the mom who sings to her kids. He was tired and thanked her as they collapsed in bed together. "Tomorrow, we'll clean up this mess."

CHAPTER 22

The Governor, 1991

It was a beautiful and quiet Sunday morning on the lake. Janet jolted awake next to Rory; she needed to get to work by noon. She jumped up out of bed and got ready. She knew she would miss the lake. Being with Rory was wonderful; they had talked all day, lounged on the beach, then barbequed dinner. Rory watched her get dressed, then drove her into town. The drive was pleasant. Janet was quiet. They planned to meet later in the day (Robel 2011).

Jason and Erin had slept in at their home in South Hill after the party. He walked out to the kitchen. It was close to 10 a.m., a bright sunny morning, when he confronted a pile of dog poop in the middle of the kitchen floor. The room was a mess. He looked at his dog, who returned a guilty expression. Disgusted, Jason yelled for Erin.

The dog was supposedly trained. That smell made the mess worse. Jason was bending down to clean it up when Erin joined him in the kitchen. He stood quickly with a peculiar look in his eye. He turned to Erin. He said, "I'm dying."

Erin helped him to the couch. Jason sat down, slowly fell over, and died.

Erin was in shock. The surprise birthday party last night . . . *Oh, God was this related? No, he could not have just died.* She called 911. She performed CPR. She called Rory. He did not answer. She tried not to panic. She loved Jason.

Erin picked up the phone and called Jason's parents. Ralph answered on the first ring. She told Ralph what was happening.

The ambulance arrived. The paramedics took over CPR and worked on Jason. A friend from the party arrived with his mom to pick up his car. They drove Erin to the hospital, where Erin and Mary sat together, waiting (Meenach 2011).

Ralph, like so many times before, was waiting in the emergency room when the ambulance brought Jason in. The paramedics continued with CPR as they came through the ER doors. Dead on arrival. The ER report from August 31, 1991, reported a collapse and seizure-like activity at home, then unresponsive. Brought in by EMT with CPR ongoing, defibrillation for bradycardia, EMD (electrical mechanical dissociation). Given were two amps of atropine and two amps of epinephrine prior to arrival.

There was nothing to do. This time, Jason was dead.

Ralph became Dr. Berg. He ordered the autopsy. It was automatic. Ralph watched Jason, covered by white sheets, go to the morgue. Rory was still not answering the phone. Ralph tried a few more times. Ralph went home. Mary, already home, sat down next to Ralph. They waited, quiet.

Rory dropped Janet off at her work. He told her, "See you later." Janet looked forward to seeing him. Rory drove home and found messages blinking on the machine. He called his parents. He heard the news from them. They were all in shock. Erin called Janet at work that morning and told her the devastating news. Numb, Janet left work, and then Rory called and told her to meet him. When Rory walked in, he put his arms around her and cried, devastated (Robel 2011).

A few days later, the autopsy findings were equally devastating for Ralph. He could not and did not talk about it. The postmortem exam showed the anatomic details that could not be known in life. Jason had died of dilated right ventricle with the dreaded EMD, now labeled pulseless electrical activity (PEA). When an additional congenital defect—correctable—was identified at the autopsy, Ralph was stunned and guilty. The undiagnosed and untreated defect haunted him. Ralph explained to me, "You learn to not talk. People are limited and do not see what you see and know."

Both Ralph and Mary were distraught. The loss of their Jason was not something either one could talk about. Not Jason's death, his heart defect, the big one, the daily diligent monitoring and struggle to maintain Jason's heart, and certainly not the autopsy. Ralph shut down. Their grief, a reflection of their love and care for Jason, was overwhelming. Ralph and Mary could not bear to think about arranging a funeral. They did not have words for their loss. It was better to not have a service (M. Berg 2011; R. Berg 2006).

Rory's daughter Estee was with her mother in Seattle. With great reluctance, Rory told her of her beloved uncle's death. It was the first death she had ever experienced and the first time she saw her father cry. She was twelve. Rory explained to her how Erin had performed CPR when Jason arrested in their home. Later she learned Jason's heart was the size of a football when he died. She could not look at a football for years without thinking of her uncle Jason and his big heart (E. Berg 2010).

Tola had loved his friend and found some small comfort that Jason's passing had happened the morning after the best night of Jason's life. Tola, living with friends, taking classes at Spokane Community College, was conflicted. Jason had never conformed. He did what he wanted. He was wild. And now Tola, not on borrowed time, was to become a father. It had been too new and unexpected for Tola to even talk about it himself. Now Tola so wanted to tell Jason about becoming a father. He wanted to share with his best friend what it meant to become a dad. Tola decided he would finish college. He would be there for his baby, no matter how difficult. He felt that way because of Jason (Rogalski 2011).

Erin chose the church, Plymouth Congregational at the corner of Maple and Seventh Avenue. She and Jason had talked of getting married there, with its big white pillars out front and a bunch of stairs leading up from the street. Friends arranged the details for the service. They put the notice in the local newspaper. On the day of the funeral, Mary had to drag Ralph to the funeral. They were late (M. Berg 2011; Meenach 2011).

Only his surgical discipline and his love of Jason kept Ralph from crumbling completely under the burden of grief and self-doubt. Why hadn't he figured out the last defect? It was obvious, looking back. Mary cried when Julie Spores walked into the church—Julie, who knew and understood their agony like no one else. She hugged Mary, who said, "I knew you would come." Julie cried with Jason's parents.

The funeral was at night. Rory stayed close to Janet as Erin stood and talked about Jason: Jason had lived well. Jason had a wonderful birthday. Jason was loved and he loved.

The friends and family that attended Jason's funeral were all deeply saddened. The reception was well attended. Cousins of Ralph attended, and they kissed him, hugged him. Andy was there with his family. Steve, now in high school, came with his parents. He had found out about Jason's death from his friends; it took several days for the word to get out. No one really talked about it. Steve met several of his cousins for the first time at the funeral. They all adored Jason (S. Berg 2011).

The longevity that Jason achieved, with his complex transposition defect and repair, was not in perspective. Everyone felt Jason had been snatched by death unexpectedly. His mother's hope and belief, set by Dr. Lang and reinforced by Ralph, had been that Jason was and would be okay.

A month later, Virginia visited Jason's beautiful cousin Cathy, who was in art school in Los Angeles, and reported she had been to Jason's funeral. It was Cathy's first notice that her special cousin had died. No one had told her; her mother had not called her. As gutted as Cathy was about it, having seen him that day in July at the lake made it easier. Jason had been happy, truly happy (C. Berg 2010).

Ralph's father, Thoralf Berg, passed peacefully in 1993. Then Ralph retired from his surgery practice at the age of seventy-three. Ralph's research fund, which had $25,000 in it when he started in 1952, had the same amount when he retired. An important priority for Dr. Berg, his dog research was the foundation for his work. He gave Sacred Heart a gift of land with the value of half a million dollars. The land was used to build a convenient hotel for patients and patient families beside the hospital.

In 1995, I returned to Spokane and started in general surgery private practice. Over the years, several former patients of Dr. Ralph Berg came to see me. They told their stories of being treated by Dr. Ralph Berg or some other interaction with him. Mr. Max Davis remembered details of his ambulance ride from Valley General to Sacred Heart as he was having his heart attack at age twenty-nine. He had been the third patient on the new two-tier protocol.

It was always a pleasure to see Ralph dressed to the nines in the surgery lounge at either downtown hospital. He was cordial to all the doctors, knew most of them, and told the greatest stories.

The inconsistencies surrounding the death of Jason were impossible for me to reconcile. Jason's longevity was stunning. A complicated blue baby who did not die right away. Yet the grief hung on, silent and painful. Curiosity kept guiding me back to Ralph to ask again, "How did you perform with your blue baby?"

To learn this history has been a gift. It would have remained hidden.

So impressive his work, and yet so closed about himself and Jason.

As an admiring niece, I drove to his house one calm, colorful fall evening in October 2006, wanting his thoughts and his approval before submitting the nomination I had written for him. Retired and full of vigor, he was always happy to visit. A child with PDA and surgical closure had come back to see him earlier that day. As an adult, this appreciative patient walked in at the chest surgery office to check up on his doctor. Ralph beamed as he told me all about the case and this procedure. "When not done correctly, Tracy, it was lethal," he stated.

He reviewed my nomination for an accolade. We sat together on the couch. Watching him as he read, I admired his laser-blue eyes. With his Viking heritage, he looked like his father, Thoralf. Then, he stiffened, and his shoulders pulled away from me. He was no longer relaxed in his white button-down shirt, open at the collar, and pale-blue jeans. Politely, he told me how nice it was. He told me it was appreciated. Then he paused, and his face changed. His whole demeanor changed, that fire ignited. That fire that used to scare me. He sternly told me that if he won, he would never accept that award, and he explained why.

With insight into what is frivolous and what is important and a profound connection to my uncle, a pioneering open-heart surgeon, I threw out the nomination, and we continued.

He explained to me how Jason, doomed, and acute heart attack patients were related by the need to preserve each patient's myocardium. I needed to know how he dealt with being a heart surgeon and father of a doomed blue baby. We connected, he explained, he sketched, he cried. A sick youngster myself inside the Berg family, I started to understand. The loss, the grief, and the passage of time brought us together, and, surgeon to surgeon, this hidden story emerged.

Jason's autopsy remained an unwelcome topic for Ralph. His reaction upon learning that his son had a repairable aortic coarctation defect at the diaphragm caused him to go silent. Over the years of developing this story to show this history in a positive way, Ralph was able to find peace in most areas—but not the governor, the aortic coarctation acting like the pulmonary band. Ralph Berg, as a parent, could not have perspective on this additional defect that decreased the workload by decreasing the peripheral circulation.

The atrial switch with a valved conduit from the left ventricle to the pulmonary artery that Dr. Kirklin installed eventually led Jason's right ventricle to dilate under the burden of the heavy systemic work. Ralph remarked, "It is now known the right ventricle does not hold up well to this task." The right ventricle, difficult to view on echo, had thinned and dilated, which presented as the EMD and Jason's death. The aortic coarctation was repairable; however, it was also the governor for Jason. The governor responsible for Jason's legs being smaller and shorter, as Rory had explained. The governor responsible for keeping a significant load off Jason's right heart, just as a governor does for any engine.

What you do not know is always so much bigger than what you do know.

Every scientific advance has a period of rejection, where the established way of thinking is resistant to the new advance. This period of rejection sometimes lasts beyond the life of the scientific pioneer. After a problem is advanced with science, several new and previously unknown problems are revealed. This is just the way it is with science. The doctors and surgeons bold and talented enough to cross into open-heart from no hope were motivated and pioneering. These young, talented surgeons came out of varied surgical training. They did not seek accolades for their accomplishments; they shared their work, with only minor lapses into competitiveness in their pursuit of intracardiac time.

Ralph Berg stayed in the game for Jason, as noted by Dr. Merendino. And every patient with coronary heart blockages benefited. People do not realize the magnitude of their work when they are in the work. Over time, open-heart surgical revascularization was replaced with PCI—percutaneous coronary interventions—like stents and clot busters. Ralph initially defended the open-heart technique, but he also knew the treatment needed to be consistently low risk, performed under sixty minutes from symptoms, and effective.

As life goes on and time heals, the ability to talk over the story and write it down has revealed the most difficult things in life. Ralph held tightly to his belief in Jason and a mystery regarding his will to live. That autopsy revealed a secret, perhaps the mystery, that both lent Jason extra time and caused his dad grief over his lack of knowledge. As an artist, Jason's life was his canvas. He never limited his art.

Grief is collective, intergenerational, and demands communal review and acceptance to settle. Ralph focused on why. Why did Mary get sick early in her pregnancy with Jason? Ralph also focused on the fix. It was sobering, but he learned he could advance but not complete the switch model in dogs., so he chose the best blue-baby repair surgeon for Jason. Ralph and Mary were parents who together and individually did their best. Each day that Jason was alive, they were able to live. When he was suddenly gone, they had to find another way to face each day. The three-way dysfunction was always spiraling, with Rory caught in the middle, protecting his brother Jason. Rory said of his parents, "They put the 'fun' in dysfunctional."

Parents never expect to bury a child. And the Berg family is not known for letting go. From July 1980—when Jason had "the big one" with the father of open-heart surgery, Dr. John Kirklin—until August 31, 1991, when Jason dropped dead after the best day of his life, Ralph raced with Jason against time. The world was silent, stunned or unaware. Yet the event, Jason's life, stands as a record—unbroken, timeless, and meaningful as father and son together willed Jason to live.

In each grief, there is opportunity. What is difficult is to stay calm and focused to find the opportunity, the way forward, through the fear and grief.

The father of chest surgery, Dr. Evarts Graham, launched young Dr. Ralph Berg into the pursuit of hearts when he placed Berg ahead of his known surgeons coming back from war. Success brought a new kind of surgeon, bold and focused, who withstood the crushing grief of failure as they focused on advancing the new heart shunts and the heart-lung machines. These rare surgeons—those who made the transition into open-heart with the machine they collectively perfected through their unique surgical camaraderie and competition—are pioneers. Their scientific devotion was taught to them in their training programs. Their collective work resulted in heart-lung machines and an explosion of technology and lifesaving operations not likely to be equaled in another era.

I am reminded of my uncle's favorite line from Alfred, Lord Tennyson: "Men may come and men may go, but I go on forever."

Share grief, and then enjoy the life you have. Men may come and men may go, but these open-heart surgical pioneers, they go on forever.

EPILOGUE

This story is a tribute to Jason, Rory, and Ralph Berg and all those who contributed to the research that revealed what a heart attack is and how to treat it. Over thirty years have passed since Jason's death at the remarkable age of twenty-two and fifty years since the first acute revascularization procedure in Spokane.

Jason's doctors told him he would not make it past age ten. Part of living on borrowed time is a keen awareness of your number being up. When your number is up, you know any day might be the day you pass. Jason made it through the big one when he was ten years old. Despite the rough and rocky experience, he made it. His eleventh birthday was a huge celebration. He claimed eleven as his number.

Dr. Ralph Berg died peacefully at ninety-six in Spokane in 2017.

Millions of lives have been saved since that first ACR procedure in 1971, where prompt revascularization by direct coronary artery bypass salvages the heart muscle and life. It forever changed the worldwide approach to the dying myocardium. Since then, the difficult repairs for complex transposition emerged, and survival of blue babies to adulthood is now over 90 percent.

Ralph helped develop this book. He read and beamed with each chapter, especially liking the chapters regarding the dog lab and heart-lung machine improvements before going live with a human patient. Fear often shackles us and keeps us from seeing clearly the path ahead. Academic and local rejection did not keep the Spokane Experience

ACR from being delivered to the world. Truth won. The love of a father for his most vulnerable son won. It was a simple choice for Ralph Berg.

My grandfather Thoralf and uncle Ralph held my interest from a young age. As a general surgeon returning to Spokane, Washington, in 1995, I regularly visited Ralph and Mary. Curious and with knowledge of Jason's amazing longevity despite his particularly difficult blue-baby syndrome, I pursued my question with Ralph. Deflection turned into talk of surgical cases with helpful insight. I returned often. When my question was answered and this story came forward that day in October 2006, I understood my uncle's desire for the Jason part of the story to remain hidden. Yet the entwined story demanded to be told.

With my uncle's directive to tell the story in a positive way, the interviews, the blue-baby survivors Linda Childs, Judy Miller Van Voorhis, and Greg, patients I met in my surgery practice who had relationships with Ralph Berg, and the large Berg family and friends fit the story together like puzzle pieces. Dr. Ralph Berg, who bore the tremendous gift of Jason and stayed steady in his course, knew myocardial preservation as the unifying concept of all heart diseases. He showed the world acute coronary revascularization while caring for Jason.

In these times, people with acute heart attacks or sudden cardiac arrest can be saved by the public—anyone who knows chest compressions, to call 911, basic airway management, and to get the defibrillator and give the shock before the ambulance arrives.

ACKNOWLEDGMENTS

To Dr. Hustrulid, my book dad, thank you for helping me with advice, getting interviews, keeping me encouraged, and keeping the members of the Spokane Experience heart teams updated and together. To Dr. Linda Harrison, Suzanne Berg, and Julie Spores for advice and editing help.

To Dr. Francis Everhart, the brilliant cardiologist who understood heart attacks, devised a scientific protocol, invited the best surgeon, Dr. Ralph Berg, to join his pursuits, and together with the Spokane Experience heart teams was able to prove what a heart attack is.

My gratitude and admiration for pediatric cardiologist Dr. Henry Lang. In early September 1969, he diagnosed and performed the initial atrial septostomy procedure for Jason to save his life and buy him time to grow. In 1974 he diagnosed my type 1 diabetes and boosted me toward health and longevity.

BIBLIOGRAPHY

Ainsberg, Thea Cooper and Arthur. 2010. *Breakthrough Elizabeth Hughes, the Discovery of Insulin, and the Making of a Medical Miracle.* Vol. 1. New York, New York: St. Martin's Press.

Bakaeen, F. MD, et al. 2018. "The Father of Coronary artery bypass grafting: Rene Favaloro and the 50th anniversary of coronary artery bypass grafting." *Journal of Thoracic and Cardiovascular Surgery* 2324-2328.

Berg, Alice, interview by Dr. Tracy Berg. 2010. *Family, PEO Chapter CL* Spokane, Washington, (December 29).

Berg, Andy, interview by Dr. Tracy Berg. 2002. *Cousin of Ralph* Spokane, Washington: Richards, Pflum, Karge, Chicago, Illinois.

Berg, Cathy, interview by Tracy Berg. 2010. *Cousin of Jason* Spokane, Washington, (May).

Berg, Ralph, interview by Dr. Tracy Berg. 2006. *Pioneering Open Heart Surgeon,* Spokane, Washington, (October 6).

Berg, Estee, interview by Dr. Tracy Berg. 2010. *Niece of Jason* Spokane, Washington, (December 10).

Berg, Mary, interview by Dr. Tracy Berg. 2011. *Mother of Jason* Spokane, Washington, (May 27).

Berg, R., S. Selinger, J. L. Leonard, R. P. Grunwald, W. P. O'Grady. 1981. "Surgical Treatment of Acute Evolving Anterior Myocardial Infarction (AEMI)." *Journal of Thoracic and Cardiovascular Surgery* 81 (4): 493-497.

Berg, Ralph. 1995. "Curriculum Vitae." *Ralph Berg, Jr., MD.* Spokane, Washington. 1-10.

Berg, Ralph. 1956. "Surgical Management of Congenital Tracheoesophageal Fistula and Esophageal Atresia." *The Journal of Thoracic Surgery* 31 (5).

Berg, Randy, interview by Dr. Tracy Berg. 2011. *Cousin of Jason* Spokane, Washington, (January 3).

Berg, RJ, Dabbs CH. 1957. "Intrapericardial bronchogenic Cysts: Report of Two Cases and probable embryologic Explanation." *Journal of Thoracic Surgery* 34 (6): 718-735.

Berg, RJ, Everhart FJ, Duvoisin GE, Kendal RW, Gangi JH, Rudy LW. 1976. "Operation for Acute Coronary Occlusion." *The American Surgeon* 42 (7): 517-521.

Berg, RJ, Kendall RW. 1971. "Surgical Management of transposition of the great vessels." *American Surgeon* 37 (8): 467-471.

Berg, RJ, Kendall RW, Duvoisin GE, Ganji JH, Rudy LW, Everhart FJ. 1975. "Acute Myocardial Infarction A Surgical Emergency." *The Journal of Thoracic and Cardiovascular Surgery* 70 (3): 432-439.

Berg, RJ, Kendall RW, Duvoisin, G. 1976. "Surgical treatment for ventricular aneurysm." *American Surgeon* 42 (7): 517-521.

Berg, Steve, interview by Dr. Tracy Berg. 2011. *Cousin of Jason* Spokane, Washington, (June 11).

Brian Berge, RN, interview by Dr. Tracy Berg. 2011. *Perspective on Dr. Ralph Berg* Spokane, Washington, (January 11).

Chaphin, AV, Yeo, CS, Cowan, SW. 2014. "Robert Edward Gross (1905-1988): Ligation of a patent Ductus Arteriosus and the Birth of a Specialty." *Surgical History*, November.

Childs, Linda Morris, interview by Dr. Tracy Berg. 2011. *Blue baby repaired* Spokane, Washington, (July 30).

Cohn, Lawrence H. 2003. "Fifty Years of Open-Heart Surgery." *Circulation* 107 (17): 2168-2170.

Cohn, Lawrence. 1993. "The first successful surgical treatment of mitral stenosis: the 70th anniversary of Elliot Cutler's mitrol

Commissurotomy." *Annals of Thoracic Surgery* 56 (5): 1187-1190.

Cooper, David. 2018. "Christian Barnard - the surgeon who dared: the story of the first human to human heart transplant." *Global Cardiology Science and Practice* (National Library of Medicine).

David K.C. Cooper, MD. 2010. *Open Heart the Radical Surgeons Who Revolutionized Medicine.* New York, New York: Kaplan Publishing New York.

Dewood MA, Spores J, Notske R, Mouser LT, Lang HT. 1980. "Prevalence of Total Coronary Occlusion during the Early Hours of Transmural Myocardial Infarction." *New England Journal of Medicine.* Vol. 303. October 18. 897-902.

Dewood, Dr. Marcus, interview by Dr. Tracy Berg. 2011. *Cardiologist and Researcher* Spokane, Washington, (May 20).

Dewood, MA, Berg, RJ. 1984. "The role of surgical reperfusion in myocardial infarction." *Cardiology Clinics* 113-122.

Dewood, MA, Leonard, J, Grunwald, RP, Berg, RJ, et al. 1989. "Medical and surgical management of early Q wave myocardial infarction II. Effects on mortality and global and regional left ventricular function at 10 or more years of follow up." *Journal American College of Cardiology* 14 (1): 65-90.

Dewood, MA, Spores, J, Berg, RJ et al. 1983. "Acute myocardial infarction: a decade of experience with surgical reperfusion in 701 patients." *Circulation* 68 (3 of 2): 118-126.

Dwight E Harkin, Paul M. Zoll. 1946. "Foreign Bodies in and in Relation to the Thoracic blood vessels and heart. Indications for the removal of Intracardiac Foreign Bodies and the behaviors of the heart during manipulations." *American Heart Journal.*

Everhart, Dr. Francis, interview by Dr. Tracy Berg. 2011. *Cardiologist* (October 31).

Everhart, F. 1975, February 25. "Angiography of the Acute evolving Myocardial Infarction." *Annual Cardiology Conference Meeting.* San Juan, Puerto Rico.

Galloway, Karla, interview by Dr. Tracy Berg. 2011. *RN* Spokane,

Washington, (October 16).

Garabedian, Dr. Hrair, interview by Dr. Tracy Berg. 2013. *Pediatric Cardiologist* Spokane, Washington.

Gayda, Margaret Berg, interview by Dr. Tracy Berg. 2011. *Sister of Ralph Berg* Spokane, Washington, (April 13).

Goran Wettrell, MD PhD. 2023. "Clarence Crafoord 1899-1984 Coarction of the aorta." *Hekeoen International A Journal of Medical Humanities*, winter.

Hendron, Shirley, interview by Dr. Tracy Berg. 2011. *family, daughter of Kitty Berg* Spokane, Washington, (April 18).

Hensley, Dr. Gerald Ross, interview by Dr. Tracy Berg. 2012. *Cardiologist* Spokane, Washington, (February 12).

Hershey, Dr. John, interview by Dr. Tracy Berg. 2011. *General Surgeon* Spokane, Washington, (May 20).

Hustrulid, Dr. Robert, interview by Dr. Tracy Berg. 2011. *MD Internist* Spokane, Washington, (March 25).

Johnson, Stephen L. 1970. *The History of Cardiac Surgery 1896-1955.* Baltimore and London, Maryland: The Johns Hopkins Press Baltimore and London.

Judge, Dr. Terrance, interview by Dr. Tracy Berg. 2012. *Cardiologist* Spokane, Washington, (January 14).

Kappen, James, interview by Dr. Tracy Berg. 2011. *RN, Operating Room Manager* Spokane, Washington, (June 3).

Katrapati, P, MD, George, J. MD. 2008. "Vineberg Operation: A review of the birth and impact of this surgical technique." *The Annals of Thoracic Surgery* November.

Kendall, Dr. Robert W, interview by Dr. Tracy Berg. 2011. *Heart Surgeon* Spokane, Washington, (October 29).

Kirklin, J, MD. 1980. *Operative Report Jason Berg.* Operative, Birmingham: University of Alabama in Birmingham Medical Center, 3.

Kirklin, John W, et al. 1955. "Intrathoracic surgery with the aid of a Mechanical pump oxygenator system (Gibbon type): Report of 8 cases." Rochester: Proceedings Staff Meetings, Mayo Clinic. 201-202.

Kleaveland, Dr. Richard, interview by Dr. Tracy Berg. 2011. *Vascular Surgeon* Spokane, Washington, (November 19).

Knauf, Larry, interview by Dr. Tracy Berg. 2008. *EMT with Spokane Ambulance* Spokane, Washington.

Larson, Donna, interview by Dr. Tracy Berg. 2011. *CRNA* Spokane, Washington, (June 4).

Legget, Hadley. 2009. *Medical Oops leads to first Coronary Angiogram, Dr. Mason Sones.* Wired, October 28.

Locati, Sister Rosalie, interview by Dr. Tracy Berg. 2012. *Sister of Province Sacred Heart Hospital* Spokane, Washington, (August 7).

Meenach, Erin, interview by Dr. Tracy Berg. 2011. *Jason Berg's significant other* Spokane, Washington, (February).

Merendino, Dr. K. Alvin, interview by Dr. Tracy Berg. 2011. *Pioneering Open Heart Surgeon* Seattle, Washington, (May 14).

Miller, G. Wayne. 2000. *King of Hearts the True Story of the Maverick Who Pioneered Open Heart Surgery.* New York, New York: Crown Publishers New York.

Mouser, Dr. Tom, interview by Dr. Tracy Berg. 2011. *Cardiologist* Spokane Valley, Washington, (July 25).

Mueller, C. Barber. 2002. *Evarts A. Graham the Live, Lives and Times of the Surgical Spirit of St. Louis.* Hamilton, Ontario: BC Decker Inc.

Murray L, Hardy Hendren W, Mayer J. 2013. ""A thrill of extreme magnety": Robert E Gross and the Beginning of Cardiac Surgery." *Journal of Pediatric Surgery* 48 (8): 1822-1825.

Myers, Maggie, interview by Dr. Tracy Berg. 2012. *CRNA* Spokane, Washington, (March 21).

Oransky, Ivan. 2005. "Obituary Wilfred Biglow." *The Lancet* 365 (9471): 1616.

Patient of Dr. Berg, interview by Dr. Tracy Berg. 2010. *blue baby Marty's mother* Spokane, Washington.

Powers, Dorothy. 1957. "Cool Heart." *Spokane Review.* Spokane,

Washington: Cowles Publishing, June 4.
—. 1955. "Deep Inside her Heart." *Spokane Review.* Spokane, Washington: Cowles Publishing, December 27.
—. 1958. "Nine Months Later." *Spokane Review.* Spokane, Washington: Cowles Publishing, February 27.
—. 1959. "Open Heart." *Spokane Review.* Spokane, Washington: Cowles Publishing, January 28.
—. 1988. *Powers: to the People.* Spokane, Washington: Cowles Publishing Company.
Providence Archives, Seattle. 1960. "Sister Mary Bede, SP, 1960, SP4367.001." *Photo of Sister Mary Bede.* Seattle, Washington: Providence Archives, Seattle.
Robel, Janet, interview by Dr. Tracy Berg. 2011. *Family, Realtor* Spokane, Washington, (January 13).
Rogalski, Tola, interview by Dr. Tracy Berg. 2011. *friend of Jason* Spokane, Washington, (September 6).
Rudolph, Abrahm, MD. 1980. "Cardiac Catheterization of Jason Berg." Heart catheter report, San Fransisco, 4.
Rudy, Dr. Lloyd William, interview by Dr. Tracy Berg. 2011. *Heart Surgeon* Spokane, Washington, (March 24).
Sallquist, Bill. 1974. "Heart Attacks Cut." *Spokesman Review Newspaper.* Spokane, Washington: Cowles Publishing, November 1. 1.
Shanewise, Dr. Jack, interview by Dr. Tracy Berg. 2011. *Anesthesiologist* Spokane, Washington, (August 12).
Shields, Dr. Paul, interview by Dr. Tracy Berg. 2011. *Cardiologist* Spokane, Washington, (March 23).
Shields, Sharma, interview by Dr. Tracy Berg. 2011. *RN Cardiology Manager* Spokane, Washington, (November 25).
Shumway, N, MD, PhD. 1996. "F. John Lewis, MD 1916-1996." *The Annals of Thoracic Surgery* 61 (1): 250-251.
Simonsen, Gary, interview by Dr. Tracy Berg. 2011. *OR technician* Spokane, Washington, (June 26).
Simpson, Dr. Carroll, interview by Dr. Tracy Berg. 2011. *Cardiologist*

Tacoma, Washington, (July 10).
Soehren, Pauline, interview by Dr. Tracy Berg. 2011. *ARNP* Spokane, Washington, (May 20).
Spores, Julie, interview by Dr. Tracy Berg. 2011. *CRNA Agatha Hodgins Award 2005, the highest award given by AANA/American Association of Nurse Anesthetists presented to "individuals whose foremost dedication to excellence has furthered the art and science of nurse anesthesia:* Spokane, Washington, (June 12).
Stephens, Nebraska, interview by Dr. Tracy Berg. 2011. *Cardiovascular Perfusionist* Spokane, Washington, (May 18).
Stimson, William. 1978. "Bypass Surgery, Spokane's Dr. Ralph Berg in Action." *Spokane Magazine*. Spokane: Cowles Publishing Spokesman Review Newspaper, March.
Swan, Henry Papers and the National Library of Medicine. n.d. "The Henry Swan Papers." In *The Cold Heart: Hypothermia and Cardiac Surgery 1949-1962*, by National Library of Medicine Profiles in Science.
Thiel, Dr. Shirley, interview by Dr. Tracy Berg. 2012. *MD Family Practice* Spokane Valley, Washington, (January 14).
Thomas, Dr. George, interview by Dr. Tracy Berg. 2010. *Merendino's Chest Fellow* Seattle, Washington, (March 31).
Thomas, Vivien T. 1985. *Pioneering Research in Surgical Shock and Cardiovascular Surgery Vivien Thomas and his Work with Alfred Blalock*. Philadelphia, Pennsylvania: University of Pennsylvania Press.
VanVoorhis, Judy Miller, interview by Dr. Tracy Berg. 2011. *Blue baby repaired* Spokane, Washington, (July 17).
W. Boehm, M. Emmel and N. Sreer. 2006. "Balloon Atrial Septostomy: History and Technique." *Images in Paediatric Cardiology* 8-14.
Wettrell, Goran MD PhD. 2023. "Dr. Ake Senning 1915-2000." *Kektoen International A Journal of Medical Humanities*, winter.
Wolfe, Dr. Charles R., interview by Dr. Tracy Berg. 2011. *MD MPH Family Practice* Spokane Valley, Washington, (July 4).

www.ingramcontent.com/pod-product-compliance
Lightning Source LLC
LaVergne TN
LVHW042250070526
838201LV00089B/103